COGNITIVE-BEHAVIORAL THERAPY
OF ADDICTIVE DISORDERS

Also from Bruce S. Liese and Aaron T. Beck

COGNITIVE-BEHAVIORAL THERAPY OF ADDICTIVE DISORDERS

Bruce S. Liese
Aaron T. Beck

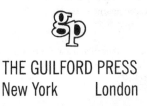

THE GUILFORD PRESS
New York   London

The authors have checked with sources believed to be reliable in their efforts to provide
information that is complete and generally in accord with the standards of practice that are
accepted at the time of publication. However, in view of the possibility of human error or
changes in behavioral, mental health, or medical sciences, neither the authors, nor the editors
and publisher, nor any other party who has been involved in the preparation or publication
of this work warrants that the information contained herein is in every respect accurate or
complete, and they are not responsible for any errors or omissions or the results obtained from
the use of such information. Readers are encouraged to confirm the information contained in
this book with other sources.

Library of Congress Cataloging-in-Publication Data is available from the publisher.

ISBN 978-1-4625-4884-2 (cloth)

About the Authors

Bruce S. Liese, PhD, ABPP, is Professor of Family Medicine and Psychiatry at the University of Kansas Medical Center and Clinical Director of the Cofrin Logan Center for Addiction Research and Treatment at the University of Kansas. Dr. Liese has served as president of the American Psychological Association Division on Addiction Psychology (APA Division 50). His scholarly work has focused on the treatment of complex mental health problems and addictions. He has published widely and is presently on three APA journal editorial boards. He has taught courses on addictions, psychotherapy, and evidence-based practice and supervised hundreds of psychotherapy trainees. In 2003, Dr. Liese received a President's Citation for Distinguished Service to APA Division 50. In 2015, Dr. Liese received the Distinguished Career Contributions to Education and Training award from Division 50, and he received an APA Presidential Citation in 2018 for service to his community.

Aaron T. Beck, MD, until his death in 2021, was Professor Emeritus of Psychiatry at the University of Pennsylvania and President Emeritus of the Beck Institute for Cognitive Behavior Therapy. Internationally recognized as the founder of cognitive therapy, Dr. Beck has been credited with shaping the face of American psychiatry and was cited by *American Psychologist* as "one of the five most influential psychotherapists of all time." Dr. Beck was the recipient of awards including the Albert Lasker Clinical Medical Research Award, the Lifetime Achievement Award from the American Psychological Association, the Distinguished Service Award from the American Psychiatric Association, the James McKeen Cattell Fellow Award in Applied Psychology from the Association for Psychological Science, and the Sarnat International Prize in Mental Health and Gustav O. Lienhard Award from the Institute of Medicine. He authored or edited numerous books for professionals and the general public.

Acknowledgments

Dr. Aaron "Tim" Beck was 100 years old when he passed away on November 1, 2021. On that day I lost a friend, and the world lost a transformative teacher and mentor. Those who *knew* Tim—and many who only *knew of* Tim—grieve the loss of this icon, the father of cognitive therapy. It was an honor and a joy to write this book with Tim. Fatefully, the final typeset page proofs arrived on the day he died. Throughout the writing process, I was awed by the energy and intellect I witnessed from this man who worked brilliantly right up to the final days of his life. Tim was deeply committed to finishing this book, even as he approached and then passed 100 years old. We both viewed this project as an important opportunity to produce a resource to improve the lives of often underserved people, whose strengths are typically underappreciated.

I also want to express my gratitude to others who have made this book possible. Certainly, I feel most grateful to my wife, Cathy, my rock and inspiration. For 7 years Cathy has been gently asking, "How's the book coming? Have you been writing lately?" I am grateful for our amazing daughters, Justine and Jessica. Justine has been the most enthusiastic and joyful fan a father could possibly hope for. And Jess has been a terrific sounding board and my favorite PhD psychologist since getting her doctorate just a few years ago.

This text was inspired by our first book, *Cognitive Therapy of Substance Abuse* (Beck, Wright, Newman, & Liese, 1993). From the time we began writing together I felt fortunate to be part of such an extraordinary partnership with Tim, Cory Newman, and the late Fred Wright. I want to express my sincerest gratitude to Dr. Cory Newman, who is one of the most honorable, principled people I know. And to Fred, one of my dearest friends ever: I sorely miss you.

I feel particularly fortunate to call Jim Nageotte a friend. As a Senior Editor at The Guilford Press, Jim has the Sisyphean challenge of "inspiring" authors like me to finish our books as enthusiastically as we start them. Month after month, year after year, Jim gracefully coached and motivated me. I'd like to claim that I dragged this project on for 7 years just to continue working with Jim. In truth, writing this book took 7 years for many reasons and Jim was supportive the entire time. I kept reminding him, "I still have a lot to learn before I can finish this book."

I'm especially grateful to Corey Monley for his help and support during the last few years of writing. Corey, now a PhD Counseling Psychology student, never tired of reading my drafts. Inevitably, our late-night discussions drifted to countless topics well beyond the scope of this text. As a result of our long, deep talks we feel more like family than friends.

I made a new friend in the process of writing this text. Victoria Wyeth was a research assistant to Tim when we first met. She and Tim would read my chapters together and provide feedback—first in writing and eventually via brief, uplifting videos starring Victoria. The final stretch was certainly easier thanks to Victoria's enthusiasm for this text.

Other people have contributed to the completion of this text, and I am grateful to them all. For example, I'd like to express my thanks to SMART Recovery founders Tom Horvath and Joe Gerstein. Tom has been a friend for more than 25 years. Tom, Joe, and their team have invested decades developing and refining the SMART Recovery program that makes cognitive-behavioral therapy-based mutual-help groups accessible to people with addictions throughout the world, regardless of their means. Three very sharp SMART Recovery teammates, Becky, Sergej, and Matt, were among those willing to read a late draft of the manuscript. Their enthusiastic and careful review helped me take this book across the finish line.

I don't want to miss this opportunity to express my gratitude to thousands of patients in recovery who, over the years, have shared their struggles and entrusted me to care for them. I can only hope that my care was helpful.

Finally, I want to thank *you* for considering this text. I hope these pages inspire you—just as so many courageous patients in recovery have inspired me—to tirelessly continue this vital work.

BRUCE S. LIESE

PREFACE

Imagine engaging in a rewarding activity for much of your life and gradually realizing that this activity is destroying everything you value. Then envision yourself trying to quit this activity and feeling unable to do so, no matter how hard you try. Next, imagine repeating this activity over and over, knowing it is contributing to your demise. Recognize that you feel compelled to do more and more of it, rather than slowing down or stopping. Then visualize your loved ones saying they won't tolerate your involvement in this activity any longer. Now add to these images, the image of an entire society stigmatizing you for engaging in this activity.

These experiences are familiar to people who struggle with addictions. Shame, guilt, ambivalence, fear, doubt, helplessness, frustration, and despair are just some of the feelings faced by many trying to abstain from addictive behaviors. It is these people who have inspired this follow-up to our original text, *Cognitive Therapy of Substance Abuse* (Beck, Wright, Newman, & Liese, 1993). Since publication of that text almost 30 years ago, we have worked with thousands of patients who have entrusted us to help them confront their addictive behaviors.

Many of our patients have entered therapy feeling desperation and despair. Many have lost all that mattered to them, including friends, family, homes, health, and careers. Some have shared desperate sentiments, for example: "I've reached the end of my rope" and "If this [therapy] doesn't work, I'm done." Much to their surprise, many of our patients have learned and applied cognitive-behavioral therapy (CBT) skills and turned their lives around. They have become healthier and happier by increasing control over their thoughts, feelings, and behaviors. Many have developed new close relationships and reestablished old relationships. Most have found steady, meaningful work. Almost all have been astonished that they could take charge of their own lives.

We have learned so much over the past 30 years. In addition to learning from our patients' experiences, we have been continually informed and inspired by the extraordinary work of our research colleagues. The results of their labors have profoundly influenced our approach, as reflected in this follow-up text. For example, we now understand that:

- People with addictions constitute an extraordinarily diverse group.
- Definitions of recovery are idiosyncratic: they differ widely from person to person.
- Patients need to determine their own outcome goals, rather than have them determined by others.
- The benefits of CBT for addictions are not limited to abstinence; they include a wide range of potential intrapersonal and interpersonal skills.
- Common psychological and physiological processes underlie the various addictions.
- Many patients need services and resources beyond those provided in psychotherapy, including mutual-help groups (e.g., 12-step programs and SMART Recovery) and medication-assisted therapies.
- Stigma about addictions is pervasive—even among health care providers—and it needs to be recognized and eliminated whenever and wherever possible.

Over the past 30 years, significant sociopolitical shifts have occurred. In this follow-up text, we discuss how these shifts influence our work with people with addictions. For example, we address potential challenges associated with legalization of marijuana in the United States (Chapter 1). We also address the impact of stigma, bias, and prejudice toward people who struggle with addictions (Chapter 4).

In this text, we acknowledge the valuable contributions of many diverse approaches to addiction treatment and highlight how we have incorporated these into CBT for substance use disorders. We emphasize the importance of conceptualizing patients thoroughly and accurately, and only then intervening with the most appropriate therapeutic actions.

In this text we do our best to outline 30 years of trends and progress in addiction research and treatment. For example, we:

- Review current evidence supporting the efficacy of CBT for treating addictions (Chapter 1).
- Apply our model to both chemical and behavioral addictions (Chapter 1).
- Introduce the syndrome model of addiction (Chapters 1 and 2).
- Review the genetic, neurobiological, psychosocial, and environmental factors associated with the development of addictive behaviors (Chapter 2).

- Propose a systematic case conceptualization method for understanding people in recovery (Chapter 3).
- Underscore the importance of research on the impact of stigma on the therapeutic process (Chapter 4).
- Explain the interrelatedness between guided discovery and motivational interviewing (Chapter 6).
- Describe 12 standardized CBT techniques for helping patients who struggle with addictions (Chapter 7).
- Apply the concepts of System 1 and System 2 thinking to the maintenance of addictions (Chapter 10).
- Introduce Dr. Aaron Beck's concept of modes and apply this concept to addictions (Chapter 11).
- Provide specific guidance regarding the facilitation of CBT group therapy (Chapter 12).

We hope you find this new material to be helpful in working with those who struggle with addictions. Throughout this text we provide many different hypothetical case examples, to demonstrate a wide range of patients with a wide range of addictions and associated problems. All case examples are composites (i.e., combinations of many actual patients we have known), and all names are fictional. We make frequent reference to the terms "substance use disorders," "addictive behaviors," and "addictions." For literary purposes, we interchange these terms, as we often do in practice. As well, when referring to singular, nongendered subjects in a sentence, we have chosen to use the pronoun "they."

CONTENTS

Contents

CHAPTER 1

OVERVIEW

The term *addiction* is ubiquitous, and we hear it applied to problematic use of alcohol and other drugs, as well as addictions that don't involve ingested substances—the so-called behavioral addictions. We hear the term used in everyday discourse, as people characterize certain habits as addictions. If you ask some people trying to lose weight why they just ate a pan of brownies, they might say, "I have a chocolate addiction" or "I'm a chocoholic." If you ask some long-distance runners why they run long distances they might say, "I'm addicted to running." But what exactly is an addiction? When is it appropriate to use this term to characterize human behavior?

In this text we focus on both chemical (or substance) and behavioral addictions. This is based on our understanding that certain cognitive, behavioral, affective, and physiological processes are analogous across addictions, as well as a substantial body of research that supports the reliability and validity of certain behavioral addiction diagnoses. We review various approaches to defining addictions, starting with the fifth edition of the *Diagnostic and Statistical Manual of Mental Disorders* (DSM-5; American Psychiatric Association, 2013). In the DSM-5, the phrase *addictive disorder* is introduced as a mental disorder characterized by behaviors that persist despite their serious problematic consequences. Relatively new to the DSM-5 (and other diagnostic standards) is the notion that an individual can have varying degrees of addictive disorders, depending on the number of symptoms that are manifest. Also, relatively new to the DSM-5 is the inclusion of gambling disorder as an addictive disorder and problematic Internet gaming under consideration as an addictive disorder.

To assist in defining *addiction*, let's consider the case of Bob, who says he drinks "just one or two beers most nights of the week." When Bob goes out to eat with his wife, Mary, he drives home despite having consumed several beers. At least once a week he wakes up with a hangover, goes to work feeling "fuzzy," and

1

finds it difficult to do his job as a project manager. He denies other alcohol-related problems (e.g., unsuccessful efforts to cut down or quit, craving, withdrawal, tolerance, health problems). Mary, on the other hand, starts drinking before noon every day, even though she has been warned by her doctor that heavy drinking may be contributing to her hypertension. When she starts slurring her words and becomes "sloppy," Bob urges her to stop drinking, which inevitably leads to arguments. When Bob tries to talk to Mary about her behaviors on a previous night, she has often forgotten (i.e., blacked out) much of the night. Though she would not admit this to Bob, Mary has tried to quit drinking after being fired from several retail sales jobs, but each time she quits she starts again because she feels restless and shaky after only a few hours of abstinence.

Bob likely has a *mild* alcohol problem. He regularly drives after consuming alcohol and his drinking results in hangovers that interfere with his work. From the information we have on Bob, it is not certain that he is addicted to alcohol. Mary likely has a more *severe* alcohol problem: She spends most of her day intoxicated, she has blackouts and has been warned to stop drinking because it is the likely cause of her hypertension, she has been unable to quit drinking, when she tries to quit she experiences alcohol withdrawal, she argues with Bob about her drinking, and she has been fired from several jobs as a result of drinking. Based on the information we have for Mary, it might be reasonable to conclude that she is addicted to alcohol.

Bob and Mary are hardly alone in having alcohol problems. In fact, when the United States Substance Abuse and Mental Health Services Administration (SAMHSA) conducted its 2019 National Survey on Drug Use and Health (NSDUH; SAMHSA, 2020), it was found that approximately 5.3% of Americans over 12 years old (14.5 million people) have alcohol use disorders (AUDs). Of particular interest when thinking about Bob (with mild AUD) and Mary (with severe AUD) is the fact that men are more likely to have AUD than women (7.8% vs. 4.1%; SAMHSA, 2017).

When our earlier text, *Cognitive Therapy of Substance Abuse* (Beck et al., 1993), was written, the United States was in the midst of a *cocaine* epidemic. Presently the United States is in the midst of an *opioid* epidemic, with almost 5% of Americans over 12 years old (approximately 12.5 million) admitting to misuse of prescription pain relievers (SAMHSA, 2017). It is likely that the primary reason for labeling the present situation as a *crisis* is the number of deaths associated with opioid misuse. In 2017, the number of Americans over 12 years old who died from all drug overdoses was 70,237. Approximately 68% of these deaths (47,600) involved opioids, which was a 12% increase from 2016 (Scholl, Seth, Kariisa, Wilson, & Baldwin, 2018). According to Scholl and colleagues (2018), the increase in all deaths was largely due to misuse of synthetic opioids (e.g., hydrocodone, oxycodone, tramadol, and fentanyl). The survey conducted by SAMHSA (2017) found that most of the 12.5 million people who misused prescription pain relievers did so to relieve physical pain (62.6%). Other reasons cited for misuse were: to feel good or "get high" (12.1%), to relax or relieve tension (10.8%), for help with sleep (4.4%), to improve problematic emotions (3.3%), to experiment or "see what it's like" (2.5%), "due to addiction" (2.3%), to increase or decrease the effect of other drugs (0.9%), and for other reasons (1.2%). Approximately 53.7% of individuals who misused opioids obtained them from friends or relatives, while 36.4% obtained their opioids with prescriptions obtained from a health care provider. Only 4.9% purchased their prescription pain relievers from drug dealers, and another 4.9% obtained their prescriptions in "some other way."

Another change that has occurred since 1993 is that (as of this writing) marijuana has been legalized for medicinal use in 35 of the United States, and for recreational use in an additional 15 states, plus the District of Columbia (Bromwich, 2020); and these numbers are continually rising. For many years it was believed that marijuana was a "safe" drug. However, over the years it has become apparent that long-term consumption of marijuana may cause substantial physical and mental problems, especially in teenagers (National Institute on Drug Abuse, 2018b; Volkow, Baler, Compton, & Weiss, 2014).

Consider the case of John, an individual with serious marijuana-related problems. John is 30 years old. He has been smoking marijuana since high school, where he learned that selling pot was a convenient way to finance his daily use. He attended college for a while and made friends with other students who enjoyed getting high daily. By the middle of his first college semester he found himself unable to keep up with the academic challenges. Or more precisely, he found himself smoking marijuana instead of studying. He met and dated women, but none were interested in a serious relationship with a man who was always high. After dropping out of college, John found a landscaping job. He was fired after being arrested for possession of four ounces of marijuana, discovered when he was pulled over by police during a routine traffic stop—while driving the landscaping company truck. With the help of his family lawyer John was able to avoid incarceration. His parents allowed him to move into their home on the condition that he look for a job, but after more than a year, John gave up efforts and eventually reunited with old friends who spent much of their time high on marijuana.

Obviously, John has a serious cannabis-use problem. Instead of using recreationally or merely habitually, John uses marijuana in ways that cause severe consequences. And yet John does not choose to stop using marijuana, the cause of these severe consequences. Many would argue that John's cannabis use has escalated to a level that would qualify as an addiction.

In comparison with John, consider the case of Jill, a 40-year-old woman with a long history of substance use disorders (SUDs) prior to her first experience with gambling. Beginning in high school, she smoked cigarettes and marijuana, used cocaine and methamphetamine, and drank heavily. Then, 11 years ago, she was arrested for assault, disorderly conduct, and possession of cocaine, after police were called during a fight with her boyfriend. Following a brief period of incarceration, Jill made a conscious choice to remain abstinent from all addictive substances. She found a job working the evening shift at a local factory, moved into an apartment, and was eventually able to purchase a car. She regularly attended Alcoholics Anonymous (AA) meetings and found them to be helpful. In fact, this is where she met Gary, whom she dated for almost a year before they were married.

Jill's gambling problem began innocently enough: She was invited by a coworker to a casino after work "just to relax and have a little fun." Upon arriving there, Jill says she "felt like a kid in a candy shop." She could not believe there was so much activity anywhere this late at night: bright lights, flashing slot machines, bells and whistles throughout the casino. Wherever she turned, people were smoking and drinking. Much to her surprise, she was more drawn to the sight and sounds of slot machines than she was to alcohol and cigarettes. Before long, she began to have what she described as "a strange experience." She began to feel the familiar rush that she had experienced so often when using alcohol and drugs. In her words, "It felt amazing!" She was able to achieve a familiar high without ingesting an addictive substance. By the end of her first night of gambling Jill knew with certainty that she was hooked. Sure enough, within a few months Jill was going to casinos most nights of the week. Though she continued to abstain from addictive substances, she described "miserable hangovers after long nights of gambling." Before long she was having some of the same problems with gambling that she had with alcohol and drugs: No amount of gambling felt like enough; she was spending all her free time at casinos; when she was not gambling she would fantasize about gambling; she was taking money out of her meager savings account to spend at casinos; she was lying to Gary about spending time with friends; and perhaps most troubling, she felt like she had lost control and was unable to stop gambling. As hard as she tried, quitting seemed impossible. In fact, she described efforts to abstain from gambling as "harder than all her other addictions." Eventually she began to have severe financial problems that ultimately led to bankruptcy and the dissolution of her marriage. As illustrated by Jill's experiences, the suffering associated with gambling disorder—a behavioral addiction—can be as punishing as that from substance addictions.

CHEMICAL AND BEHAVIORAL ADDICTIONS: MORE ALIKE THAN DIFFERENT

Howard Shaffer has made an important contribution to the field of addictions by studying gambling disorder and pioneering *the addiction syndrome* (Shaffer, 2012; Shaffer & Hall, 2002; Shaffer et al., 2004). Shaffer and his colleagues describe the addiction syndrome as a complex pattern that underlies all addictive behaviors. Instead of viewing individual addictions (e.g., alcohol, marijuana, opioids, gambling, gaming) as unique and separate, all addictions are understood to have similar distal (past) antecedents, proximal (recent) antecedents, and consequences (e.g., expressions, manifestations, and sequelae). According to this model, the various addictive behaviors and chemicals are mere *objects* that have the capacity to "shift subjective experience reliably and robustly" (Shaffer, 2012, p. xxxi). These chemical and behavioral *shifters* activate similar reward centers of the brain. The addiction syndrome provides an integration of neurobiological elements, shared psychosocial elements, and shared experiences: The brain's reward system is similarly activated by addictive substances and behaviors; individuals with addictions tend to have similar psychological problems, and the course of addictive behaviors tends to be similar across addictions. Thus, the model emphasizes commonalities among the various addictive processes.

It is important to understand that the early consequences of addictive behaviors are positive, which is why people initially engage in them. Alcohol has the potential to relax, excite, and disinhibit; marijuana has potential to mellow; amphetamines have the potential to energize; opioids have the potential to relieve pain; and gambling has the capacity to generate excitement about the prospect of big winnings. It is important to understand that these effects in persons who are addicted overshadow the negative consequences of engaging in them—at least initially. As long as individuals believe positive consequences will outweigh negative consequences of addictive behaviors, they will be tempted to engage in them.

Obviously, there are numerous negative consequences associated with addictive behaviors. Shaffer and colleagues (2012, 2004) conveniently divide these into two categories: those that are unique to each addictive behavior and those that are shared across addictive behaviors. Examples of *unique* consequences include liver disease (alcohol), pulmonary and cardiovascular disease (smoking), financial problems (gambling), legal problems (illicit drugs), and death from overdose (opioids). Examples of *shared* negative consequences include tolerance, withdrawal, relapse, psychiatric comorbidity, object substitution, social drift, criminal behavior, stigma, and more. A major aim of CBT for addictions is to help individuals acknowledge the negative consequences of their addictive behaviors, while also understanding that their anticipation of positive consequences serves to maintain their addictions.

Another way to conceptualize both substance and behavioral addictions has been proposed by Mark Griffiths, who has done extensive research and published hundreds of scientific papers on behavioral addictions. Griffiths (2005) explains that "most official definitions [of addiction] concentrate on drug ingestion" (p. 192). He recommends the use of six components that focus primarily on addiction processes or patterns, rather than on any particular substance or activity:

1. *Salience:* For a substance or behavior to be addictive, it has to be salient or important to an individual. Salience might be reflected in excessive use or engagement, or it might be reflected in frequent or intense thoughts about the substance or behavior. A high degree of salience might also be viewed as an obsession or preoccupation with the addictive behavior.

2. *Mood modification:* For a substance or behavior to be addictive, it has to impact emotions, feelings, or mood. For some individuals the sought-after mood might involve feeling more "up" (i.e., exhilarated or energized), while for others the sought-after mood might be "down" (i.e., mellow or relaxed). And for many individuals, mood modification is experienced as decreased physical pain, anxiety, depression, anger, or withdrawal.

3. *Tolerance:* Individuals who need greater amounts of a substance or behavior to experience the same effects have developed a tolerance, which is a strong indicator of addiction.

4. *Withdrawal:* Many people who try to quit addictive behaviors experience negative physical or psychological consequences, or withdrawal. The nature and degree of withdrawal depends on various factors; among them is frequency and quantity of the addictive behavior, but also the specific substance or behavior involved. For example, alcohol withdrawal can result in seizures and death, opioid withdrawal can feel like a terrible bout of influenza, and abstinence from gambling may result in anxiety or depression.

5. *Conflict:* The term *conflict* brings to mind a disagreement between two individuals. However, in the context of addictions this term relates to both interpersonal conflict (between people) and intrapersonal conflict (within oneself). Simply stated, the most common such intrapersonal conflict involves the thought, "I really shouldn't be doing this."

6. *Relapse:* Trying to change, reduce, or quit addictive behaviors is not easy, and perhaps that is why many consider relapse the hallmark of addiction.

We find the Griffiths model to be simple and easy to explain to patients. For example, when John (from the case example above) initially came in for therapy he asked his therapist, "Do you think I am an addict?" In response his therapist explained Griffiths' six components, and John agreed: "They all kinda' sound like me."

The approaches to SUDs and addictive behaviors described above are all useful, and there is substantial overlap among them. We suggest that therapists familiarize themselves with each one, since they all provide a unique and useful perspective. For example, the DSM-5 (American Psychiatric Association, 2013) provides specific diagnostic criteria; the addiction syndrome (Shaffer et al., 2004; Shaffer, 2012) provides a unique, evidence-based theoretical and developmental perspective; and Griffiths' (2005) model relates to chemical and behavioral addictions in a way that is straightforward and easily understood by most patients.

As mentioned earlier, throughout this text we interchange the terms *addiction, substance use disorder,* and *addictive behavior.* We advocate for using terms that *minimize the stigma* associate with negative labels. For example, we avoid terms like *drug addict* and *alcoholic,* instead using phrases like "a person who has problems with [alcohol, drugs, gambling, etc.]." We even avoid terms like *dirty urine,* with the understanding that they may be pejorative (Kelly, Wakeman, & Saitz, 2015).

CBT FOR ADDICTIONS

Misconceptions of CBT are common (Gluhoski, 1994). In fact, during workshops we often hear participants say, "This CBT is different from what I've learned about CBT." So before describing our approach to CBT for addictions, we thought it important to underscore what CBT *is not.* The following are some misconceptions regarding CBT:

- CBT is merely a collection of standardized techniques, like a bag of tricks.
- CBT is mechanical and linear, to be followed like a cookbook recipe.
- CBT minimizes the importance of patients' early life experiences, and especially childhood experiences.
- CBT minimizes the importance of patients' interpersonal relationships (e.g., family and friends).
- CBT minimizes the importance of the therapeutic relationship.
- CBT is necessarily brief, or short-term.
- CBT aims exclusively for abstinence from addictive behaviors without regard for other psychological problems.
- CBT is so effective that clinicians should expect all patients to resolve their addictions and experience substantial benefits from therapy.

Most stereotypical images of CBT portray therapists more as robots or computers than as real people. This has been the case stretching all the way back to the early days of CBT (Beck, Rush, Shaw, & Emery, 1979):

> Cognitive and behavioral techniques often seem deceptively simple. Consequently, the neophyte therapist may become "gimmick-oriented" to the point of ignoring the human aspects of the therapist-patient interaction. When this occurs, [the therapist] may relate to the patient as one computer to another rather than as one person to another. Some young therapists who are most skilled in applying the specific techniques are perceived by their patients as

mechanical, manipulative, and more interested in the techniques than in the patient. It is important to keep in mind that the techniques . . . are intended to be applied in a tactful, therapeutic, and human manner by a fallible person— the therapist. (p. 46)

In reality, CBT employs a complex process, described briefly here and in much more detail in later chapters. Addictions tend to be chronic, self-reinforcing problems, characterized by intermittent relapses. Hence, CBT for SUDs and addictive behaviors often requires long-term patient engagement (McLellan, 2002; McLellan, Lewis, O'Brien, & Kleber, 2000). Of course, the length of engagement is dependent on many individual and contextual variables. Furthermore, addictive behaviors tend to occur in vicious cycles, initiated for the purpose of regulating emotions, but eventually causing emotion dysregulation that perpetuates and exacerbates the original addictive behaviors. As a result, treatment is rarely linear, with a distinct beginning, middle, and end. Instead there are often ups and downs for patients recovering from substance use problems. To be effective, CBT requires an accurate understanding (i.e., case conceptualization) of each patient. To be useful, the case conceptualization should include relevant information about early and current life circumstances (i.e., context). Unless we have such context, it is difficult (if not impossible) to understand an individual's addictive behaviors and barriers to change. For example, without knowledge of a patient's family history of addictions or close relationships with other addicted individuals it may be difficult to comprehend the intractability of their addictions. In addition, the absence of a thorough case conceptualization and collaborative therapeutic alliance increases the likelihood that a patient will disengage from therapy (Brorson, Arnevik, Rand-Hendriksen, & Duckert, 2013; Liese & Beck, 1998).

There is no single, definitive approach to CBT. In fact, many knowledgeable CBT practitioners and researchers refer to CBT in the plural form (i.e., cognitive-behavioral therap*ies*). The following CBT approaches have all been successfully applied to the treatment of addictive behaviors: acceptance and commitment therapy (ACT; Hayes, Strosahl, & Wilson, 2012), behavioral activation (BA; Daughters et al., 2018; Daughters, Magidson, Lejuez, & Chen, 2016), contingency management (CM; Petry, 2012), community reinforcement and family therapy (CRAFT; Meyers & Squires, 2001), dialectical behavior therapy (DBT; Linehan, 2015), mindfulness-based relapse prevention (Bowen, Chawla, Grow, & Marlatt, 2021; Witkiewitz, Marlatt, & Walker, 2005), and more.[1]

---

[1]We especially wish to credit Alan Marlatt for introducing relapse prevention (Marlatt & Gordon, 1985), which sowed the seeds of CBT for addictions. Dr. Marlatt and these other scholars have greatly advanced CBT for addictions, and we acknowledge that our work has been profoundly influenced by their vital contributions.

Five Major Components of CBT for Addictions

Since publishing *Cognitive Therapy of Substance Abuse,* we have been modifying and refining our approach to both individual and group CBT (Liese, 2014; Liese, Beck, & Seaton, 2002; Liese & Tripp, 2018; Wenzel, Liese, Beck, & Friedman-Wheeler, 2012). We find it helpful to view CBT as consisting of five major components: (1) structure, (2) collaboration, (3) case conceptualization, (4) psychoeducation, and (5) standardized techniques. In fact, we have observed that all CBTs place emphasis on these components, though to varying degrees. These components are briefly described in the following paragraphs, and then discussed in detail throughout this text.

Structure is best thought of as the process necessary for staying focused throughout a therapy session. Most therapists (and indeed many patients) have had the experience of being in the midst of a session wondering, "How is this conversation relevant to the presented problem?" or "Why are we talking about all these details and not the main problem?" When it is done well, CBT keeps the discussion in a session on track. By design, it is a structured, focused approach to helping people with addictions.

Structure also involves organizing sessions in such a way that problems are defined and addressed. Our approach to CBT can be conducted in individual, family, or group modalities. When provided individually, we start each session by setting an agenda. This process can be either formal or relaxed, depending on the patient and other circumstances. For example, patients who are generally well organized and in minimal distress might prefer sessions that are highly structured, while patients who are less organized or in substantial distress might benefit from a more flexible structure. Agenda setting is followed by a mood check, reflections from last session(s), prioritizing agenda items, and then problem solving. In group CBT, patients share their names, addictions, status of their addictions, goals, and contexts in which their addictions take place. Again, the structure of individual and group CBT will be discussed in detail in later chapters.

Collaboration is typically thought of as key to the therapeutic bond, alliance, or relationship. The ability to form alliances across a wide range of patients is essential to therapist effectiveness, and certain interpersonal skills enable such alliances to be established (Wampold, Baldwin, Holtforth, & Imel, 2017). We strongly advocate for therapists' attention to their own interpersonal skills, which are needed to the fullest extent possible when practicing CBT. While this may seem simple and straightforward, many therapists find it difficult to be warm and empathetic with patients who struggle with lapses and relapses.

Mutual goal setting and goal achievement are also vital to the therapeutic relationship. The process of agreeing on goals is often more complex than most therapists expect. Many patients feel uncomfortable committing to goals they have failed to achieve in the past. Given the reinforcing nature of addictions, many patients also find it difficult to maintain motivation to change. From minute to minute, day to day, week to week, patients' enthusiasm for achieving particular goals may wax and wane, corresponding with their moods, circumstances, and so forth. In order to maintain collaborative alliances with patients, it is important that therapists avoid being emotionally reactive to patients' goal-related failures and successes.

Case conceptualization involves the identification, organization, and integration of patients' thoughts, beliefs, schemas, triggers, predominant emotions, and behaviors—with close attention paid to how these have developed. Essential contextual components of the case conceptualization may include friends, family, and the communities in which patients live. Other components may include underlying medical, psychological, or psychiatric problems that might contribute to or exacerbate addictive behaviors. For example, many patients use addictive behaviors to self-medicate anxiety, depression, bipolar disorder, and schizophrenia—or opioids to treat physical pain. In order to develop accurate case conceptualizations, therapists must possess highly effective listening skills and the ability to accurately empathize with patients who often behave in self-defeating ways. Additionally, therapists must be able to formulate hypotheses regarding the etiology and function of addictive behaviors in patients' lives—and then test these hypotheses during their clinical encounters with patients.

Psychoeducation involves transmitting knowledge or skills: either directly, through modeling, or by the process of active, *reflective* listening. Sometimes it is appropriate for the therapist to explain CBT concepts or processes, while at other times doing so might be perceived by patients to be untimely or irrelevant. The determination of when it is most appropriate to teach CBT concepts is an essential part of the case conceptualization and collaborative therapeutic relationship.

Standardized techniques are formal activities designed to guide cognitive, behavioral, or affective changes. Just a few examples of CBT techniques are advantages–disadvantages analysis, automatic thought records, and functional analysis. These and other standardized techniques will be described in detail in Chapter 7. As mentioned earlier, one of the most pervasive misconceptions of CBT is that standardized, *cookbook-like* techniques are at the heart of therapy. In fact, choosing the right standardized techniques for patients requires careful consideration and attention to the case conceptualization and collaborative therapeutic relationship.

How Does Our Approach to CBT Compare to Others?

Years ago, Dr. Aaron Beck walked into a restaurant, looked around, saw that everything was run well, and said, "They must be doing cognitive therapy here." When asked what he meant by this Dr. Beck explained, "Regardless of setting, good work requires good thinking." We submit that all effective therapies facilitate "good thinking." For example, ACT therapists facilitate acceptance, behavioral activation therapists facilitate the identification of personal values and associated behaviors, mindfulness-based relapse prevention therapists facilitate greater mindfulness, and so forth. Strangers to 12-step programs might be surprised to learn many 12-step slogans involve good thinking that you might expect to learn in CBT, for example in the recurring reminders, "This too shall pass," "Live and let live," "Cultivate an attitude of gratitude," and "Your worth should never depend on another person's opinion" (12step.org, 2018).

Most clinicians are familiar with the process of motivational interviewing (Miller & Rollnick, 2012) and the stages of change model (Norcross, Krebs, & Prochaska, 2011; Prochaska, DiClemente, & Norcross, 1992; Prochaska & Norcross, 2001). These terms have become commonplace in the treatment world because they are useful and relevant to all approaches to treating addictive behaviors. Simply stated, motivational interviewing (MI) is an approach to helping people that *meets them where they are* in order to facilitate change. MI requires active listening, empathy, flexibility, collaboration, and effective interpersonal communication. The stages of change model (also known as the transtheoretical model of change) provides a framework for understanding a person's readiness to change, ranging from precontemplation (not yet considering change) to maintenance (life after change).

It is our position that all cognitive-behavioral therapists should have MI skills (e.g., effective listening, accurate empathy, collaboration). We also maintain that cognitive-behavioral therapists should have a keen awareness of patients' readiness to change. In fact, an individual's readiness to change should be part of the case conceptualization and influence how therapists decide to structure sessions, engage in psychoeducation, and facilitate standardized techniques. A therapist who attends to readiness to change is most likely to apply structure, psychoeducation, and techniques in ways that enhance collaboration, while a therapist who ignores a patient's readiness to change may do irreparable damage to the therapeutic relationship.

One of the authors, Dr. Bruce Liese, was facilitating a workshop on CBT for addictions several years ago. During a break, one of the participants approached him and boldly stated, "You are teaching and demonstrating MI." Dr. Liese responded by asking, "What makes you say that?" The participant explained that she was systematically rating his role-play demonstrations with the Motivational Interviewing Treatment Integrity scale (MITI; Moyers, Manuel, & Ernst, 2014), and all demonstrations received high MI scores. Examples of positive anchors on this motivational interviewing scale include:

- Uses structured therapeutic tasks as a way of eliciting and reinforcing change talk
- Does not miss opportunities to explore more deeply when client offers change talk

- Strategically elicits change talk and consistently responds to it when offered
- Rarely misses opportunities to build momentum of change talk
- Genuinely negotiates the agenda and goals for the session
- Indicates curiosity about client ideas through querying and listening
- Facilitates client evaluation of options and planning

The lesson to be learned here is simply that effective CBT incorporates basic MI skills.

Differences between our approach and other cognitive-behavioral approaches are minimal, but essential. We offer unique structure for individual CBT sessions (see Chapter 5) and group CBT sessions (see Chapter 12), which sets us apart from most other approaches. We also stress the mantra: "To do good CBT, it is necessary to *think* like a cognitive-behavioral therapist." Highly effective therapists perpetually ask patients questions like:

"What was your thought when you made that decision?"
"What is the evidence for that thought?"
"What is your belief about [fill in the blank]?"
"How did you develop that belief?"
"What are the advantages and disadvantages of that choice?"

The goal of asking these questions is not solely to influence change. These questions are also intended to expand therapists' understanding of patients, in order to facilitate patients' self-understanding. Patients who continually hear therapists ask, "What were you thinking when . . . ?" and "What are your beliefs about . . . ?" come to understand that these questions are important, and they eventually develop the habit of asking themselves these questions as they strive to make effective decisions and solve life problems.

WHAT ARE THE GOALS OF CBT FOR ADDICTIONS?

People with serious addictions are at risk for many problems, including social, interpersonal, vocational, health, legal, and financial difficulties. To the extent that addictions have caused, exacerbated, or maintained these problems, the goal of CBT is to help people to abstain. However, many individuals seeking help for addictions do not wish to abstain from their addictive behaviors. Furthermore, most people who attempt to abstain from addictive behaviors experience multiple relapses prior to achieving sustained abstinence. In an excellent review of the recovery literature, Witkiewitz and her colleagues (2020, p. 9) remind us that there are "multidimensional and heterogeneous pathways to recovery." So even though abstinence might be a goal to strive for, therapists must be careful to avoid passing judgment on or of becoming frustrated with patients who do not abstain.

We strongly discourage debating with patients regarding abstinence versus control of addictive behaviors. Instead we suggest therapists encourage patients to set their own goals in a deliberate, intentional manner, and then review these goals over the course of therapy. We also emphasize that *failing to meet goals* (e.g., experiencing relapses) provides opportunities for patients to learn about themselves. To complicate matters, complete abstinence from some potentially addictive behaviors is not possible or realistic (e.g., a person who binge eats cannot completely abstain from eating food).

Understanding the principles of the harm reduction is especially helpful for therapists whose clients reject abstinence as their goal. In the spirit of harm reduction (Marlatt, Larimer, & Witkiewitz, 2012), we encourage collaborative goal setting that goes beyond addictive behaviors to include all changes that improve the quality of patients' lives. We offer a detailed discussion of harm reduction in Chapter 13.

It is also important to note that *medication-assisted treatment* (MAT) is among the evidence-based modes of therapy for addictions. For example, methadone, buprenorphine, and naltrexone are all used as medications for opioid use disorder (MOUD). It is reasonable to view these medications as harm-reduction approaches. And yet, many treatment programs do not accept the use of these medications as part of therapy, and many therapists still believe any drug use is wrong and bad.

Given the demonstrated efficacy of certain medications for certain addictions, it is important for cognitive-behavioral therapists to understand their mechanisms of action (i.e., why they are effective), and support patients whose goals include MAT. Supporting this goal is another way for therapists to express support for patients. In many cases, MAT provides a level of relief that enables patients to address other, perhaps more important, goals (e.g., the acquisition of skills). Therapists can find extensive detailed information about MAT and MOUD on the website of the National Institute on Drug Abuse (NIDA; https://www.drugabuse.gov).

SUMMARY

We often detect frustration in clinicians who treat people with addictions. This frustration may result from unrealistic and sometimes even judgmental beliefs about patients who engage in addictive behaviors (see Chapter 4). Frustration results also from unrealistic expectations regarding the clinical course of addictive behaviors. Therapists who hold negative, judgmental beliefs about people with addictions will inevitably experience frustration, irritation, and disappointment as they try to provide treatment. And therapists who expect the clinical course of addictions to be brief are also likely to find themselves disappointed.

Yet helping people with addictions can be deeply rewarding. When CBT for addictions goes as planned, patients have better lives than they may have imagined possible. They realize that life without addictive behaviors is full of possibilities. And when all does *not* go as planned, and yet the therapeutic relationship remains strong, patients are often eternally grateful for the help and support they receive from therapists who have played an extraordinarily important role in their lives.

We hope you find this book helpful for conducting CBT with people who have chemical and behavioral addictions. And we hope you find this work as rewarding as we do.

CHAPTER 2

THEORETICAL MODEL

At the heart of CBT is a theoretical model that enables therapists to understand addictive behaviors—in order to help patients who struggle with them. This model is essential for conceptualizing patients who engage in potentially life-threatening addictive behaviors despite the risks they face. Our model encompasses some fundamental cognitive processes. We begin this chapter by focusing on these processes, which are essential for understanding the development and maintenance of addictive behaviors and SUDs.

THE COGNITIVE PROCESSES
UNDERLYING ADDICTIVE BEHAVIORS

Cognitive processes are mental activities that take many forms. They can be rigid or flexible, brief or enduring, deep-seated or incidental, self-enhancing or self-defeating. Cognitive processes discussed in this section include three broad categories: basic beliefs, addiction-related thoughts and beliefs, and automatic thoughts. We also describe several specific cognitive processes relevant to addictive behaviors: self-efficacy, outcome expectancies, permissive beliefs, and instrumental thoughts.

Broad Categories of Cognitive Processes

We use the two terms *thoughts* and *beliefs* throughout this book. Generally speaking, we define a *thought* as an idea or image that may manifest as an impression, prediction, judgment, memory, plan, and so forth. Examples of thoughts include: "I'm getting wasted on Saturday night," "I can't wait to eat that grilled salmon," or "I'm going to buy $150 running shoes today." *Automatic thoughts* are especially brief, spontaneous, and "not the result of deliberation or reasoning" (J. S. Beck, 2021, p. 29). Examples of automatic thoughts include: "Party time!" or "I need relief."

Beliefs, on the other hand, are more enduring cognitive processes that develop over time and *give rise to thoughts*. For example, the thought above about getting wasted might stem from the belief that, "The best way to spend a Saturday night is to get very drunk." The thought regarding grilled salmon might grow out of the belief that "Salmon is a healthy food that tastes good." In fact, a single thought may be the result of multiple beliefs. For example, the thought above regarding running shoes might reflect the two beliefs, "Running is an essential part of my life" and "It is necessary to purchase expensive running shoes to run my best." (Chapter 10 provides a detailed discussion of thoughts and beliefs associated with addictive behaviors.)

Basic beliefs (also referred to as *core beliefs*) are principles, ideas, or values that are central to a person's identity. They include at least the following content domains: self, world, future, others, and relationships. Examples from each domain are presented in Table 2.1. Basic beliefs are largely responsible for individuals' recurrent emotions and behaviors, including addictive behaviors. For example, individuals who believe they are worthwhile and lovable are likely to feel more joy and fulfillment than those who believe they are unworthy and unlovable. Individuals who believe the world is safe and predictable are more likely to feel free and take healthy risks out in the *real world* than those who believe that the world is unsafe and unpredictable. In contrast, individuals with pervasive negative beliefs about themselves, their personal worlds, futures, other people, and relationships are more prone to developing depression and anxiety (Clark & Beck, 2010; Beck et al., 1979).

TABLE 2.1. Positive and Negative Basic Beliefs about Self, World, Future, Others, and Relationships

Domain	Positive basic belief	Negative basic belief
Self	"I am a worthwhile, lovable person."	"I am unworthy and unlovable."
World	"The world is safe and predictable."	"The world is unsafe and unpredictable."
Future	"I am hopeful."	"I am hopeless."
Others	"People are trustworthy."	"People are untrustworthy."
Relationships	"I will be nurtured in relationships."	"I will be hurt in relationships."

Negative beliefs put people at risk for addictive behaviors in several ways. For example, those who have pervasive negative beliefs and corresponding emotional distress may seek relief from their distress by using addictive substances and behaviors. This process has often been labeled "self-medicating." Furthermore, negative basic beliefs are likely to include helplessness or hopelessness (e.g., "I can't do anything right" and "Nothing matters"), consistent with failure to control addictive behaviors and relapse.

It is well known that people with addictions and SUDs are at risk for co-occurring mental health problems. In fact, according to the National Institute of Drug Abuse (NIDA), "about half of people who experience a mental illness will also experience a substance use disorder at some point in their lives and vice versa" (NIDA, 2018a). These people find themselves in vicious cycles that involve negative basic beliefs, leading to negative emotional states, including depression and anxiety (see Figure 2.1). As already noted, many people use drugs and addictive behaviors at least partly to seek relief from these negative affective states. But instead of finding enduring comfort they find only momentary relief, with more severe long-term addiction-related problems that exacerbate their preexisting mental health problems.

Addiction-related thoughts and beliefs are simply thoughts and beliefs associated with addictive behaviors (see Table 2.2). Form 2.1 at the end of the chapter can be reproduced and used with clients. For example, individuals who consume alcohol, tobacco, other drugs, or food specifically to regulate emotions, typically hold addiction-related thoughts and beliefs that correspond with their chosen addictive behaviors. For example, a cigarette smoker might believe, "Smoking is satisfying" or "I need smoke breaks to slow down and relax." A person with a drinking

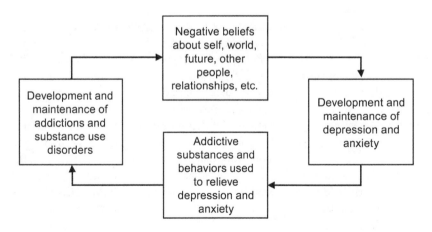

FIGURE 2.1. Vicious cycle involving addiction and co-occurring depression and anxiety.

TABLE 2.2. Addiction-Related and Self-Control Thoughts and Beliefs

Addiction-Related Thoughts and Beliefs	Self-Control Thoughts and Beliefs
"Smoking is satisfying."	"Being healthy is more satisfying than smoking."
"I need smoke breaks to slow down and relax."	"I can slow down and relax without smoking."
"Drinking makes it easier to be myself."	"When I drink, I'm not really myself; I'm just a drunk version of myself."
"Life is more fun when people are buzzed."	"I'm learning that I can have fun without being buzzed."
"Concentrating on anything while I'm hungry is impossible."	"Binge eating and overeating do not help me concentrate but they do help me gain weight."
"If I keep gambling, I will eventually win back all my losses."	"I will never win back my losses; everyone knows the house always wins."
"I just love the sights and sounds of a casino."	"I just love the sight of money in my bank account."

problem might believe, "Drinking makes it easier to be myself" or "Life is more fun when people are buzzed." A person who overeats or binge eats might believe, "Concentrating on anything while I'm hungry is impossible" or "Eating a big meal is the best way to celebrate." A person with gambling disorder might believe, "If I keep gambling, I will eventually win back all my losses" or "I just love the sights and sounds of a casino."

In contrast to addiction-related thoughts and beliefs, there are self-control thoughts and beliefs. Self-control thoughts and beliefs are central to the recovery process. Examples include "Being healthy is more satisfying than smoking," "When I drink, I'm not really myself; I'm just a drunk version of myself," and "I'm learning that I can have fun without being buzzed" (see Table 2.2). People who struggle with addictions (and their therapists) often underestimate the time and effort it takes to develop new self-control thoughts and beliefs. They sometimes forget that addiction-related thoughts and beliefs may take decades of repetition to develop and preserve. As a result, they may find themselves frustrated with the slow progress associated with formulating self-control thoughts and beliefs that are more salient than addictive thoughts and beliefs. Patients and therapists alike are encouraged to be patient and perseverant as they work on this challenging transition together.

Automatic thoughts (ATs), mentioned earlier, are fleeting words, phrases, or images that rapidly enter and exit a person's awareness. ATs are profoundly influential and yet most people do not recognize when they occur. Examples of ATs leading to addictive behaviors might include "Smoke break!" (prior to smoking a cigarette), "I'm starving!" (prior to eating), or "Party!" (prior to using a drug for celebrating). ATs are particularly insidious for at least four reasons: (1) they seem to appear spontaneously, out of nowhere; (2) they disappear as quickly as they appear; (3) they may appear as images, rather than words; and (4) they have the potential to trigger powerful urges, craving, lapses, and relapses. For example, the image of lighting a cigarette and taking a puff would most likely trigger craving in a heavy smoker. The image of ice clinking in a glass might trigger craving in a heavy drinker. Imagining a hit from a joint, pipe, or bong might trigger craving in a heavy marijuana smoker. The image of biting into a favorite food might trigger craving for that food, even in the absence of actual physiologic hunger. Imagined sights and sounds of a casino (e.g., slot machines, card tables, roulette wheels) might trigger intense urges, craving, lapses, or relapses in a gambler.

Given the power of addiction-related thoughts and beliefs, a major role of the cognitive-behavioral therapist is to help patients identify and address these thoughts and beliefs before they lead to lapses and relapses. Among the many ways to identify and address these is through functional analysis. Functional analysis (also known as chain analysis), carried out by therapists retrospectively, involves asking for a chronological accounting of triggers, thoughts, beliefs, feelings, and actions leading up to addictive behaviors. Functional analysis is a foundational CBT technique, and it will be described in detail later in Chapter 6.

Specific Cognitive Processes Relevant to Addictive Behaviors

When *Cognitive Therapy of Substance Abuse* came out, there was little research on the role of specific thoughts or beliefs in addictive behaviors. However, over the past 30 years, hundreds of publications have focused on at least three addiction-related cognitive processes: self-efficacy, positive outcome expectancies, and negative outcome expectancies.

Self-efficacy is best understood as individuals' appraisals of their abilities to accomplish specific tasks or achieve specific goals. Self-efficacy is not the same as self-esteem or self-confidence. The latter two concepts involve a more global sense of self, whereas self-efficacy is more like self-confidence regarding a specific skill or outcome. In the context of addictive behaviors, self-efficacy might involve individuals' beliefs about their abilities to achieve abstinence, or to pursue substance-free activities, for example. The concept of self-efficacy was initially applied to addictive behaviors by Marlatt and Gordon (1985) in their classic *Relapse Prevention* text. According to Marlatt, individuals who perceive themselves to possess effective coping skills and self-efficacy are most likely to effectively control their substance use; those who do not perceive themselves to possess effective coping skills are at greatest risk for relapse. Self-efficacy (or the lack of it) can manifest as a deeply held belief (e.g., "I can easily stop eating when I start to feel full" versus "When good food is put in front of me, I just can't stop eating"). Self-efficacy may also manifest as an automatic thought (e.g., "I can" or "I can't").

Outcome expectancies have been extensively studied, and psychometric instruments have been developed to assess outcome expectancies for alcohol use (e.g., Nicolai, Demmel, & Moshagen, 2010), marijuana use (e.g., Buckner, Ecker, & Welch, 2013), prescription pain medication use (e.g., Ilgen et al., 2011), gambling (e.g., Wickwire, Whelan, & Meyers, 2010), and Internet activity (e.g., Brand, Laier, & Young, 2014). Studies of outcome expectancies provide empirical support for some of the most essential CBT principles regarding thoughts, beliefs, emotions, and addictive behaviors. As the term implies, *outcome expectancies* are thoughts and beliefs about the consequences associated with specific addictive behaviors. In *Cognitive Therapy of Substance Abuse* we referred to outcome expectancies as *anticipatory thoughts and beliefs*. We continue to find this terminology to be useful and interchange these terms throughout this text.

Positive outcome expectancies include basic beliefs and ATs involving good or desired outcomes resulting from engagement in addictive behaviors. Obviously, these positive outcome expectancies increase the likelihood of engaging in addictive behaviors. As just a few examples:

"Drinking makes it easier for me to express my feelings."
"Smoking a cigarette will calm my nerves."
"I get more done when I do a line of cocaine."
"I always feel better after a good meal."

It should be obvious that a major goal of CBT is to recognize and challenge positive outcome expectancies that lead to lapses and relapses (Li & Dingle, 2012). Strategies and standardized techniques for doing so will be presented later in Chapters 6 and 7.

Negative outcome expectancies include thoughts and beliefs about problematic or undesired outcomes resulting from addictive behaviors. These negative outcome expectancies reduce the likelihood of engaging in addictive behaviors. The following are just a few examples of negative outcome expectancies:

"If I drink too much, I'll do stupid things."
"Cigarette smoking will make me stink of tobacco."
"Overeating will lead to health problems."
"Buying drugs on the street will land me in jail."

Consider the case of Rick who is morbidly obese and recently learned that he has diabetes. Rick has always had positive outcome expectancies regarding his favorite foods, believing strongly that certain foods provide a great sense of comfort. In fact, like many people, Rick labeled these his "comfort foods." In stark contrast to Rick's positive views of comfort foods were his negative views, recently triggered by his diagnosis of diabetes: "Eating these foods will ruin my health." Rick also had negative outcome expectancies triggered when thinking about looking in the mirror each morning: "Eating like I do will make me less and less attractive." Furthermore, each time he noticed that formerly loose clothing fit more tightly, he thought: "If I keep eating like this, none of my clothing will fit me." Eventually, Rick's negative outcome expectancies caught up with his positive outcome expectancies, which led to profound ambivalence.

In reality, most people with addictions experience *ambivalence* about their behaviors. Like Rick, they have competing positive and negative outcome expectancies. When this occurs, individuals make decisions based on their most salient thoughts and beliefs at the time. A variety of CBT techniques (e.g., decisional balance and advantages–disadvantages analysis) focus on cognitive dissention between negative and positive outcome expectancies. These techniques, aimed at decreasing the salience of positive outcome expectancies, are presented in Chapter 7.

Perhaps one of the most prominent CBT concepts is that people generally prefer *immediate* or *instant* gratification over *delayed* gratification. In other words, their positive outcome expectancies are greater when rewards are immediate, versus when they are delayed. Depending on the individual, addictive behaviors provide instant gratification in the form of more comfort or less *dis*comfort. For example, a large scoop of ice cream *right now* in Rick's mind is more comforting than waiting weeks, months, or years to experience benefits associated with physical fitness. This process (a preference for instant versus delayed gratification) has been the focus of research on *delay discounting,* defined as the process of discounting, or reducing the perceived value, of events that happen in the distant future. Years of research in the field of behavioral economics support this concept (see reviews by Bickel, Johnson, Koffarnus, MacKillop, & Murphy, 2014; Reynolds, 2006).

Prior to leaving this discussion of addiction-related beliefs, we review two more cognitive processes central to understanding addictive behaviors: *permissive beliefs* and *instrumental thoughts.*

Permissive beliefs are important because they occur at vulnerable moments when people are likely to be ambivalent about their addictive behaviors. Permissive beliefs may be the "last straw" before a lapse or relapse. Recall the case of Rick, from above. Given an opportunity to eat unhealthy foods, Rick's negative outcome expectancies might include, "Eating this pizza will make my diabetes worse" or "Eating this pizza will make my clothing fit tighter." Opposing these thoughts and beliefs are permissive thoughts and beliefs like, "One slice of pizza won't kill me" or "I'll start my diet tomorrow." Some have referred to permissive beliefs as rationalizations, justifications, or excuses. We prefer the term *permissive beliefs* because it reduces stigma associated with the other terms, and it more closely conveys the cognitive dynamic of *giving oneself permission.*

Instrumental thoughts are also important, as they guide the logistics or mechanics of addictive behaviors. Instrumental thoughts and beliefs involve the "how to." For example, if Rick decides to eat pizza tonight, this decision will be followed by instrumental thoughts about how he will order and consume this pizza so that he is not embarrassed about eating in public. For example, he might think, "I'll get a large pizza from the Acme Pizza Company and eat at home on the couch, watching my favorite TV shows." He might then add a permissive belief: "I'll only eat two or three slices and save the rest for later in the week." It helps to identify instrumental thoughts because, if caught in time, they can be replaced by thoughts about alternative behaviors that divert individuals away from their addictive behaviors.

THE CBT MODEL IN ACTION

From the earliest days of CBT, the basic "ABC" model in Figure 2.2 has prevailed. According to this most basic model, antecedent internal and external triggers (e.g., cues, situations, circumstances, stimuli) activate beliefs and thoughts, which directly impact emotions, behaviors, and physiological responses.

Antecedents or *triggers* are stimuli that activate thoughts and beliefs such as those described in the previous paragraphs. Marlatt and Gordon (1985) labeled triggers "high-risk situations." Triggers can be internal or external. Internal triggers may involve physical or emotional sensations, like anxiety, depression, urges, craving, and pain. External triggers include the people, places, and things that are associated with addictive behaviors. Most important about triggers is the fact that they activate thoughts and beliefs that potentially lead to lapses and relapses. For example, exposure to an external trigger, like an unfinished pack of cigarettes found in the seat of a car, might certainly activate thoughts about smoking in

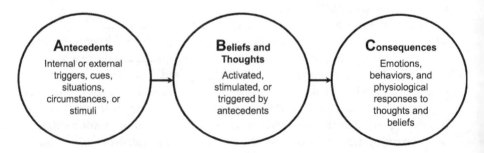

FIGURE 2.2.   The ABC model.

an ex-smoker. An internal trigger, for example emotional distress, may activate thoughts about taking prescription pain medication in a person who had been addicted to pain medications in the past.

Behaviors are actions or activities meant to accomplish a goal or achieve an outcome. Purchasing a pack of cigarettes, opening the pack, taking out a cigarette, lighting it, inhaling the smoke, and eventually snuffing out the butt, are all behaviors associated with smoking. Each behavior is initiated in order to accomplish some goal unique to smoking. For some smokers, the ultimate goal of smoking is to relieve stress, while for others the goal is to stop uncomfortable nicotine withdrawal symptoms. As noted earlier, addictive behaviors aim to increase comfort and decrease discomfort.

Over time, most daily behaviors become repetitious. For example, getting out of bed, getting ready for the day's activities, eating meals, texting friends, traveling from place to place, returning home, and getting ready for bed—all tend to be repetitious. As we repeat behaviors, they become habitual, mediated by automatic thoughts. We don't think much about them; they just seem to happen. Of particular interest is that people experience specific automatic thoughts in response to specific triggers. For example, when we wake up in the morning, especially if it's light outside (both waking and light are triggers), we realize, "It's time to get up" (the automatic thought), and we climb out of bed (the behavior). The automatic nature of behaviors is particularly poignant in addictive behaviors; they, too, become automatic and habitual. The cigarette smoker does not give much thought to purchasing or lighting a cigarette. The person with an active opioid use disorder does not give much thought to opening the medicine cabinet and swallowing a pain pill or two with a gulp of water. Behaviors must become automatic so we can function throughout the day and not need to give careful, deliberate thought to activities like showering or starting the car.

An important feature of the ABC model is its logic and simplicity, particularly as a system for explaining psychological processes to patients. Many patients misattribute their emotions, behaviors, and physical feelings to external phenomena (i.e., situations and circumstances). When talking to patients about these phenomena, we explain, "It's your thoughts and beliefs that most impact your feelings and behaviors; not the circumstances around you. You have the freedom to interpret your world and therefore behave however you choose." We emphasize that people, in general, do not have much control over the external world, but they may develop healthy control over their thoughts and beliefs, which in turn impact their behaviors and emotions.

While it is understood that behaviors are activated by thoughts and beliefs, it is important to realize that behaviors also function as triggers that activate thoughts and beliefs. For example, a person with alcohol use disorder, shopping in a grocery store and standing in front of a beer display, thinks, "I have no beer at home. I need to pick some up." This thought leads to picking up a six-pack of beer and placing it in a grocery cart (i.e., the behavior resulting from the preceding thought). The act of placing beer in the grocery cart (a behavior) triggers the thought, "I'd love to pop one open and drink it right now!" This kind of thinking may (unfortunately) lead to paying for the groceries, walking to the car, opening the beer, drinking it in the car, and then driving home. The functional (or chain) analysis illustrating this process, is presented in Figure 2.3.

Emotions, sometimes referred to as feelings or moods, are subjective experiences intricately linked to addictive behaviors. It is universally acknowledged that people strive to maximize positive emotions and minimize negative emotions. Those who have difficulty regulating their emotions are likely more vulnerable to addictive behaviors than those who effectively regulate their emotions. Evidence for this premise is the fact that people with mental health problems are at higher risk for addictions. As we mentioned earlier, many people who engage in addictive behaviors do so to increase positive emotions or decrease negative emotions. In other words, many individuals turn to addictive substances and behaviors to self-medicate.

The CBT model of addictive behaviors and SUDs is presented in Figure 2.4. This model does not differ much from the model we presented in *Cognitive Therapy of Substance Abuse.* In fact, more than a quarter century of helping addicted individuals has only reinforced our original view of addictive behaviors. According to this model, addiction lapses and relapses are part of a vicious cycle that begins with internal and/or external triggers, activating addiction-related thoughts. These thoughts inevitably lead to urges and craving to engage in addictive behavior. Following these urges and craving, individuals have an opportunity to abstain from their addictive behaviors. However, if they instead grant themselves permission to engage, they most likely will lapse back into their addictive behaviors.

It is important to understand that a single lapse has the potential to function as the new antecedent event, triggering a flood of addiction-related thoughts and beliefs that perpetuate addictive behaviors. Marlatt and Gordon (1985) introduced the phrase *abstinence violation effect* (AVE) to denote a set of thoughts and behaviors that perpetuate a full relapse. The AVE begins as the thought, "I violated my commitment to abstinence, so I might as well keep using." Or, framed as an automatic thought, it might just be, "The hell with abstinence!"

THE DEVELOPMENT OF ADDICTIVE BEHAVIORS

It is essential for cognitive-behavioral therapists to understand how patients develop their addictive behaviors. By doing so, therapists are likely to acquire vital clues regarding treatment. For example, if a patient's heavy drinking is precipitated by a history of social anxiety, we understand the importance of addressing this anxiety while treating the drinking problem. If a patient with an opioid use disorder

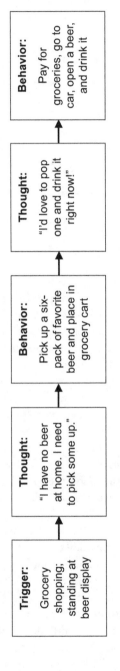

Trigger:

Grocery shopping; standing at beer display

Thought:

"I have no beer at home. I need to pick some up."

Behavior:

Pick up a six-pack of favorite beer and place in grocery cart

Thought:

"I'd love to pop one and drink it right now!"

Behavior:

Pay for groceries, go to car, open a beer, and drink it

FIGURE 2.3. Functional analysis illustrating how behaviors become triggers.

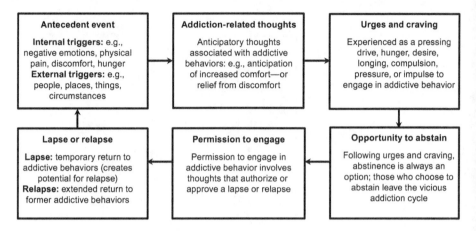

Antecedent event	Addiction-related thoughts	Urges and craving
Internal triggers: e.g., negative emotions, physical pain, discomfort, hunger **External triggers:** e.g., people, places, things, circumstances	Anticipatory thoughts associated with addictive behaviors: e.g., anticipation of increased comfort—or relief from discomfort	Experienced as a pressing drive, hunger, desire, longing, compulsion, pressure, or impulse to engage in addictive behavior

Lapse or relapse	Permission to engage	Opportunity to abstain
Lapse: temporary return to addictive behaviors (creates potential for relapse) **Relapse:** extended return to former addictive behaviors	Permission to engage in addictive behavior involves thoughts that authorize or approve a lapse or relapse	Following urges and craving, abstinence is always an option; those who choose to abstain leave the vicious addiction cycle

FIGURE 2.4. The cognitive-behavioral model of addictive behaviors and SUDs.

has a history of childhood trauma, we understand the importance of determining whether opioids are being taken to address painful consequences of such trauma. If a patient is struggling with any addictive behavior, it can be helpful to identify a family history of addictions, in order to help that patient understand the important role genetics or early life experiences may play in their addiction.

We cannot overemphasize the importance of understanding how addictive behaviors develop. In formulating individual case conceptualizations, we first collect information about current triggers, addiction-related thoughts, beliefs, emotions, and behaviors. But following this initial process we assess how addictive behaviors have developed *for each individual patient.* In this section, we focus on some of the many risk factors, including early life experiences, that may contribute to or even cause patients' addictive behaviors. Influenced by the work of Shaffer and colleagues (2012; 2004), we also label these risk factors distal antecedents. Distal antecedents include genetic, neurobiological, psychosocial, and environmental factors (see Figure 2.5).

The importance of *genetic* factors (i.e., heredity) should not be underestimated when assessing and treating addictive behaviors. In fact, addictions have been described as being "among the most heritable of psychiatric disorders" (Goldman, Oroszi, & Ducci, 2005, p. 522). Researchers have estimated that between 39% and 72% of addictive behaviors are attributable to heredity, depending on the drug (Bevilacqua & Goldman, 2009; Goldman et al., 2005). Besides the high likelihood that genetics play a direct role in addictions, genetics may also play a direct role in other mental health problems that may precipitate or perpetuate addictive behaviors. For example, people with a family history of depression and other potentially heritable mental health problems are at greater risk for addictions than those who do not have a family history of mental health problems. It is important for therapists to understand these processes so they can help patients gain an understanding of their addictions.

The development of addictions is also directly attributable to early life *psychosocial* and *environmental* factors (again, see Figure 2.5). A thorough review by Enoch (2011) found that alcohol and drug problems may be linked to early life stressors, including maltreatment (e.g., physical and emotional abuse, neglect, sexual abuse) and stressful life events (e.g., parental divorce, family violence, economic adversity, parental death, and mental illness). Many people with addictions, and professionals who provide treatment to them, identify addictive behaviors with *self-medicating* (Bolton, Robinson, & Sareen, 2009; NIDA, 2010). For example, growing up in an abusive, neglectful, chaotic environment, or in a family, community, or social environment where drug use is routine, places individuals at risk for developing addictions themselves. We use the term "vulnerability" to explain this phenomenon. It is understood that the adverse distal antecedents listed above lead to cognitive, behavioral, and affective vulnerabilities. And then exposure, experimentation, and continued engagement in addictive behaviors reinforce the thoughts and beliefs that perpetuate addictive behaviors.

Now consider the case of Bill, a 36-year-old man. Bill's wife, Brenda, became concerned when Bill grew sullen and withdrawn soon after the birth of their first

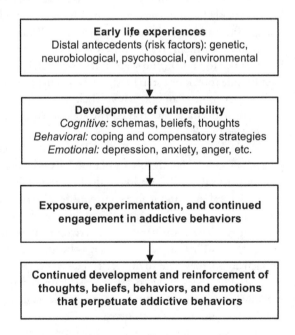

FIGURE 2.5. Development of addictive behaviors.

child, Samantha. Eventually, Brenda made an appointment for a conjoint session with a cognitive-behavioral therapist recommended by their family physician. By conducting a thorough history, Bill's therapist recognized the pattern that developed after Samantha's birth. Bill would come home and find Brenda busy with Samantha. Feeling lonely, he would mix himself a strong martini and sit in front of the television. At dinner and then afterward, Bill would drink another martini and then another, until he eventually passed out in front of the television. Sometimes it was difficult for Brenda to wake and escort him to the bedroom. Bill's therapist helped Bill understand that he had developed a vicious cycle in which he would feel lonely, drink alcohol, spend time alone, become lonelier, drink more, and then pass out. In the morning Bill regularly woke up feeling hung over, guilty, and angry at himself. Eventually this pattern led to Bill lapsing into a major depressive episode that he "just couldn't shake."

As he began to treat Bill's depression and alcohol use, the therapist asked Bill about his past. Bill's responses resembled the responses of many patients before him. He claimed, "I had a great childhood"; "We went on lots of vacations"; "My parents came to all my games"; "My mom was really sweet." Fortunately, the therapist, skillful at taking a thorough history, asked about any family history of mental health problems, including addictive behaviors. Bill responded by explaining that his mother went through some dark times, but his father never drank. He then added, somewhat defensively, "I certainly don't drink too much: maybe one or two cocktails a night." It quickly became apparent that Bill's wife, Brenda, would be helpful in the first and future sessions, because she offered additional information. She stated, "Bill, I think your mom was depressed and I think your dad stopped drinking because he drank too much, and your mom eventually gave him an ultimatum." And then Brenda took it one step further: "Bill, don't get angry at me for saying this, but you drink more than one or two cocktails a night. It's more like two, three, or even four drinks a night. You go through at least one of those big bottles with a handle every week."

Bill's therapist asked many more questions about Bill's background and learned that Bill had a substantial family history of mood disorders and addictions. Several men on his father's side died from likely alcohol-related health problems. On his mother's side, several men and women suffered from serious mood disorders. Based on this information, Bill's therapist knew he would benefit from psychoeducation regarding the genetic influences of affective and addiction disorders.

Patients' reports of early life trauma, or abuse, may be unreliable. And instead of overestimating such abuse, they tend to underestimate it (Fergusson, Horwood, & Woodward, 2000). Therapists need to ask precise, targeted questions (e.g., "What do you mean when you say that your mother went through a dark period?" and "What factors led to your father's decision to abstain from drinking?"). Otherwise, therapists will have vague, generalized information about patients, rather than precise, relevant details.

As we will discuss later, perhaps the most important component of CBT is the case conceptualization. The conceptualization of addictive behaviors necessarily includes the acute symptoms, including associated thoughts, feelings, and behaviors, but it also includes the development of these. And learning about the development of each patient's addictive behaviors is an essential part of the case conceptualization process.

THE MAINTENANCE OF ADDICTIVE BEHAVIORS

We presented our basic CBT model earlier in Figure 2.4. To reiterate, addictive behaviors inevitably function as self-sustaining vicious cycles. The decision to engage or not engage begins when individuals are exposed to triggers. This exposure activates learned addiction-related thoughts and beliefs that naturally lead to urges and craving. Prior to engaging in addictive behaviors, individuals have an opportunity to abstain from doing so. However, abstaining almost inevitably leads to substantial discomfort. When an individual abstains, it is likely because that individual generates control-related thoughts and beliefs (e.g., "If I don't partake I'll feel so much better tomorrow" and "I don't want to break my promise to myself"). Those who fail to generate control-related thoughts are likely to give themselves permission to engage in addictive behaviors, leading to continued engagement. This engagement is highly reinforcing, and it becomes a trigger for continued use, resulting in the vicious cycle of addictive behaviors. Put simply, people choose addictive behaviors because they *anticipate* some benefit from doing so. Addiction-related thoughts, feelings, and behaviors become so automatic that they are almost imperceptible by the addicted person, who develops the belief, "I'm out of control and will never be able to stop this behavior." CBT helps such individuals by providing them with a deeper understanding of this vicious cycle and guiding them to decide how they want to break this cycle.

A major factor in maintaining addictive behaviors is the common belief that discontinuing the behavior will produce intolerable side effects. In reality, these effects vary enormously from person to person and from substance to substance, and the impact is greatly enhanced by the psychological meaning attached to the withdrawal symptoms. These meanings are often more salient than the actual adverse physiological sensations in determining the intensity of withdrawal symptoms. Hence, a common goal of CBT for addictions is to help patients change the meaning of withdrawal from "This discomfort is my punishment for being so stupid!" to "This discomfort means I'm doing important work to better my life."

In the earlier example, Bill's potential for having a lapse or relapse began when he arrived home from work (see Figure 2.6).

Careful examination of Bill's thoughts, feelings, and behaviors helps us understand how he maintained his drinking pattern, despite potentially severe

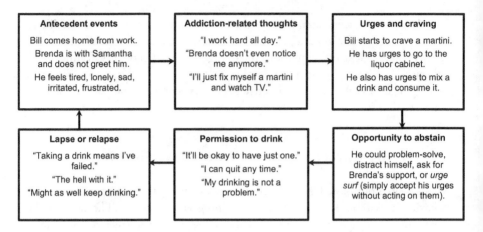

FIGURE 2.6. CBT model of addictions applied to Bill.

negative consequences. His addiction to alcohol involved a vicious cycle that was self-sustaining. After repeated use, he developed thoughts and beliefs regarding the necessity of continued drinking, and physiologic dependence on alcohol. Attempts to stop drinking resulted in withdrawal symptoms, which triggered thoughts and beliefs about the necessity of continued drinking.

Bill's therapist helped him to accept and then overcome the discomfort he felt from reducing his alcohol consumption, so he could focus on his loneliness and troubled marriage. This process of accepting discomfort is vital to recovery from addictive behaviors. Marlatt and Gordon (1985) coined the term *urge surfing* to reflect this process of accepting discomfort. We will discuss urge surfing in much more detail later in this text.

Thanks to his wife's support and urging, Bill eventually decided to completely abstain from drinking. He was also helped by his therapist to articulate that he felt abandoned by Brenda when their baby was born. Upon hearing this, Brenda actually cried and reassured Bill of her love. At the end of therapy Bill reviewed the progress he had made: "It was so hard to admit that drinking was a problem. I just wasn't ready to give it up. Brenda and Samantha's love sure feels better than any bottle of booze I've consumed, and their love doesn't give me a hangover."

THE COURSE OF ADDICTIVE BEHAVIORS

When we talk about the course of addictive behaviors, it is especially helpful to focus on the ups and downs experienced by people with addictive behaviors. These ups and downs have the potential to profoundly impact the ebb and flow of treatment.

This is where the transtheoretical (stages of change) model can be especially useful (Norcross et al., 2011; Prochaska et al., 1992; Prochaska & Norcross, 2001). The stages of change are complex, dynamic, and to some extent unpredictable—rather than simple, static, or predictable. Furthermore, the term *stages* can be misleading. It is rare that people with addictions experience recovery as occurring in a linear, staged fashion. Instead, lapses and relapses are common. People commonly reach one stage, only to return to an earlier one, often several times, before resolving their addiction. In presenting these concepts here, we focus on the thoughts and behaviors associated with each stage of addiction and recovery.

Prochaska, DiClemente, Norcross, and colleagues describe five stages of change experienced over the course of addictive behaviors. These stages include precontemplation, contemplation, preparation, action, and maintenance. An understanding of these stages enables both clinicians and clients to anticipate the challenges and successes related to addiction treatment. The transtheoretical model addresses issues related to motivation and lends itself easily to approaches to change. Furthermore, the transtheoretical model focuses on the interplay between thoughts, feelings, and behaviors that are central to the CBT model of addictions. Let's begin by defining each stage.

The *precontemplation stage,* just as the name implies, involves the time before contemplation has begun. It may or may not include an awareness of an addictive behavior, but it certainly does not include a desire or plan to change. It is reasonable to assume that the beliefs held by a person in precontemplation might be:

"I don't have a problem."
"I have a problem but I'm not at all interested in making changes right now."
"My behavior is fully under my control."
"I'm not worried about my behavior."
"I don't care if my behavior is a problem, I enjoy things just as they are."

The *contemplation stage* is when individuals begin to consider whether or not it is time to change their behaviors. Earlier in this chapter we discussed ambivalence. Ambivalence is typically most salient in the contemplation stage. By this, we mean that it is likely that people in contemplation will go back and forth regarding whether or not it is the right time to quit, whether they need to quit, how they might quit, and why maybe they should not yet quit. For many people with addictions, contemplation is a difficult time, riddled with self-doubt and self-criticism. Examples of thoughts of someone in contemplation might be:

"I know I should quit, but I'm not sure I'm ready."
"I don't like what my addiction is doing to me, but I could probably continue for a while longer without causing much damage."
"I want to quit but I don't know how."

"I don't want to quit, but I should."
"Maybe I can quit this week, or maybe not."

The *preparation stage* is sandwiched between contemplation and action. It is a time when individuals have begun to take action. Earlier in this chapter we described instrumental thoughts as the *how to* process. The preparation stage of change is the time when individuals are thinking about *how to* stop engaging in their addictive behaviors, rather than thinking about how they might continue. Thoughts of a person in the preparation stage might be:

"I'm throwing out all of my cigarettes today."
"I'm going shopping, so I can fill my refrigerator with only healthy foods."
"I'm deleting my dealer's phone from my phone and blocking his number."
"I'm going to my doctor to find out about medication-assisted treatment—so I can stop taking all these prescription pain pills."
"I'm telling all my friends that I won't be drinking with them anymore."

The *action stage* is the time when an individual has made desired changes, but only relatively recently. Research suggests the action stage continues for six months after change has been initiated. Some have argued (and we tend to agree) that the action stage is when individuals are most vulnerable to having a lapse or relapse. Here are some of the thoughts of a person in the action stage:

"I can't believe I've gone for 30 days without using."
"I wonder why I'm not craving."
"I hope I can keep this up."
"I wake up feeling more energetic."
"I wonder if I'll ever go back to [the old addictive behavior]."

In the *maintenance stage,* individuals have integrated changes into their lives and their new lifestyle feels "normal." Some people in the maintenance stage say they miss their old addictive behavior, but most do not. The primary risk during this stage and the action stage is that some individuals begin to think that they can return to their past addictive behavior now that they have good control over it. This thinking is illustrated in some of the thoughts below:

"I can't believe I used to be a [drinker, smoker, etc.]."
"I don't even think about using anymore."
"I feel pretty good without [the addiction] in my life."
"Maybe someday I'll be able to [eat/drink/smoke] like a normal person."
"I'll have to just wait and see."

There are important implications of these stages of change; namely, individuals in the various stages of change think and act differently, so their needs are different. For example, a person contemplating change may benefit from a review of the advantages and disadvantages of their addictive behaviors. In contrast, a person in the action stage of change might benefit most from a discussion of triggers that might present challenges to the patient's changes. Perhaps more importantly, the thoughts that correspond with their readiness to change will determine their receptivity to interventions. For example, a person in the precontemplation stage who thinks, "I don't have any problems in need of fixing," is unlikely to respond well to an invitation to do an advantages–disadvantages analysis of their addictive behavior.

SUMMARY

A theoretical model is vital for understanding addictive behaviors. It enables cognitive-behavioral therapists to identify mechanisms and targets for change. Our experiences with addicted individuals have been that they enter CBT with little knowledge regarding the interplay between their thoughts, feelings, and behaviors. They attribute many of their problems to circumstances beyond their control. For example, they believe that other people make them angry, rather than understanding that their thoughts and beliefs play a more important role in their feelings.

It has been our experience that people with addictions find our model to be helpful. While it was initially developed for therapists' understanding, we have found patients greatly appreciate a model for understanding their own problematic behaviors. In the chapters that follow we discuss strategies and techniques for helping people with addictive behaviors. All of our strategies and techniques are based on the CBT model. Understanding that antecedent events trigger addiction-related beliefs reminds us that it is important to encourage patients to be aware of these triggers and take steps to avoid high-risk situations. Realizing the power of addiction-related thoughts and beliefs helps us to emphasize that patients will need to change many of these thoughts and beliefs. Reminding patients that there is a moment when abstinence is possible, as long as they do not give themselves permission to use, is potentially helpful to patients who might otherwise relapse.

Instructions: In the left column, write thoughts and beliefs likely to lead to your addictive behaviors. In the right column, write thoughts and beliefs that argue against the addiction-related thoughts and beliefs in the left column. Be sure to make them realistic and consistent with the thoughts you want to have as your own.

Addiction-Related Thoughts and Beliefs	Self-Control Thoughts and Beliefs
Examples: *"I need to take a drink to have fun." "I need to smoke to calm down." "I need to gamble to win back my money."*	Examples: *"I can have fun without drinking." "I can calm down without smoking." "I need to save my money instead of giving it to the casino."*

CHAPTER 3

CASE CONCEPTUALIZATION

No two people with addictions are exactly alike. People with addictions vary in the severity of their problems, their readiness to change, mental health, socioeconomic status, personal resources, social support, cultural practices, and perhaps most importantly their thoughts, beliefs, behaviors, and emotions. Because people differ, their treatment needs and plans must differ. Each individual's case conceptualization serves as a foundation for their individualized treatment plan. Accurate case conceptualizations enable therapists to understand the complexity of each patient's problems so they can help patients successfully resolve these problems. By weaving together each person's unique past and present thoughts, beliefs, schemas, feelings, behaviors, strengths, weaknesses, coping strategies, high-risk situations, and other processes, therapists can effectively understand the development and maintenance of addictive behaviors and ultimately assist patients in developing strategies to overcome their addictions. In this chapter we explain how our theoretical model is woven into the case conceptualization of individuals who struggle with addictions. The case conceptualization helps answer many essential questions, for example:

- How and why did *this* particular person develop addictive behaviors?
- How did this person's addictive behaviors escalate to their present level?
- How effectively did this person function prior to becoming addicted?
- What triggers precipitate this person's addictive behaviors (or relapses)?
- What unique schemas, thoughts, or beliefs maintain this person's addictive behaviors?
- What role does the environment play in this person's addictive behaviors?
- What barriers have prevented this person from stopping addictive behaviors?
- Do any other mental health problems contribute to this person's addictive behaviors?

Guided by questions like these, the cognitive-behavioral therapist is able to structure sessions and formulate strategies and techniques. Without a current, accurate case conceptualization the therapist is like a ship without a rudder, drifting aimlessly through the session.

10 ESSENTIAL ELEMENTS
OF THE CASE CONCEPTUALIZATION

In this section we present 10 elements that we consider essential to the case conceptualization. These elements provide a structure for organizing and integrating vast amounts of background information gathered from patients. While some information is deliberately collected at the beginning of therapy, much is collected over time as the therapist learns more and more about the patient. Thus, the case conceptualization is a collaborative and ongoing process between therapist and patient. The 10 essential elements of a case conceptualization are as follows:

1. *Primary problems:* SUDs/addiction; related mental and physical health conditions
2. *Social/environmental context:* Current living situation, close relationships, sociocultural factors, minority status, economic circumstances, any legal or safety concerns
3. *Distal antecedents:* Neurobiological, genetic, psychosocial, environmental influences
4. *Proximal antecedents:* Current internal and external cues, triggers, high-risk situations, circumstances, relationships
5. *Cognitive processes:* Relevant schemas, beliefs, thoughts; cognitive distortions, System 1 and System 2 thinking (described in Chapter 10)
6. *Affective processes:* Predominant emotions, feelings, moods, physiological sensations
7. *Behavioral patterns:* Adaptive versus maladaptive behaviors; coping skills versus compensatory strategies
8. *Readiness to change and associated goals:* Stages, from precontemplation to maintenance for all problem areas; short-term and long-term goals for all problems
9. *Integration of the data:* Salient processes; significant patterns; causal relationships between context, thoughts, beliefs, schemas, emotions, and behaviors
10. *Implications for treatment:* Identification of the most appropriate cognitive and behavioral strategies and techniques, based on the data collected

Primary problems include past and present SUDs/addictions, psychiatric diagnoses, and associated physical or medical concerns. As described in earlier chapters, it is common for individuals to have multiple addictions, consecutively or concurrently, and it is certainly common for individuals to have mental and physical health conditions that coexist with their SUDs and addictions. For example, it is particularly common to encounter patients with opioid use disorder (OUD) who struggle with pain and depression. In fact, many patients with OUD are first introduced to opioids by physicians who have prescribed them for physical pain, and many who become addicted have discovered that these drugs also provide relief from psychological suffering. As another example, it is common in clinical settings to encounter patients who are obese and depressed, and who struggle with binge eating. These individuals may also be addicted to tobacco and have numerous associated health problems (e.g., diabetes, hypertension, heart disease, pulmonary disease, and so forth). In fact, many smokers say they smoke in part to reduce overeating and prevent further weight gain.

When asking about primary problems, it is important to obtain accurate, detailed information. For example, when collecting information about alcohol and drug use it is important to learn about quantity, frequency, timing, and route of administration. Learning about quantity can help determine addiction severity. Obviously, someone who smokes two or three cigarettes per day is less addicted than someone who smokes two or three packs of cigarettes per day. Quantity is also important because it is associated with tolerance. For example, a person who says they "can easily drink between a pint and a fifth of vodka in a day" has certainly developed an alcohol tolerance that likely reflects a severe alcohol problem. Regardless of the drug of choice, it may be beneficial to ask about the route of drug administration (i.e., whether the drug is smoked, snorted, injected, inhaled, or chewed). This information has the potential to impact treatment plans because many individuals describe feeling addicted to the route of administration (e.g., injecting or inhaling) as much as to the chemical itself. It is just as important to collect accurate, detailed information about behavioral addictions. For example, time of day, location, surrounding atmosphere, social environment, amount of money won or lost, and the impact of losses are all essential when working with someone with gambling disorder.

Social/environmental context includes an individual's current living situation, close relationships, sociocultural factors, economic circumstances, legal or safety concerns, friends or family that may also have addiction problems, and so forth. The U.S. Office of Disease Prevention and Health Promotion (ODPHP) defines social determinants of health (SDOH) as conditions in which people "live, learn, work, play, worship, and age." They specifically list five key areas of SDOH: (1) economic stability; (2) education; (3) social and community context; (4) health and health care, and; (5) neighborhood and built environment. SDOH have the potential to profoundly influence individuals' thoughts, feelings, and behaviors, as well as their resources for making personal changes. Simply stated, a person living in a safe, secure environment with a supportive social structure has access to resources that are not available to a homeless person who moves from shelter to shelter and is in regular contact with people who also suffer from mental and physical health problems, social problems, and addictions.

When collecting information regarding an individual's social/environmental context, the following questions may be pertinent:

"Where and with whom do you live?"
"Do you feel safe and secure in your current living situation?"
"Do you have the necessary material resources to meet your basic needs?"
"How would you describe your social support system?"
"Do you view yourself as a member of a minority group (e.g., racial, ethnic, gender)? If so, how has this impacted your life?"
"Do you have close relationships with people who struggle with addictions or mental health problems? If so, what is the impact of these relationships?"

It is well known that people's living situations can profoundly influence their health and addictive behaviors. For example, people who live with heavy drinkers or smokers are more likely to drink or smoke. Consider the case of Mary and Rita, who are married and live together. Both struggle with problem gambling and cigarette smoking. Worried about her health and finances, Mary decides to simultaneously quit smoking and gambling. Thinking she should do the same, Rita commits to making these changes, though only half-heartedly. Weeks later, Rita receives an *Invitation-Only Special,* exclusively for casino card holders, that promises "great entertainment, discounted rooms, and a free all-you-can-eat buffet on Saturday night." Rita excitedly shares this opportunity with Mary, who reluctantly agrees to spend the weekend at the casino. Predictably, both women resume gambling and smoking, and years pass before they consider abstinence again.

Sociocultural factors also play an important role in the development and maintenance of SUDs and addictive behaviors. People who are socioeconomically disadvantaged or from certain minority groups (e.g., people of color, sexual and gender minorities) are more likely to struggle with addictions than those who are not (e.g., Keyes, Hatzenbuehler, Grant, & Hasin, 2012). An empirically supported explanation for this association is that these people experience greater stress as a result of being marginalized and stigmatized for their membership in these groups. Carefully assessing the impact of cultural factors (e.g., membership in a minority group) is important, especially since they impact individuals differently and to different degrees.

Distal antecedents include genetic, neurobiological, psychosocial, environmental, and cultural factors likely to contribute to the development and the maintenance of addictive behaviors. As explained in Chapter 2, a person with a family history of addictions is at significant risk of developing addictions. This increased risk might be a result of genetic, psychosocial, or environmental factors, or all of these. As therapists develop their case conceptualizations, they might ask any of the following questions:

"How and when did you begin to [smoke, drink, gamble, use drugs, etc.]?"

"How and when did you begin to realize you had a problem with [smoking, drinking, gambling, using drugs, etc.]?"

"Who else in your immediate or extended family [smoked, drank, gambled, used drugs, etc.]?"

"How did your early life experiences impact your current addictive behaviors?"

"How did your early life experiences influence the person you are today, beyond your addictions?"

"For example, what beliefs did you develop about yourself, the world around you, other people, relationships, and your future?"

While developing a case conceptualization a therapist might be told, "I was the only person with a *drinking problem* in my family." Upon hearing this, the therapist might explain that addictions take many forms, and then ask about any family history of *other addictive behaviors,* including tobacco use, gambling, street drugs, prescription drugs, and so forth. Searching for relevant distal factors and family history is not always as straightforward as it might seem. For example, the following exchange between a therapist and a 23-year-old patient demonstrates that retrieving relevant information sometimes requires focused and determined questioning:

THERAPIST: So, you're concerned about your drinking?

PATIENT: Yeah, I guess I drink too much. At least that's what my parents think.

THERAPIST: Tell me about your drinking, but also about your living situation.

PATIENT: I've lived with my parents for the past few months, since graduating from college. It's just until I find a decent full-time job and can support myself.

THERAPIST: Do you have a family history of problematic drug or alcohol use?

PATIENT: No, I'm the only one in the house who drinks.

THERAPIST: How about other family members?

PATIENT: My parents aren't alcoholics, if that's what you mean.

THERAPIST: No, it's just that sometimes people don't realize that family members might abstain because of past problems with alcohol or even other addictions.

PATIENT: I can't think of any family members with drinking problems.

THERAPIST: Any idea why your parents don't drink?

PATIENT: My dad once said something about how it nearly killed his dad.

THERAPIST: What do you think that's about?

PATIENT: Well, I guess it means my grandfather had a drinking problem. Maybe it scared my father into not drinking.

THERAPIST: Are you sure your father never drank?

PATIENT: I guess he did say something once about drinking when he was my age.

THERAPIST: How about your mom?

PATIENT: Well now that I think about it, both my mom and dad were cigarette smokers.

THERAPIST: It sounds like you may have some addictions in your family.

PATIENT: Maybe.

Given that many people with addictions come from families with addictions, it is important to consider the various ways that addictions impact family members. Therapists might explore whether family members modeled addictive behaviors. They might also ask about trauma caused or perpetuated by a family member's addictive behaviors. In many families with addictions, people develop beliefs like "alcohol takes the edge off" or "getting wasted is the only reliable way to escape." Some addicted patients come from volatile homes where they have been harshly treated, or where their worth is dependent on perfect behavior. These patients are at risk for developing core beliefs such as, "I'll never be good enough," "I can't do anything right," or "I might as well quit trying." Thoughts such as these have the potential to lead to feelings of depression, anxiety, and potentially addictive behaviors aimed at self-medicating.

Proximal antecedents (or triggers) include current circumstances and the full spectrum of problems faced by people with addictions, including relationship problems, unemployment, health problems, legal problems, unstable living arrangements, and more. As therapists conceptualize these various life problems, it is helpful to determine which problems *contribute to* addictive behaviors, which are *consequences of* addictive behaviors, and which are *both* contributory and consequential problems. CBT for addictions is incomplete without a treatment plan to address these problems, especially since many problems trigger addictive behaviors.

Proximal antecedents include immediate *external* circumstances in which addiction-related beliefs become activated. For example, consider the case of Joe, who has a history of severe alcohol use disorder. Joe has been abstinent for several months—until he is invited to an event where alcohol is served, people are drinking heavily, and everyone appears to be having fun. Watching these people, he starts to think, "This is not fair. I want to have as much fun as they're having." These thoughts activate strong alcohol-related beliefs, such as "Just a few beers would give me a great little buzz." This thought activates strong urges and craving. While experiencing these feelings Joe next has the permissive thought, "Just a few can't hurt me." Not surprisingly, this leads to one beer, and then a second beer, and a third, until finally Joe has had so much to drink that he can't see straight.

Proximal antecedents also include *internal* triggers, including emotions and physical sensations. People with addictions describe numerous internal sensations that trigger addiction-related beliefs and ultimately urges and craving. These include but are not limited to boredom, restlessness, sadness, frustration, anger, irritation, disappointment, worry, fear, loneliness, joy, excitement, surprise, exhilaration, tension, pain, numbness, restlessness, and fatigue. From this list, it should be obvious that both negative and positive sensations can lead to addiction-related cognitive processes.

Cognitive processes are fundamental to our model of addictive behaviors, and therefore the case conceptualization should focus intensely and tirelessly on these processes. As discussed in Chapter 2, cognitive processes include basic beliefs, automatic thoughts, self-efficacy, outcome expectancies, permissive beliefs, and instrumental thoughts. Most people are not aware, conscious, or mindful regarding their thoughts or beliefs. In other words, *people generally do not think about how they think*. As a result, it is often necessary to probe for cognitive processes. The following is a list of potential questions that might be asked in an effort to elicit cognitive processes:

"How would you describe or view yourself?"
"What are your most deeply held values, beliefs, principles, or ideals?"
"What are some thoughts or beliefs you have about people, and especially those close to you?"
"What are your predictions about your near and distant future?"
"How do you understand (or explain) your addiction?"
"How do you view (or understand) the process of change?"
"How do you understand your relapses?"
"When you relapse, what are the precipitating thoughts?"
"How likely are you to succeed at reaching your goals for change starting *today*?"

These questions are aimed at discovering patients' schemas, basic beliefs, automatic thoughts, self-efficacy, outcome expectancies, and permissive thoughts.

This process of discovery is likely to be helpful to the patient. As mentioned earlier, *people generally do not think about how they think,* so this process enables patients to identify and label their thoughts (i.e., think about how they think). It should not surprise therapists when patients cannot easily or readily describe their thoughts. In fact, sometimes it is necessary to offer multiple-choice answers to these questions. For example, consider the following dialogue between a patient and therapist:

> THERAPIST: How would you describe yourself, or how do you see yourself?
>
> PATIENT: What do you mean?
>
> THERAPIST: I mean if someone asked you to describe yourself, what would you say?
>
> PATIENT: I don't know. Nobody has ever asked me that question.
>
> THERAPIST: I guess I'm asking whether you think you're a nice person, a responsible person, a good person, a smart person.... That's what I mean.
>
> PATIENT: Oh, then I'd say that I'm okay. [*Takes a long pause*] Actually, I think of myself as *an addict.* I don't believe anyone would think of me as responsible.
>
> THERAPIST: What about being a good person or a smart person?
>
> PATIENT: No, I don't think I am good or smart. There was a time when I thought I was a good guy and maybe even smart. But not anymore.

As patients share thoughts and beliefs like these, it is recommended that therapists reflect them back to patients (i.e., paraphrase or restate them), in order to establish that patients have been accurately heard. It is also recommended that therapists maintain a written list of patients' evolving thoughts and beliefs, so case conceptualizations are comprised of current and accurate cognitive processes. At various times throughout sessions these lists should be shared with patients, explaining, "I am writing your thoughts and beliefs as you share them, in order to best understand how they lead you *toward* or *away from* your addictive behaviors."

Automatic thoughts stem from the activation of basic or core beliefs, conditional beliefs, and addiction-related beliefs. Some typical automatic thoughts of people with addictions are: "I can't stand these cravings," "Just a little bit won't hurt," "Go for it," "You deserve it," and "It's been long enough." These automatic thoughts often potentiate urges, cravings, and ultimately plans to engage in addictive behaviors.

Basic beliefs and schemas may best be viewed as profound, deeply held cognitive processes that develop early in life and become more durable over time; perhaps this is why basic beliefs are often referred to as core beliefs. Whereas basic beliefs take the form of actual words and sentences (e.g., "I am a good/bad person" or "I am a worthwhile/worthless person), schemas are best defined as cognitive structures for "coding, screening, and evaluating" oneself and one's personal world (Beck, 1967, p. 283). Basic beliefs and schemas generally fall into two categories: lovability and adequacy. It is important to note that basic beliefs and schemas might not necessarily be described by patients with these exact words, but they are often derivatives or correlates of lovability and adequacy. For example, the belief that "I am unlovable" might be expressed as, "I'm fat," "I'm ugly," "No one would want me," or "I've given up on love." Beliefs associated with inadequacy might be expressed as, "I can't do anything right," "Nothing I do works out," "I'm helpless," "I shouldn't even bother," or "I might as well give up." Basic beliefs and schemas like these have the potential to cause substantial psychological suffering, which may lead to a desire for relief in the form of an addictive behavior (i.e., self-medicating). And some negative schemas and basic beliefs involve helplessness or hopelessness, which may lead to giving up on healthy goals. For example, an individual who has been abstinent for several months might relapse after thinking, "Nothing has changed since I stopped getting high and nothing ever will, so I might as well go back to my old ways." Therapist should be aware of clients' thoughts related to hopelessness, especially if they become more intense or frequent. Such hopelessness may precipitate engagement in harmful behaviors such as drug use, self-harm, and suicide.

Conditional beliefs are thought processes that take the form of "if . . . then . . ." (with or without the actual words *if* and *then*). For example, "If I quit drinking, then life will be boring," or, "If I keep smoking, I'll get cancer." Conditional beliefs may involve predictions made about the outcome of certain choices, or they may involve rules to be followed. A person who grows up in a home that emphasizes competition, for example, may have the conditional belief "if I am not the very best, I'm nothing." A person who has a dependent personality might hold the conditional belief "if I don't conform to others' demands and expectations, I'll always be alone and lonely." Conditional beliefs are neither innately good nor bad. Some conditional beliefs lead directly to *engaging in* addictive behaviors (e.g., "If I get high today, I'll have fun") and other conditional beliefs lead to *abstaining from* addictive behaviors (e.g., "If I get high today, I'll regret it tomorrow").

Again, an accurate, current case conceptualization is vital for effective treatment planning, and (from our perspective) the most important element of the case conceptualization is an accounting of thoughts, beliefs, and schemas that lead *toward* and *away from* addictive behaviors. However, in addition to focusing on cognitive content (i.e., actual thoughts, beliefs, and schemas), it is important to focus on cognitive patterns (i.e., the manner in which thoughts, beliefs, and schemas arise and are maintained). The terms *System 1 thinking* and *System 2 thinking* have been coined by the Nobel prize-winning scientist and author Daniel Kahneman (2011). We have found these concepts to be extremely helpful in understanding the maintenance of problematic thoughts, feelings, and behaviors. System 1 thinking is automatic, rapid, and effortless. In contrast, System 2 thinking is slow, deliberate, and effortful. In fact, most daily human functioning involves System 1 thinking. For example, most people get out of bed, get dressed, and brush their teeth in the morning without much deliberate thought. Similarly, people find their way to work or school without much effort—all with System 1 thinking. It is only when System 1 is not achieving desired aims that we turn to System 2 for help. System 2 thinking is slow, deliberate, and necessary for solving complex problems, and especially for making meaningful personal changes. It might be helpful to understand System 2 thinking as a *mindful* process—in contrast to System 1, which is relatively *mindless*.

The implications of System 1 and 2 thinking for understanding addictions are profound. As with other repetitive behaviors, addictive behaviors eventually become automatic and effortless. It is only when they become problematic that System 2 thinking is needed to make changes. As part of the case conceptualization, it helps to understand that addictive behaviors are perpetuated by System 1 thinking, while System 2 thinking is vital for learning to abstain from addictive behaviors. For example, Ed is a cigarette smoker who wants to quit smoking. Ed explains that he often reaches for a cigarette, lights it, and starts smoking without being aware of these behaviors. This occurs because each action is facilitated by System 1 thinking. When Ed quits smoking, he will need to implement deliberate and mindful coping strategies with System 2 thinking in order to overcome temptations to smoke.

Fortunately, repetition of new thoughts and behaviors (i.e., changes driven by System 2 thinking) results in their evolving into System 1 thinking. In other words, the new, healthy thoughts and behaviors will eventually become automatic through repetition. When Ed began smoking, each step (purchasing, carrying, lighting, and smoking) was new and therefore required deliberate (System 2) thinking. However, as smoking became habitual for Ed, all of these steps became automatic and effortless (System 1). Now that he wants to quit smoking, he will have to endure sustained, deliberate effort initially, but through repetition, his thoughts as a nonsmoker will be automatic, governed by System 1 thinking. Instead of seeing smokers and automatically thinking, "I need a cigarette," Ed will think, "That used to be me."

Affective processes involve emotions, feelings, moods, and physiological sensations that usually follow automatic thoughts or beliefs. As mentioned earlier, most people are unaware of the cognitive processes that precede emotions such as anger, anxiety, or sadness. Similarly, they are typically unaware of (or at least unable to label) emotions they feel or moods they experience. In addition to recognizing their cognitive processes, an essential aim of the case conceptualization is to help patients become more aware of (and be able to label) emotions associated with addictive behaviors.

In order to elicit emotions and help patients to label them, the therapist might consider the following questions:

"How do you define or understand the term *emotions?* Or *feelings?*"
"During the course of an average day, how would you describe your typical emotions or feelings?"
"Over the course of a single day, how often do your emotions or feelings change?"
"How would other people describe your typical emotions?"
"What functions do your emotions serve? Or what impact do they have?"
"When you feel good, how would you describe the actual emotions?"
"When you feel bad, how would you describe the actual emotions?"
"What makes you happy? Sad?"
"How effective are you at changing your emotions?"
"What strategies do you use to change your emotions?"
"What emotions are you feeling right now, as we talk?"

Many people have identified addictive behaviors as self-medicating, meaning they are initiated to reduce discomfort or increase comfort. This is important to keep in mind as we consider the role of emotions in addictive behaviors. Often, a person will engage in an addictive behavior to modify their emotions. If, during the case conceptualization process, it is determined that this is the case for a particular patient, it is essential for the therapy to consider addiction-free strategies for increasing pleasure or reducing (physical or emotional) discomfort.

Behavioral patterns include repetitive actions that may be more or less adaptive versus maladaptive. Adaptive behavioral patterns are those that lead to outcomes consistent with goals, values, and aspirations. For example, most people value independence, and therefore actions that hinder independence (like incarceration) might be understood to be maladaptive, while those that lead to independence would be adaptive.

It is also helpful to identify coping strategies versus compensatory strategies. Coping strategies involve behaviors that resolve problems with few or no negative consequences. Compensatory strategies, on the other hand, resolve problems momentarily, but often with long-term negative consequences. For example, getting "blind drunk" with friends might temporarily reduce painful anxiety, but it might also result in negative consequences that last a lifetime (e.g., driving drunk and injuring innocent people). On the surface, compensatory strategies seem to work, but they are often limited by being compulsive and inflexible. Furthermore, compensatory strategies do not effectively resolve self-doubt, insecurities, fear, and inadequacies. Typical compensatory strategies for people with addictions involve the use of alcohol and drugs, however there are many other behaviors that are compensatory (e.g., emotional and physical aggression, binge eating, compulsive shopping, and more).

Ultimately, all emotions and behaviors can be understood as links in a chain of proximal antecedents, activated beliefs, automatic thoughts, and consequences—where triggers lead to addiction-related thoughts, thoughts trigger addictive behaviors, behaviors trigger more addiction-related thoughts, and so forth—as problems escalate. For example, a man might get in an argument with his wife. This argument might trigger thoughts like, "I can't stand when she nags me," which might trigger feelings of anger, which might trigger the thought, "She can't tell me what to do," which might trigger the thought, "I'll show her," which might trigger drinking, which might trigger the thought, "I'm going to give her a piece of my mind," which might trigger hostile behaviors toward her, which might very well trigger heightened anger, drinking, and increasingly serious problems requiring police intervention. These chains have also been viewed as cycles where links in the chain continue to activate each other in a continually reinforcing manner.

Readiness to change and associated goals are closely related. Originally formulated by Prochaska, DiClemente, and Norcross (1992), readiness manifests in stages on a continuum from *not at all ready* (i.e., precontemplation) to *sustained change* (i.e., maintenance). As discussed in Chapter 2, Prochaska and colleagues labeled the stages precontemplation, contemplation, preparation, action, and maintenance. Clinicians often make the mistake of assuming that these stages are static or linear rather than dynamic and fluid. In fact, readiness to change can vary from moment to moment. Each stage is comprised of corresponding thoughts, beliefs, emotions, and behaviors. For example, the stage of contemplation is often characterized by concern, ambivalence, and doubt, while a person is still engaged in an addictive behavior. The action stage is often characterized by hope, confidence, pride, and (for some) self-doubt and substantial discomfort, all while the individual is abstinent from the addictive behavior.

In reality, a person can vary in readiness to change from minute to minute, hour to hour, day to day, week to week, and so forth. It is not uncommon for a patient to shift back and forth in a single therapy session as therapist and patient discuss the advantages and disadvantages of using. Readiness to change typically correlates with individuals' goals. For example, individuals in precontemplation are likely to have few or no goals regarding behavior change while individuals in the action and maintenance stages aim to make or maintain changes.

While formulating the case conceptualization it is important to ask about the patient's history of motivation over time, rather than focusing exclusively on current motivation to change. The following are some questions that might elicit the process of change over time:

"On a scale from 0 to 100%, how ready are you to change right now?"
"What are your current thoughts about the pros and cons of changing?"
"How often have you tried to make similar changes in the past?"
"During past efforts to change, how has your motivation shifted over time?"
"In other words, when you have relapsed in the past, how has your motivation been up and down, like a roller-coaster?"

We cannot overemphasize the fact that readiness might change from moment to moment. In fact, as we noted in Chapter 2, Marlatt and Gordon (1985) talked about the *abstinence violation effect* (AVE), which occurs when a person in the action or maintenance stage has a single lapse that activates helpless, hopeless thoughts more reflective of the contemplation stage of change. For example, after hearing about an opioid overdose death in the news on Monday, Annie decides to stop taking her oxycodone. However, on Tuesday she wakes up feeling anxious and depressed, and decides to take an oxycodone from a bottle remaining in her medicine cabinet. As soon as she swallows the pill she feels regret, so she does not take any more pills that day. However, on Wednesday she decides to take several more pills, believing that she has "fallen off the wagon" the previous day and is no longer able to achieve her goal of abstinence. This is a classic case of the AVE. Annie's motivation shifted back and forth and back again in just a few days: from ready, to not ready, to ready, to not ready to change.

Integration of the data is the most challenging and most important step in the ongoing process of conceptualizing the patient's life and problems. Here, therapists synthesize all background information into a cohesive, data-based narrative that explains the patient's difficulties and leads to treatment recommendations that make sense. For example, the therapist might posit the following:

Jeff is a 40-year-old married man who has stimulant (methamphetamine) use disorder. Jeff's wife recently demanded that he move out of their house. The couple has two children, and she insisted on separating because Jeff was becoming erratic and threatening at times. Jeff discloses that he has had long periods of depression in the past. He explains that he began regular use of meth after discovering that it made him feel less depressed and more able to function at work. Jeff now lives with his brother, who is single and a heavy drinker. As a plumber, Jeff makes just enough money to pay his household expenses, which is why he lives with his brother rather than getting his own apartment. Jeff explains that he and his brother grew up in a loud, volatile home, where both of his parents were heavy drinkers. He was introduced to meth at work, where several of his coworkers regularly use. His dealer is one of his coworkers, who often reminds Jeff that he has "some really good stuff." Jeff is triggered by multiple internal and external cues (e.g., depression, fatigue, coworkers who use, and easy access). He has always seen himself as "just short of a loser" and "never surprised when things go wrong." These thoughts lead to thoughts that trigger his meth use: "What the hell," "I need a boost," "My family will never know," and "I need to contact my dealer." When he is not using, Jeff feels depressed, and has little in his life that makes him feel better. Prior to getting separated from his wife, he at least found satisfaction from making money to support his family. He says he is "willing to change" now (to fully abstain from using meth), but he adds, "It's mostly to get my family back."

Implications for treatment is where CBT strategies and techniques are planned. The case conceptualization provides essential, well-integrated information regarding the patient's problems, background, triggers, thoughts, beliefs, emotional struggles, and so forth. It also provides information about the severity, motivation to change, goals, and barriers to change. Treatment strategies and techniques should be chosen according to their importance and patients' abilities to address problems that have been uncovered. For example, if it is determined that a patient is using marijuana to reduce social anxiety, CBT should focus on cognitive and behavioral strategies to reduce anxiety. If it is determined that cocaine is being used as an antidepressant, CBT should focus on reducing depressive symptoms. If alcohol is being used to induce sleep in a person with insomnia, CBT sleep hygiene strategies should be introduced. In cases where an individual is using addictive behaviors simply to stop urges and cravings, urge surfing techniques might be taught.

Returning to Jeff, above, the therapist understands that the treatment plan needs to include multiple facets. First and foremost, Jeff's therapist will focus on Jeff's motivation to change. The therapist will do so by helping Jeff to carefully examine the advantages and disadvantages of continuing versus discontinuing use of meth. Second, Jeff's therapist will assist Jeff in understanding and controlling his urges and cravings to use. Third, the therapist will help Jeff understand and master his thoughts, feelings, and behaviors—by both helping him to understand that he developed extremely self-defeating schemas and beliefs as a child and guiding him to discover his strengths and capabilities as an adult. The therapist will also help Jeff to clarify his values and identify how he will make behavioral changes that will enable him to live according to his most deeply held values.

CASE EXAMPLE: CAROL

Throughout this chapter we have provided brief examples of individuals who struggle with addictive behaviors to illustrate each element of the case conceptualization. In this final section we introduce a new patient and focus on all 10 elements to conceptualize this patient. We recommend that therapists use all 10 elements to conceptualize patients, as we demonstrate here.

Carol is a 45-year-old woman who began therapy at the insistence of her husband, Jim. The couple had been married for 20 years and Jim threatened divorce if Carol did not "make some big changes." Jim accompanied Carol to her first session to offer his perspective on Carol's problems. He insisted, "her gambling is the reason we have a terrible marriage." During their first visit, the tension between them was palpable as they bickered in response to most of the therapist's questions. For example, when Carol described Jim as "always angry," Jim argued that it was Carol who was always angry. When Carol accused Jim of letting their two teenage kids "get away with murder," Jim responded by saying that Carol regularly belittled and demeaned them. When Jim accused Carol of losing their entire savings on gambling, Carol responded by saying, "My gambling is no different from your wasting our money on that damn motorcycle of yours." During subsequent visits Carol returned alone, and the therapist asked many more questions in order to conceptualize her. The therapist explained that this process of gathering and integrating background information would be time well spent, and it would enable them to choose the most appropriate goals and strategies moving forward.

• **Primary problem(s):** In her first two visits Carol was reluctant to admit to any serious personal problems, beyond having a "terrible marriage." However, by her third visit she was more open and began to describe her problem gambling. Carol was first introduced to gambling by coworkers at her current job, approximately 10 years ago. She gambled mostly on weekends after work but said she would gamble every day if she could afford to. She played only slot machines and found herself fixated on the sounds and images of everything surrounding one particular machine. She estimated losing an average of $500 during each trip to the casino, even after calculating the occasional times when she would win. She said it felt like a "gigantic obsession" since she now found herself thinking about gambling all the time. Carol's gambling losses had escalated from the time she first started gambling, and she estimated that she lost as much as $50,000 over 10 years. Money spent on gambling came from family savings, her children's college fund, and cash withdrawals on credit cards. On occasion Carol tried to stop gambling, but the resulting distress was so unbearable that she resumed gambling immediately. Carol denied feeling depressed, but said she often felt desperate before, during, and after gambling. When asked about other possible addictions, she denied ever drinking more than a couple of drinks at any one time and said she had never regularly used tobacco or any other psychoactive drugs.

• **Social/environmental context:** Carol continues to live with Jim and their children, Caleb (12 years old) and Sara (14 years old). She works as the night manager at a popular local restaurant and Jim works as an electrician. She appears ashamed as she explains that she never considered attending college after graduating from high school. She spends most of her free time with coworkers from the restaurant, and states, "Jim is so boring. We don't have anything in common anymore." Most of Carol's socializing takes place at a casino where she and her coworkers play slots from the time they leave work until the early morning hours. Until recently the couple was financially stable, with a mortgage as their only debt. However, without Jim's knowledge Carol depleted all of their savings accounts (including their children's college fund) and reached the spending limits on all of their credit cards.

• **Distal antecedents:** Carol grew up in a household with parents who argued often. Carol explains that she rarely saw her parents discuss anything important and the word *love* was certainly never used in their home. She had only one sibling, a younger brother, who died at 23 years old in a motor vehicle accident. There were no other vehicles involved so Carol believes he must have been driving under the influence. She remembers her father drinking and smoking cigarettes every night, but no one ever discussed whether he had a diagnosable alcohol problem. Her mother is still alive, but her father died of lung cancer at 57 years old. Carol doubts that anyone else in her family has ever stepped foot into a casino. She does not recall any mental illness in her family but says, "It sure wasn't a happy place to be."

- **Proximal antecedents:** Carol states that she thinks about gambling all the time, and only stops thinking about gambling when she is "really busy at work." At one point in therapy she joked, "My biggest trigger is being alive." She recognizes that the strongest urges and cravings begin early in the evening, especially on Friday or Saturday, when she knows she will gamble later on. When asked about any internal feelings that trigger craving, she readily identifies boredom, restlessness, irritation, anger, frustration, and tension—especially as she thinks about going home to her family.

- **Cognitive processes:** Carol has some schemas and basic beliefs that are likely related to her gambling. For example, she does not think of herself as particularly loveable or adequate. She has gained 40 pounds since her wedding day and often says, "I used to be attractive enough, though you wouldn't know it looking at me now." She has distinct regrets about not attending college: "I probably should have gone to college. It might have been a ticket out of the hell hole I live in now." She does not believe that close family relationships can possibly be rewarding, and obviously thinks that her relationship with Jim is toxic. She has viewed Jim as more of an adversary than a friend for much of their marriage. She says she likes her coworkers, though she adds, "I would never tell them the kinds of things I'm telling you."

Prior to visiting the casino, and while Carol is there, she has many thoughts and beliefs common to people with gambling disorder, for example:

> "If I keep gambling, I'll eventually beat the house."
> "I've lost so many times; I must be due to win soon." [The infamous "Gambler's Fallacy"]
> "This time my luck will be better."
> "I'm not spending that much money."
> "This will be my lucky day."
> "I'll eventually get good at this."
> "I can't afford to stop now."
> "I'm doing this to win back the money I've lost."

- **Affective processes:** Carol says she never feels joy or happiness, but she also denies prolonged feelings of depression or anxiety. As noted above, she often feels desperation associated with gambling. She admits that her most salient emotions include anger, irritation, tension, and frustration, triggered by her marital relationship.

• *Behavioral patterns:* Carol has never developed interests or skills associated with maintaining healthy close relationships. She is a reliable, hard worker and her coworkers say she is a good manager. At home though, she only minimally interacts with her husband and children, except for functional reasons or to argue with Jim. She typically sits at her computer and surfs the Web for hours at a time. She admits that she would gamble online, but Jim has blocked all gambling websites. She has no other hobbies, pastimes, or chores except occasionally preparing meals, light housework, and doing laundry.

• *Readiness to change and associated goals:* Carol feels resigned to quitting gambling. She anticipates that she will soon be unable to gamble, as Jim has blocked her access to their money, and their credit cards are at their limit. She honestly admits, "I do not *want* to quit gambling, I am being *forced* to quit gambling." She has also commented, "If I could get out of this crappy marriage, I'd be able to gamble as much as I want."

• *Integration of the above data:* Carol has a severe gambling disorder (meeting at least six DSM-5 symptoms). She has a family history of SUDs, including some family members who were heavy drinkers and cigarette smokers. She has severe marital problems but does not have the knowledge or skills to solve these problems. Gambling is clearly the only activity that provides Carol relief from her unhappy existence. Her triggers mostly involve negative emotions, and these emotions trigger a whole host of gambling-related thoughts. She is willing to contemplate change, but certainly not prepared for or committed to making substantial changes to her life.

• *Implications for treatment:* In order to help Carol, it will first be essential to collaboratively establish that: (1) she has a problem, (2) she would benefit from making changes, and (3) she will be able to acquire the necessary skills for doing so. In other words, it will be vital for her to believe: "It's best for me to quit gambling," and "I am capable of quitting." Carol will be taught the full CBT developmental model and helped to understand how it applies to her. She will be helped to understand that her family history suggests that she may always be at risk for addictive behaviors. She will be helped to identify internal and external triggers, and how she might respond to these triggers. She will be assisted in identifying her own goals, for example: (1) stop having obsessive thoughts about gambling, (2) find new hobbies, (3) stop fighting with Jim. She will also be encouraged to identify potential barriers to accomplishing these goals and methods for overcoming these barriers. While focusing on gambling cessation, Carol will also be taught cognitive-behavioral skills for regulating her mood, and she will be encouraged to learn behaviors that are more fulfilling.

As noted earlier in this chapter, the case conceptualization evolves over the course of CBT. Some patients only reveal previously undisclosed, often deeply personal problems as they learn they can trust the therapeutic process and relationship. Also, as patients achieve insights and behavior change, they are likely to discover problems that underly and relate to their addictions. For example, an individual who smokes marijuana several times a day may discover upon abstaining that the marijuana use was motivated by severe anxiety. Of course, as the case conceptualization evolves, so should the treatment plan. As patients and therapists uncover previously unrecognized problems, they work together to formulate new CBT strategies for addressing these problems.

It is helpful to anticipate that many individuals with addictions may have their own self-conceptualizations, influenced by prior life experiences and addiction treatment modalities (e.g., medically oriented treatment facilities, 12-step programs, etc.). These individuals may worry that their existing ideas about addictions will clash with newly introduced CBT concepts. For example, since many professionals and lay people consider addiction a disease, some individuals may worry that CBT rejects the disease model of addiction. Our answer to this dilemma is simple: The disease model has been useful to many people, for many years, and for many reasons. In fact, some highly effective CBT practitioners view addiction as a disease. We encourage therapists to learn about each patient's self-conceptualizations as they formulate their own conceptualization of each patient. With experience and practice, most cognitive-behavioral therapists learn that there are more similarities between the various models of addictions than there are differences.

SUMMARY

In this chapter we have focused on the 10 essential elements of the case conceptualization, and we have used various case examples to illustrate the importance of each of these elements. We hope readers will adopt this approach to conceptualizing addictions, since we have found it to be so helpful.

As we noted earlier, the case conceptualization is just one of the five components of effective CBT. The other four components are structure, collaboration, psychoeducation, and structured techniques. These four other components are most likely to be effective when they are based on a thorough, accurate case conceptualization. That is, sessions will most likely be appropriately structured, therapist and patient goals will be aligned, psychoeducation will be well timed, and structured techniques will have the greatest positive impact when the case conceptualization is thorough and accurate.

CHAPTER 4

SHAME, STIGMA, AND THE THERAPEUTIC RELATIONSHIP

Shame, guilt, fear, helplessness, frustration, and despair are just some of the emotions felt by people who struggle with addictions. To make matters worse, addicted individuals experience the contempt of a society that stigmatizes them, until they eventually self-stigmatize and become their own worst critics (Kelly et al., 2015; Schomerus et al., 2011; van Boekel, Brouwers, van Weeghel, & Garretsen, 2013). Naturally, these processes of social stigma and self-stigma further complicate already complex therapy relationships. In this chapter we discuss relationships between therapists and addicted patients, with emphasis on maintaining strong therapeutic alliances and overcoming the negative impact of patients' shame and stigma.

Empathetic therapists who understand the impact of stigma and self-stigma are well positioned to help patients with addictions, recognizing that addicted patients perpetually struggle with internal and external judgment and disdain. Such therapists strive to create a positive atmosphere of support and collaboration as they serve patients who struggle with addictions. In fact, such positive, supportive, collaborative psychotherapy relationships are vital to effective treatment (e.g., Miller & Rollnick, 2013; Norcross & Lambert, 2018; Wampold, 2015). The impact of social stigma and self-stigma on psychotherapy relationships is often underestimated. As a result of stigma, patients may choose to conceal their concerns and try to appear as though *everything is okay*. They may have no basis for trusting strangers with their problems and may assume that *all therapists will judge them*, as others have. They may also be *too ashamed* to talk openly about addictive behaviors. Hopefully, when they do seek help, they find therapists who are receptive to these potential thoughts and feelings about being in therapy.

Dynamics That Adversely Impact Therapeutic Relationships

We begin this chapter by discussing the impact of psychosocial dynamics that adversely influence the therapeutic relationship. We have chosen these particular dynamics because we often observe them in patients who find it difficult to engage in therapy:

- Pressure to enter treatment
- Feelings of shame
- Tendencies to minimize addictions or lack of motivation to change
- Being stigmatized by professionals in the past
- Stereotypical views of therapy and therapists
- Fear that self-disclosure will result in punishing consequences

Consider the following three case examples: *Arnold,* whose wife is threatening to divorce him if he continues to drink; *Becky,* who will be fired from her job if she has another positive drug screen; and *Charlie,* who is on probation and mandated to treatment for possession of marijuana. These three people have thoughts and feelings that will potentially impact any therapy relationship they enter into. They are likely to feel resentful, ashamed, fearful, irritated, frustrated, or worse about being coerced or mandated to therapy—and these feelings can easily get in the way of their accepting help. These case examples will serve to illustrate the dynamics listed above. In discussing these dynamics, we offer essential therapist skills and attitudes that facilitate engaged therapy relationships. These skills and attitudes include reflective listening, accurate empathy, eliciting feedback, guided discovery, genuine caring, immediacy, authenticity, and much more.

Patients May Feel Under Pressure to Enter Treatment

As noted earlier, Arnold's wife has threatened to end their marriage if he does not stop drinking. She has also demanded that he seek treatment. Hence, he feels substantial pressure to pursue therapy. The following dialogue between Arnold and his therapist is presented as an example of accurate empathy and the skill of eliciting feedback:

THERAPIST: Hello Arnold, I'm glad you're here. What would you like to work on with me?

ARNOLD: I'm not sure. I'm here because I don't want to lose my wife.

THERAPIST: Please tell me more.

ARNOLD: We've been married for 30 years. We have two grown-up kids and four beautiful grandkids. I don't understand how she could throw that all away.

THERAPIST: You really care about your wife and your family.

ARNOLD: I don't want to lose what I've worked so hard for.

THERAPIST: You really want to save your marriage and your family. What makes you think your wife might "throw it all away?"

ARNOLD: She says she's done with me if I don't stop drinking.

THERAPIST: What's led to her concerns about your drinking?

ARNOLD: I don't know. She's always complaining that her father was a drunk and says she doesn't want to be married to one.

THERAPIST: She thinks of you as a drunk?

ARNOLD: Yeah, and she's wrong. I'm nothing like her father. I'm home every night. I never do the stupid things her father did. He was a mean drunk. I enjoy a few drinks once in a while, and it just sets her off.

THERAPIST: Arnold, it sounds like you're under a lot of pressure to be here, in therapy. From what I can tell, you're here because you really care about your wife and family, and you don't want to lose them.

ARNOLD: Yeah, that's about right.

THERAPIST: Have you ever reached out to anyone like you're doing now, by coming here?

ARNOLD: No, I never thought I had a problem.

THERAPIST: How does it feel to be here?

ARNOLD: I don't know. Not great. I don't like asking for help with anything. And to be honest, I think my wife and I can solve our own problems.

THERAPIST: Let me make sure I understand. You genuinely want to solve your marital problems. You'll do just about anything to keep your family together. And it doesn't feel right being here, because it's just not your nature to ask for help. And you're not concerned about your drinking like she is.

ARNOLD: That's right.

THERAPIST: Well, I understand all that and appreciate your honesty—even about not wanting to be here.

ARNOLD: It's not you that's the problem. It's just that I'm a private person. Always have been. Growing up in my family . . . we just didn't talk about our problems.

THERAPIST: Thank you for telling me that. I assure you that I'll do my best to be helpful.

In this exchange, it is clear that Arnold did not think he had a drinking problem, and he did not feel comfortable talking to strangers about personal matters. He came to therapy to save his marriage, rather than to change his drinking habits. He may occasionally contemplate that his drinking is a problem, or even try to slow down or stop his drinking, but he certainly was not forthcoming about these things. Hence, it will likely take time for him to trust his therapist and openly reflect on the extent and severity of any personal problems. His therapist realized this and invited Arnold to share any concerns about being in therapy. After carefully listening to Arnold's concerns, his therapist accurately reflected them back in a supportive, empathetic manner. Arnold's therapist understands that Arnold will eventually need to focus on his own personal problems—but only when Arnold is ready to do so.

Patients May Feel Ashamed of Their Addictive Behaviors

Shame is a powerful motivator. As people acknowledge that they struggle with addictions, many, if not most, feel shame. And most who feel shame prefer to keep their addictive behaviors a secret. However, when patients keep secrets from therapists, they are not likely to obtain benefits from therapy. They might also be at risk for dropping out of therapy before it can be helpful. Effective therapists understand the potential impact of shame and they engage in guided discovery with great sensitivity, acknowledging that questions about addictive habits can be difficult to answer, and that the patient's accuracy in responding to these questions is greatly appreciated and respected.

Becky began taking pain medication, prescribed by her physician, following a biking accident. She had broken three ribs, and the medication substantially reduced her physical pain. But Becky also noticed that taking this medication improved her moods. When her prescription ended, she called her doctor, who told her she needed to transition to nonnarcotic pain medication. Becky panicked and called a friend, who provided an "alternative" source of narcotics. Becky's job required random drug screening, and when Becky's time came, she was found to have opioids in her urine. When confronted by her supervisor she argued that she took narcotics for pain. However, she was unable to produce a current prescription verifying this claim. She was put on probation at work and advised to seek professional help for addiction. The following exchange occurs in her first session with a cognitive-behavioral therapist:

THERAPIST: Good to meet you Becky. How can I help you?

BECKY: I'm required to be here for work.

THERAPIST: What's gone on at work that's resulted in your having to see me?

BECKY: It's a long story. I got in a bike wreck and broke some ribs. I was in a lot of pain. For a while, every breath was painful. The doctors gave me pain medication and then took it away before I was ready to stop. A friend lent me some of her medication and I got busted by HR after peeing in a cup at work. Now I have to come here.

THERAPIST: I'm sorry to hear about your bike wreck and problems at work. I hope I can be helpful. What do you think we can work on together?

BECKY: I have no idea. I can't believe I'm sitting here. It feels like I've been called to the principal's office.

THERAPIST: You feel like you're being punished?

BECKY: All I know is that you're a shrink who treats addicts, and at my job they think I'm an addict. [*Takes a long pause and then becomes tearful.*] So maybe I am. This whole mess is really embarrassing. Yeah, I feel like I'm being punished for taking pain medication. It's really humiliating.

THERAPIST: Becky, I understand that it's embarrassing for you to be here. You said it feels like punishment. But you also suggested that you might have a drug problem. What makes you think that?

BECKY: You want the truth? My job is difficult. I don't like it, but I need an income. Someone has to support my kids and me. That medication made going to work each day a little more bearable.

THERAPIST: Do you mind if we start this process by just getting to know each other? I'd like to learn about you without making any premature assumptions. I also welcome any questions you might have for me.

BECKY: What do you want to know?

THERAPIST: Let's just start with some basics. Maybe you can tell me some things about yourself or your life that you feel good about.

BECKY: Like what?

THERAPIST: Like anything positive about yourself, your interests, your kids, or other things. I want to begin our work together by thinking of you as a human being, rather than starting out with the label, "drug addict."

Becky's therapist immediately recognized that Becky was ashamed of being referred for therapy, especially given her reference to being called to the principal's office. In response, her therapist expressed greater interest in other aspects of Becky's life. Later in the course of therapy, Becky directly admitted that she was "overwhelmed with guilt and shame" upon realizing she had become addicted to pain medication. She shared that the therapist's treating her like a "whole person" rather than "an addict" was an important turning point in her recovery.

Patients May Minimize Addictive Behaviors or Lack Motivation to Change

Some people believe they are being unjustly criticized when others, including therapists, inquire about behaviors such as drinking, smoking, overeating, gambling, online gaming, or drug use. It is important for therapists to be aware of this dynamic and understand that individuals' readiness to change is likely to occur in stages over time (Connors, DiClemente, Velasquez, & Donovan, 2013). Premature attempts to coerce patients into acknowledging addictions will most certainly be counterproductive. Further, the use of labels such as "addict" or "alcoholic" may be experienced as offensive. In broaching the topic of addiction, it may be best for therapists to first talk about patients' general thoughts and beliefs about their behaviors, and then later inquire about advantages and disadvantages of these behaviors. In some cases, this process can be framed as "causes and effects" of behaviors. For example, "When you do x (e.g., drink), the result seems to be y (e.g., miss work), and I wonder if you have concerns about that?" As we will discuss later in this chapter, *words matter,* and criticizing or prejudging patients can result in the early dissolution of the therapeutic relationship.

Charlie, introduced earlier, provides an excellent example of an individual who minimizes his marijuana use. In the following exchange during Charlie's second visit, his therapist works hard to discuss problems associated with Charlie's marijuana use:

THERAPIST: Welcome back Charlie.

CHARLIE: Yeah, thanks.

THERAPIST: What do you want to put on the agenda today?

CHARLIE: What is this, some kind of business meeting?

THERAPIST: [*Therapist chuckles.*] No, sorry, that's just the way I start therapy sessions. It's my way of inviting you to talk about what's on your mind.

CHARLIE: What's on my mind is getting this over with.

THERAPIST: I know you'd rather not be here. You were clear about that from the first moments we met. But I would like to be helpful in some way, while we're together.

CHARLIE: Look, like I told you last time, I smoke weed like other people have a cocktail. We just happen to be in a state where it's illegal. It's legal in lots of other states. Our politicians are just a bunch of conservative hypocrites. They sit around drinking expensive booze, and I sit in your office on probation for possession of twenty dollars' worth of weed.

THERAPIST: I agree that this whole marijuana legalization process is hard to understand. There are lots of unknowns and causes for confusion.

CHARLIE: That's a weird way of saying the whole thing sucks. I just don't get it. I really do smoke weed like most people drink alcohol. The only problem I have is that I got busted and I'm not one of those rich people who can buy their way out of legal trouble. Smoking weed is one of few things I do that relaxes me, and I'm not about to start drinking again. That was my real nightmare.

THERAPIST: Charlie, you've said a lot there. Do you mind if I ask you about your history with weed and alcohol? I know you quit drinking, but I don't know exactly what led to that decision or why you call it a nightmare. And I know you smoke weed, but I don't know how much, or when, or what you mean when you say it's one of the few things that relaxes you.

CHARLIE: Go ahead and ask your questions. We might as well do something with the time we have. Otherwise, the time is just going to drag on.

Charlie was obviously unhappy about being in therapy and he freely shared his frustration with his therapist. If he had any private concerns about his marijuana use, he was certainly not ready to share these concerns. However, his therapist was patient, and willing to take all necessary time to learn more about Charlie's alcohol and marijuana use. If Charlie's therapist were to act with urgency, or aggressively pursue this line of questioning, Charlie would certainly shut down or possibly even reciprocate by aggressively challenging the therapist.

Patients May Have Been Stigmatized by Professionals in the Past

Disparaging portrayals of people with addictions are abundant in society and therefore stigma is pervasive. Ideally, professionals who encounter people with addictions would be immune to stigmatizing them, but unfortunately this is not always the case. Despite extensive training, many professional counselors, psychologists, physicians, nurses, social workers, and others, view people with addictions in negative terms. They persist at using terms like "addict" and "alcoholic." Some use even more derogatory terms like "druggie" and "drunk" to describe people with drug and alcohol problems.

By their third session, Arnold (introduced earlier as having marital problems) seems willing to talk about his alcohol consumption, and his therapist learns he drinks as many as six beers per night, every night of the week. Arnold's therapist wants to learn more about Arnold's drinking, but he hopes first to learn about potential barriers to doing so. In other words, he wishes to determine whether Arnold feels comfortable enough in their relationship to discuss the negative consequences of his drinking:

THERAPIST: Arnold, I appreciate your willingness to talk more about your drinking.

ARNOLD: I figure if I have to keep coming here, I might as well tell you what you want to know.

THERAPIST: You still seem a little reluctant to open up, so I want to respect your boundaries.

ARNOLD: What do you mean?

THERAPIST: I mean I don't want to be pushy and ask any questions that are offensive to you.

ARNOLD: I'm not offended by your questions. I just don't want you to get the wrong impression of me. You know what I mean?

THERAPIST: No, I'm not sure. Explain.

ARNOLD: Early in our marriage my wife insisted that we get counseling. I agreed, but after the first visit we never went back.

THERAPIST: What kept you from going back?

ARNOLD: Well, my wife told her side of our story and I told mine. Then the counselor looked at me and asked whether I understood that my wife didn't want to live with a drunk like her father. It was like he looked me right in the face and called me a drunk. Then, you know what he did next? He said if I really loved her, I would quit drinking that day.

THERAPIST: Wow, sounds like a difficult experience. From what you just told me, you felt accused of being a drunk and you were then ordered to quit drinking... *or else.*

ARNOLD: I didn't just *feel* like I was accused. I *was* accused!

THERAPIST: Again, it sounds like it was pretty difficult. You can be sure that I'll never call you a drunk, and I'll never order you to quit drinking.

ARNOLD: Then what am I here for?

THERAPIST: My job is to help you define your problems accurately and decide what solutions will work best for you.

Arnold's therapist actually found it disturbing to learn that a professional had labeled his patient a drunk, though he was not terribly surprised. Nor was he surprised that a professional had ordered his patient to quit drinking. He now better understood why Arnold had been reluctant to pursue therapy, and he was again reminded that stigmatizing people is more likely to alienate them than promote change.

Patients May Have Stereotypical Views
of Therapy or Therapists

There are many public portrayals of psychotherapy and psychotherapists that are unflattering, unfavorable, and inaccurate. As a result, some potential patients may imagine that therapists are judgmental, detached, privileged, eccentric, or even deeply troubled themselves. Even when this is not the case, some believe talking about their problems does not solve them. Others believe no one, not even therapists, could possibly understand, or even care about how they feel. Many patients who admit to addictive behaviors are skeptical about therapists who are not in recovery themselves, believing only someone who has suffered as they have can help them.

After learning more about Becky in their first session (described earlier), Becky's therapist returns to a statement made by Becky at the beginning of their session:

> THERAPIST: Becky, earlier you described me as "a shrink who treats addicts." I'm curious about your thoughts about therapists and therapy.
>
> BECKY: Oh, I'm really sorry that I said that. I didn't mean to offend you.
>
> THERAPIST: Don't feel bad. I assure you that I wasn't offended. That statement gave me an opportunity to learn more about your views of therapy and therapists.
>
> BECKY: Well, you are different from what I expected when I was told I had to come here.
>
> THERAPIST: What were you expecting?
>
> BECKY: First of all, I thought I'd have to lie on a couch. Second, I thought I'd have to do all the talking. And third, I thought you'd be kind of stuffy. You know, like from a world very different from mine. . . . [*Suddenly pauses and appears embarrassed.*] I'm sorry, I can't believe I'm saying all these things. I probably got these ideas from therapists on TV or the movies.
>
> THERAPIST: No, please don't feel bad. This is very helpful. Your honesty actually makes me optimistic about us working together.
>
> BECKY: I just didn't imagine that you'd understand what I had to say about myself. But you do . . . seem to understand, that is.

This moment proved to be a turning point in the session, as it contradicted many of Becky's negative expectations regarding therapy. Specifically, she never expected to be this honest with her therapist, particularly in their first session. She did not expect her therapist to be *authentic* with her. And she certainly did not think their meetings would involve mutual exchanges. She expected their encounters to be much more formal, structured, and *clinical*.

Patients May Believe Self-Disclosure Will Result in Punishing Consequences

In addition to being stigmatized, some addictive behaviors may involve illegal or socially maligned behaviors. To some extent, this should be addressed before therapy begins—that is, patients need to be told about mandated reporting and the limits of confidentiality. Only with that information can patients effectively decide what they are willing (or not willing) to disclose.

Therapists should emphasize that their highest priority is to help patients, though patients reassured by such statements might actually disclose thoughts or behaviors that create dilemmas for therapists. For example, patients might admit to stealing, prostitution, driving under the influence, sale of illegal drugs, embezzlement, or other illegal behaviors related to their addictions. Or more commonly, they might disclose illegal drug use or possession. Depending on the policies and statutes in their particular setting, a therapist may or may not be required to report such behaviors to authorities. Hence, therapists are urged to be fully knowledgeable about institutional, local, state, and federal laws regarding mandated reporting. Furthermore, therapists who know they will encounter illegal or socially sanctionable behaviors should commit themselves to working in a manner that is nonjudgmental and nonthreatening.

From time to time, therapists are likely to discover that patients have been less than fully honest or transparent in therapy, out of fear that the consequences will be punishing. Therapists may learn this from contradictory patient statements, where at least one of the statements must be untrue. They may learn through public, commercial, or social media outlets that patients have been engaged in behaviors never disclosed in therapy, for example when a patient is in the news for committing a crime never disclosed to the therapist. And occasionally therapists are contacted by friends, family members, or other professionals to report that a patient is engaged in behaviors never disclosed to the therapist. The following interaction between Charlie and his therapist demonstrates how concern about punishing consequences might become relevant in a session:

THERAPIST: I understand your reluctance to discuss your marijuana use, especially given the consequences you've experienced in the past.

CHARLIE: Then you don't blame me for clamming up with you.

THERAPIST: I don't blame you at all. It's just hard to know what's okay to ask and what's off limits.

CHARLIE: You can ask me whatever you want. Just don't expect me to answer all of your questions ... [*laughs*] ... at least honestly.

THERAPIST: You mean you won't always tell the truth?

CHARLIE: You got it.

THERAPIST: Would you be willing to say you don't want to answer a question, instead of not telling the truth?

CHARLIE: I guess that would be okay, but I can't promise.

THERAPIST: What's your biggest concern about telling me the truth?

CHARLIE: That you will tell my probation officer. Isn't that part of your job? Like being a snitch?

THERAPIST: Actually, no. As I explained when we first met, I don't know that I will ever have any reason to talk to your probation officer. All he expects from me is my signature on that paper you have me sign at the end of each visit. At this time, I don't have your consent to talk to anyone but you.

CHARLIE: Okay, well maybe that makes a difference. We'll just have to see.

It is apparent in this exchange that Charlie preferred not to disclose certain behaviors at that time, for fear of punishing consequences. Remarkably, Charlie was more honest than most patients about his reluctance to share certain matters with his therapist. Fortunately, Charlie's therapist did not need to know all of Charlie's secrets to be helpful in therapy. In the meantime, it was important for Charlie and his therapist to discuss topics that were germane to his therapy, and that he felt secure his therapist would maintain confidentiality.

HOW WORDS MATTER

When conducting therapy, language is important. Some words can be helpful, and some words can be hurtful. To complicate matters, there are words that are considered by some patients to be helpful, while those same words are considered by others to be hurtful. For example, some individuals in recovery find it helpful to label themselves "drunks," "alcoholics," and "addicts," while others are deeply disturbed by these labels. Generally speaking, cognitive-behavioral therapists are encouraged to use terms that do not risk alienating patients. Instead, they are encouraged to use clinical phrases like "a person with a substance use disorder" or "a person with alcohol use disorder," rather than an "addict" or an "alcoholic."

When a therapist tells a patient to avoid certain terms and phrases associated with addictive behaviors, they can expect mixed reactions. Consider, for example, this exchange between Charlie and his therapist:

CHARLIE: You should have seen me back when I was a drunk. It wasn't pretty.

THERAPIST: I notice that you often refer to yourself as a drunk when you talk about your drinking history.

CHARLIE: Yeah, I was a stinking, falling-down, drunk. There's no two ways about it.

THERAPIST: How does it make you feel to use language like that when talking about yourself?

CHARLIE: I hadn't given it any thought. It's just the way I talk.

THERAPIST: I often think labels like "stinking" and "drunk" can be hurtful instead of helpful.

CHARLIE: Actually, I think it helps me to think about my drinking that way. It helps me to think that drinking turns me into a stinking, falling-down drunk.

THERAPIST: What would be the disadvantage of simply thinking that drinking is really bad for you? Instead of thinking that you were a bad drunk.

CHARLIE: I guess I could think that way, but I don't know why I would.

THERAPIST: You didn't like it when you were accused of being a "drug addict" because you smoke marijuana. You felt like you were being judged. I thought you might consider putting an end to all self-labeling when you talk about your behaviors. Instead, you could just label the behaviors.

CHARLIE: You're losing me. I'm not sure I understand.

THERAPIST: Your drinking behaviors caused you problems, so you stopped drinking. It was the behavior that was bad for you, but you didn't think of yourself as bad.

CHARLIE: I'm starting to get it. I'm not sure it'll help to change my vocabulary, but I'll think about it some more.

John Kelly and his colleagues have done some of the most important work in this area. Kelly et al. (2015) point out that even terms like *clean* versus *dirty* can adversely impact relationships between well-meaning providers and their patients. They urge professionals to stop using "tough, punitive language" that implies "willful misconduct" (p. 8). In other words, therapists should label *behaviors* as problematic, rather than labeling the *people* who struggle with addictive behaviors.

INITIAL THERAPY SESSIONS

Initial interactions with patients entering therapy are extremely important (Spencer, Goode, Penix, Trusty, & Swift, 2019). Even self-referred patients may feel ambivalent about pursuing treatment for an addiction problem. From the start, most patients attempt to determine whether therapists are competent, trustworthy, sincere, caring, and even likeable. Early negative experiences with therapists often result in premature (if not immediate) termination from therapy.

Introductory CBT sessions should be guided by the dual aims of establishing a positive collaborative alliance and setting mutual process and outcome expectations (Curreri, Farchione, & Wang, 2019; King & Boswell, 2019). The basic therapeutic tasks of listening, reflecting, and projecting genuine interest and positive regard are essential for achieving these goals. Therapists are urged to understand patients' perspectives. When they do, and they can convey that understanding, patients believe, "*You actually get me.*" While it is useful to describe the CBT model during initial early sessions, in the first session or two it is important to minimize psychological jargon and formal language and stay as close as possible to ordinary language. This will help apprehensive patients to relax and view the therapist as an *authentic* person.

Consider the following therapist's introduction to CBT: "We are going to be examining your cognitive distortions and maladaptive behaviors so we can modify your dysfunctional addictive behaviors." Instead, a preferable introduction might be: "I'd like to know what you hope will happen when we meet for cognitive-behavioral therapy sessions. I also want to answer any questions." Depending on the patient's response to statements like these, a therapist might continue, "In our sessions I will try to understand how you think about yourself and your life right now. I'll be interested in what's working well and what's not working so well for you—so we both understand what you're going through. I especially want to know what you hope to get out our time together, and what you would like to change in your life. What are your thoughts about all this?"

In the second statement, the therapist does not go into depth about the CBT model, but instead lays some groundwork by making statements like, "We try to understand how you think about yourself." Furthermore, the therapist does not emphasize addictions per se, but talks more broadly about goals, and about what works and what does not work. When patients experience therapists to be competent, trustworthy, and likeable, they tend to open up in the first session and return for additional sessions. And when they return for additional sessions, many opportunities exist for teaching about the CBT model.

Patients struggling with addictions may feel especially ashamed or fearful of being judged during initial sessions. Indeed, sometimes it is challenging for therapists to be empathetic toward patients as they learn of behaviors that may have caused harm to innocent family members or society. Therefore, therapists need to monitor their own thoughts and verbal behaviors, so they do not project disapproval or condemnation in therapy. Especially during initial sessions, it is strongly recommended that therapists relate to addictive behaviors as problems to be solved, rather than moral, legal, societal, or character failings.

Therapists can begin to develop positive collaborative relationships during initial CBT visits by establishing that they are interested in the quality of patients' lives, and not just motivating them to abstain from addictive behaviors. Since many patients with addictions are in treatment as a result of personal crises (Kosten, Rounsaville, & Kleber, 1986; Ramsay & Newman, 2000; Sobell, Sobell, & Neirenberg, 1988), many are likely to have coexisting mental health problems (Casteneda, Galanter, & Franco, 1989; Evans & Sullivan, 2001; Nace, Davis, & Gasperi, 1991; Newman, 2008). Therefore, it is appropriate to address such concerns as depression, anxiety, anger, financial stress, minority status stress, family relationships, friendships, vocational problems, and so forth. In doing so, therapists show that they are interested into getting to know the patient as a person, not simply as an "addict." They also improve their chances of calling patients' attention to addictions as principal causal factors in their overall emotional, interpersonal, and physical distress. In short, a positive approach is likely to positively influence patients' receptiveness to therapy and motivation to change.

As noted earlier, an important relationship-building strategy is to *ask patients for their thoughts about entering therapy.* Questions may include asking about their doubts and concerns, as well as their hopes, expectations, and goals. These questions communicate a willingness to hear patients' views and demonstrate that they will have input throughout CBT. Also, these questions allow therapists to communicate that certain thoughts (e.g., skepticism or doubt about therapy) can lead to corresponding emotions (e.g., tension, fear, frustration) and behaviors (e.g., missing appointments or dropping out of therapy) that profoundly impact the therapeutic relationship. After openly discussing patients' skepticism or doubt, therapists can share alternative ways of viewing therapy that are more hopeful or uplifting. For example, a therapist might say: "Starting therapy, despite your doubts, reflects courage and a willingness to try difficult and uncertain challenges." The following dialogue between Charlie and his therapist illustrates this process:

CHARLIE: How many times do I have to come here, to these sessions?

THERAPIST: Well, as I understand it, for as long as we both believe therapy is helping you. We can meet until the end of your probation, or until we think you're no longer in need of regularly scheduled sessions. What are *your* thoughts on this subject?

CHARLIE: I don't have any thoughts. I don't have any choice.

THERAPIST: That's actually a thought right there . . . that you don't have any choice. Your thought is that this therapy is being forced on you.

CHARLIE: Yeah. No offense, but I'm tired of this whole thing. [*Long pause.*]

THERAPIST: I'm listening. Tell me what you're tired of.

CHARLIE: I'm on probation. I'm supposed to be free, but this isn't freedom. I have to check in with my probation officer constantly, I have to pee in a cup, I can't drive without blowing into my interlock ignition device, and I have to come see a shrink. I'm always under a microscope. I'm sick of it.

THERAPIST: Is that what therapy feels like to you? Another threat to your freedom? Another way of being watched and controlled? Like you're under a microscope?

CHARLIE: That's what it *is*. You have to report about me to my PO.

THERAPIST: I can see how it would feel that way to you. Having to be here and having to get my signature on your paperwork every week probably feels demeaning and humiliating. Honestly, I've been impressed with how open you've been with me so far. I find you to be honest about your feelings and I appreciate that. I hope to help you learn skills that will provide you more freedom in the long run. I don't think of my job as checking on you, because that's not what I'm here for.

CHARLIE: I have to come here, but I don't have to like it.

THERAPIST: You'll be the final judge of whether this therapy is helpful, but I'd like to think we're working together to benefit you. Instead of thinking that this is an annoying obligation, I hope you'll eventually think our time together has value, and that this can help you achieve at least some personal goals. Can you think of *anything* you'd like to get out of our sessions that might make therapy more than just part of a mandatory sentence?

At this point, Charlie and his therapist might have an opening to talk about Charlie's goals, which might lead to some initial points of agreement and a greater sense of collaboration. In fact, Charlie eventually offered the goal of "Not getting busted again," and his therapist agreed this was an excellent goal. Near the end of this session Charlie's therapist offered a summary of their appointment and emphasized that Charlie's negative thoughts about therapy contribute to his feeling resentful about being there. In contrast, when Charlie considers possible benefits of therapy, including "Not getting busted again," he starts to feel somewhat engaged. This eventually began a path toward educating Charlie about the CBT model.

As is evident in dialogue above, therapists need to hear patients' concerns and complaints about therapy, especially during initial sessions, without feeling personally attacked, defensive, or avoidant. A sensitive elicitation of patients' thoughts, followed by authentic involvement by relaxed questioning and direct, honest feedback, increases the likelihood of building rapport. Additionally, therapists can give new patients positive feedback for simply attending initial sessions and participating. Therapists' positive comments can help patients have more favorable expectations of therapy, but all such comments should be made only if they are sincere—or patients will see new therapists as insincere, disingenuous, or even patronizing.

BUILDING, MAINTAINING, AND REPAIRING TRUST

Throughout this chapter we have asserted that common correlates of addictions are social stigma and self-stigma, where people with addictions feel harshly judged by others, and eventually judge themselves. When stigma plays a role in therapy patients may feel ashamed and inadequate as they share their most private thoughts, feelings, and behaviors. Or they may choose not to share them at all. Stigma typically leads to mistrust, and mistrust has the potential to promote disengagement (Miller & Rollnick, 2013). And naturally, secrecy tends to hamper the therapeutic relationship and deter progress in therapy. Consider the following examples of patients who are untruthful because they do not trust therapists or the therapy process:

- A college student says, "My drinking is fine. I only drink a couple of beers with my buddies on Friday and Saturday nights." In reality, he gets blackout drunk from Thursday through Sunday night, and then finds it impossible to function when he occasionally attends classes on Fridays and Mondays.
- A patient fails to show up for her Monday morning therapy appointment and later tells the therapist she did not realize they had an appointment that day. In actuality, she overslept the morning after a weekend of heavy cocaine use.
- A patient tells her therapist that her two most recent urinalyses came back positive for opioids, but she swears she has not been using opioids, and insists the positive result "must be from eating a muffin with poppy seeds."
- In family therapy a mother says her unemployed son is stealing money from her. The son denies doing so, expressing great indignation that she would accuse him. The mother cries, saying she has proof, and it breaks her heart to hear her son lie.
- A woman in therapy for depression describes regular trips to the casino. Although she has a well-paying job, she often worries about paying her bills. In an attempt to address this problem, the therapist asks how much money the patient has been losing as a result of gambling. The patient responds, "I always break even."

Generally speaking, therapists want to believe their patients and not question their honesty. Nonetheless, many patients do not trust therapists and therefore do not share important details regarding their problems or their lives. Therapists need to develop strategies for establishing trust with all patients, especially given scenarios like those depicted above. Such strategies must involve honest, supportive, compassionate—but also direct—communication. By engaging in this fashion, therapists are most likely to establish and maintain trust.

Clearly, it does little good for therapists to say to patients, "Don't worry, you can trust me." Only through consistent empathy, caring, authenticity, and reliability can patients begin to realize that therapists truly wish to help them. We say *begin to realize* because trust is a process that is often difficult to establish, but easy to damage or lose.

Therapists should bear in mind that early life experiences (i.e., distal antecedents) contribute to patients' lack of trust. For example, some patients may have been raised in emotionally unstable, volatile homes where traumatic events occurred on a regular basis. Others may have grown up in families where one or both parents had addictions and perhaps lied about anything associated with their addictive behaviors. Other patients may have lived in settings or communities where deception was the norm. Yet other patients may have had legal problems and been treated unfairly in the judicial system, resulting in mistrust toward the system. It is easy to understand how patients with such backgrounds might believe others cannot be trusted, and especially those in positions of authority.

The Potential Role of Schemas in the Therapeutic Relationship

An understanding of *schemas* is especially important when helping people with addictions. A schema is a pattern, structure, or framework for organizing deeply held assumptions about one's self, others, relationships, one's personal world, and the future. Schemas are mostly developed during childhood, as a result of early life experiences, and can be positive or negative. In fact, most individuals have some positive and negative schemas. For example, some might have positive schemas related to their abilities to succeed at work, while having negative schemas related to feeling unlovable as a spouse, parent, or other family member. It should be noted that schemas are different from basic, or core, beliefs. Schemas begin to form so early in childhood that they do not necessarily require words. Again, they are better described as patterns, structures, or frameworks (e.g., a pattern that involves personal adequacy or lovability). Basic (or core) beliefs on the other hand, can be expressed with words and sentences (e.g., "I am terribly inadequate or unlovable.") It may be helpful to think of schemas as being the garden from which a variety of plants (i.e., basic beliefs) grow.

One example of a negative schema is the *mistrust schema* (see Beck, Davis, & Freeman, 2015; Young, Klosko, & Weishaar, 2003). This schema manifests as pervasive mistrust of others and the withholding of thoughts and feelings associated with vulnerability. The mistrust schema is common to certain personality disorders (e.g., borderline, narcissistic, and paranoid personality disorders), and is likely to have developed as a result of the early life experiences described earlier. Effective therapists are aware of the influence of this schema and how it develops, and therefore do not take offense when patients mistrust them. Instead, they accurately conceptualize patients' problems and base clinical decisions on each patients' case conceptualization. They also do their best to offer a safe, nonjudgmental environment to their patients in order to avoid activating mistrust schemas.

Specific Strategies for Building and Maintaining Trust—and Repairing Therapy Ruptures

Certain therapist behaviors contribute to building and maintaining trust by consistently demonstrating their authentic involvement and commitment to the therapeutic process. Examples of these behaviors include: (1) being available for therapy sessions on a regular basis, (2) being on time for sessions (even if the patient generally is not), (3) returning patients' telephone calls in a prompt manner, (4) being available for emergencies (or having accessible backup coverage), (5) showing concern and a willingness to contact patients when they miss appointments, and (6) remaining in contact with patients (and available for the resumption of sessions) if inpatient hospitalization, detoxification treatment, halfway house rehabilitation, or reincarceration takes place during the course of therapy.

Despite even the most rigorous and sincere efforts to develop and maintain trust, therapy relationships inevitably develop ruptures, and therapists need to be skillful at recognizing and repairing ruptures (Eubanks, Burkell, & Goldfried, 2018; Eubanks, Muran, & Safran, 2018; Safran, Crocker, McMain, & Murray, 1990). A therapeutic rupture is defined as a breakdown or strain in the therapeutic alliance (Eubanks, Muran, & Safran, 2018), but it may also be understood as a process wherein trust is damaged. Ruptures may occur for many reasons and under numerous circumstances, related to events initiated by either therapists or patients. The following are hypothetical examples of therapeutic ruptures:

- A patient is late for an appointment and his therapist jokes about it. The patient becomes withdrawn for the remainder of the session, thinking his therapist has made a mockery of the serious situation that caused his lateness.
- A patient says she has not consumed alcohol for a week, but the therapist smells alcohol on her breath. The therapist clearly feels irritated and the patient notices.
- During a session, a patient commits to abstaining from cocaine but has a relapse before his next scheduled visit. He decides not to return to therapy

until he has been abstinent for several weeks. When he returns, he worries the therapist will be disappointed in him. He talks only about mundane topics to avoid discussing his cocaine use.

• After an extended break from therapy a patient says she has resumed cigarette smoking. Her therapist asks, "After doing well for so long, why would you ever go back to smoking?" The patient experiences that as a judgmental statement, rather than a sincere inquiry, and feels hurt.

These are just some examples of the countless potential ruptures that might occur in a therapeutic relationship. It is important for therapists to detect and discuss ruptures when they first happen, rather than avoiding them. Ideally, therapists state their objective observations (e.g., "You grimaced when I made that comment") and express a sincere desire to resolve the rupture (e.g., "I want to make sure my comment wasn't offensive to you"). When therapists do this openly, empathetically, and nondefensively, trust in a ruptured relationship can be restored. Unresolved ruptures in therapeutic relationships are likely to be corrosive to patient trust and ultimately lead to patient disconnectedness or premature termination from therapy. The following is an exchange between Charlie and his therapist, discussing a current rupture in their therapeutic relationship:

THERAPIST: Hello Charlie, what do you want to work on today?

CHARLIE: I'm doing pretty good. I can't think of anything. Maybe it's time for us to wrap things up.

THERAPIST: I'm glad you're doing pretty good. What do you mean, "wrap things up"?

CHARLIE: I mean it might be time for us to part ways.

THERAPIST: How did you decide that it might be time to part ways?

CHARLIE: In our last session you said you didn't think I had *real serious* problems.

THERAPIST: Wow, I sure didn't mean to say you don't have *real* or *serious* problems. Do you remember my exact words?

CHARLIE: Yeah, I remember clearly. I was telling you that I was pissed off about my neighbor's barking dog and you asked whether that was a *real serious* problem.

THERAPIST: Oh, I remember now. It was at the beginning of the session. Do you mind if I explain what I meant by that question?

CHARLIE: Do what you need to do.

THERAPIST: Does that mean it's okay for me to explain?

CHARLIE: Sure, go ahead.

THERAPIST: We were setting our session agenda and you were talking about your neighbor's barking dog, and how angry you felt, and I was trying to figure out if it was a problem you wanted to discuss in therapy or if you were just mentioning it. I'm sorry I said it in a way that implied I didn't take you seriously.

CHARLIE: I don't know what to say about that. I heard what I heard.

THERAPIST: I hope you'll give me another opportunity to show that I take you seriously.

CHARLIE: [*After a long pause.*] Well I'm here, so we might as well use the time for something.

THERAPIST: Thank you. I hope you know I welcome your feedback and especially appreciate your honesty with me.

Charlie was obviously reluctant to talk about the rupture when it occurred. In general, patients avoid directly confronting therapists. Some do not become upset until well after the rupture occurs, as they reflect on the session. Some realize they have negative feelings at the time of the rupture but have strong reservations about sharing immediately, for fear of the consequences. Regardless, it is the therapist's responsibility to identify ruptures as they occur and enlist patients' help in resolving them and moving forward. Fortunately, many patients do return to therapy after a therapeutic rupture, hoping that the rupture will be resolved.

RESISTING THE TERM *RESISTANCE*

Clinicians often use the word *resistance* when their best efforts to help patients are unsuccessful. This term is problematic for several reasons. First, *resistance* implies patients actually know *what* and *how* to change, but *intentionally* avoid doing so. Second, therapists who believe patients are *resistant* risk blaming their patients for their problems and stigmatizing them as others do. Third, the term *resistance* is imprecise. For example, does *resistance* mean patients intentionally sabotage therapy? Does it mean patients want to remain addicted? Does it mean patients are stubborn? Does it mean they do not want to be in therapy? The term *resistance* does not readily lend itself to problem solving. Instead, viewing patients as resistant may lead to counterproductive therapist responses such as frustration, irritation, apathy, and ultimately rejection.

As noted earlier, some patients will be reluctant to share the full extent of their struggle with addictive behaviors. Rather than viewing this reluctance as *resistance,* therapists should be sensitive to patients' suffering, and how this suffering might make the entire therapy experience difficult for patients. As discussed earlier in this chapter, patients may fear honesty will lead to judgment, abandonment, or even punishment. Therapists should avoid thinking patients intentionally resist change, as such judgmental thoughts are likely to cause tension in both therapists and patients. Instead therapists should continually understand that change (including therapy) is difficult, and empathy (rather than judgment) enhances the process of change (Miller & Rollnick, 2013).

While we stress the importance of empathy throughout this chapter, it is important to acknowledge that empathy alone may not be sufficient to motivate openness in therapy or actual change. Nonetheless, we maintain that a strong alliance, made possible by therapist empathy, maximizes the likelihood that patients will eventually be more receptive to change.

The following scenarios are common in therapy with addicted patients. Each has the potential to activate therapist beliefs about patient *resistance:*

- Patients who say they are committed to change, but regularly relapse
- Patients who say they can't think of anything to work on in therapy
- Patients who repeatedly describe barriers to change (e.g., "I can't . . . because . . .")
- Patients who miss sessions or regularly come late to them
- Patients who seem disinterested or detached during sessions

These are just some of the countless scenarios that might trigger therapists' negative, critical thoughts, and especially those associated with the concept of *resistance.* As noted earlier, such thoughts lead to negative feelings that are likely to undermine therapy and limit outcome. In addition to being empathetic, therapists should use case conceptualization skills to understand patients' reasons for engaging in the scenarios above.

ESTABLISHING BOUNDARIES AND SETTING LIMITS

Therapists need to establish boundaries and set limits but, needless to say, this is easier said than done. First, therapists need to ask themselves, *"What are my boundaries and limits as a therapist?"* or *"What patient behaviors can I tolerate, and what behaviors do I find intolerable?"* In fact, boundaries and limits vary from therapist to therapist. For example, some therapists welcome patients who have used alcohol or drugs prior to sessions, while others do not. Some therapists insist on ending sessions if they smell alcohol on a patient's breath, while others wait to determine patients' capacity to engage in the therapy process. Furthermore, some behaviors are *objectively* more tolerable than others. For example, most people would agree that threats of violence toward therapists are intolerable, while occasional lateness to appointments is tolerable. Consider the following list of patient behaviors:

- Recurrent relapses
- Nondisclosure of relapses
- Regularly missing appointments
- Showing no evidence of improvement
- Noncompletion of homework
- Frequent crisis phone calls
- Engaging in nonviolent crimes to support an addiction
- Engaging in violent crimes to support an addiction

Therapists vary in their reactions to each of these behaviors. Some might be repulsed by patients who admit to criminal behavior, while others might be impressed with patients' willingness to be honest about such activity. Thus, therapists should carefully reflect on the values and beliefs that determine their boundaries and limits, and be able to clearly communicate these to patients, so patients can make informed decisions about what they want to share in therapy—and even whether they want to see a particular therapist.

Caring therapists genuinely want to help their patients, but they also need to recognize that some requests for help may actually be invitations to cross boundaries. For example, some patients will inquire about ongoing communication outside of therapy (as they might expect with an AA sponsor). While it might be uncomfortable to say "no" to a patient who requests attention between sessions, the relationship only becomes more uncomfortable when patterns develop that cross a therapist's boundaries. It is occasionally necessary to say *no,* but it can be said in a caring, supportive manner, for example: "I understand your need for support, but lengthy phone calls between sessions could easily lead to your dependence on me. It is important for you to develop sources of support outside of our sessions, so you have the support you need whenever you need it."

As another example of setting limits, we present the following exchange with Charlene, who calls her therapist for help with a domestic problem:

CHARLENE: I'm glad I caught you before you left the office. I need your help with something. I'm on my way home from an AA meeting but my husband is going to accuse me of messing around and he's going to kick me out. Could you call him and let him know that I've been to a meeting and that everything is cool? I give you my permission.

Before saying anything, many thoughts race through the therapist's mind. First, he knows he cannot validate Charlene's attendance at a meeting he did not attend. Second, Charlene is asking him to intervene in a situation outside of their therapeutic relationship. And third, she is asking him to do so immediately and urgently, providing no time for his careful consideration. Charlene's therapist continues their conversation as follows:

THERAPIST: Charlene, I am committed to helping you in therapy, but I'm afraid this is a problem I can't help you with.

CHARLENE: What do you mean? [*Sounding annoyed.*]

THERAPIST: You're asking me to do something I really can't do. Perhaps if you had been in my office for a session and you gave formal consent to talk to your husband, I would have you call him and then agree to get on the phone to confirm we were together. But this is a different situation altogether.

CHARLENE: So, what you're saying is that you're not going to help me? So that's the way it's going to be? Okay, fine, thanks for being such a helpful therapist.

THERAPIST: Charlene, I'm more than happy to help you deal with this problem, but I can't make it go away. Instead, I would prefer to do some problem solving with you.

CHARLENE: That's what I'm asking you to do. Help me solve this problem!

THERAPIST: I'll do all I can under these circumstances. Do you want to schedule an appointment for tomorrow so we can discuss this matter at length?

CHARLENE: I don't know. [*Still sounding disgusted, though less so.*]

THERAPIST: If you want to see me, just let me know. I'll look at my schedule and call you back.

CHARLENE: I don't know. Okay, I guess so.

In this brief dialogue, Charlene's therapist did his best to be warm, caring, and collaborative—while also maintaining boundaries and setting limits. Another way for therapists to set limits is by deferring decisions until such requests can be given more careful consideration. Doing so sets limits regarding the timing of clinical decisions. It also reminds patients that they are interacting with a professional who must adhere to a set of standards.

MAINTAINING CREDIBILITY

Many patients who struggle with addictions believe therapists can't possibly understand their problems or be credible resources. So how can a therapist establish credibility? Credibility is related to trust, but there are subtle differences between the two. We view credibility as the degree to which patients view therapists as *skillful* and *knowledgeable*, whereas trust involves patients' perceptions of their *reliability* and *integrity*. To establish credibility, therapists need to understand human behavior generally and addictive behavior specifically. They also need to implement appropriate, effective treatment strategies that are helpful to people with addictions. But more importantly, credibility requires an accurate understanding of each individual patient—and this is only accomplished through empathy and thorough, accurate case conceptualizations.

An important factor that contributes to credibility is therapists' willingness to admit to their limitations. For example, when patients say they are using new designer drugs unfamiliar to therapists, it is important for therapists to admit to their lack of familiarity with these particular drugs. Furthermore, therapists may explain that they are eager to learn from their patients. Thus, it is advisable for therapists to manifest humility and a spirit of collaboration. For example, a therapist might state, "You know a lot about your life and your addiction, and I know a lot about cognitive-behavioral therapy. It is my hope that we work as a team and learn from each other, in order to come up with goals and plans that serve you well."

As noted above, some patients believe that only others in recovery are credible recovery resources. As a result, they may assume they can only be understood or helped by therapists who have struggled with past addictions. Indeed, some therapists know more about addictions as a result of their own personal addiction experiences. However, some therapists in recovery are at risk for being less understanding, or even less helpful, believing they have experienced "*the* right way" to recover from addictions. Such therapists might feel uncomfortable when patients take a different path to recovery. For example, a therapist who has been successful with AA or SMART Recovery might be tempted to insist that patients attend these groups. Along the same lines, therapists in recovery who have chosen abstinence, without ever attempting to moderate their own substance use, may balk at a patient who says their recovery plan involves reduced substance use. To avoid such problems, it is recommended that therapists in recovery be aware of such biased thoughts and be especially careful not to impose them on patients.

Related, is the inevitable question asked by many patients: "Are you in recovery?" or "Have you ever been addicted?" Treatment models vary in the responses they recommend when therapists are asked this question. Some models recommend deflection, with such responses as "Why is that important to you?" or "I'd be happy to share that with you at some point in the future." We recommend that cognitive-behavioral therapists simply give a straight, honest answer, such as: "Yes, I've been in recovery for several years and feel privileged to be helping others in recovery" or "No, I've never had an addiction, but I've learned so much from helping people like you who have struggled with addictions." Of course, these are simply suggestions. Other than recommending that therapists be honest and direct, we advise therapists to choose responses that feel most authentic to them.

MANAGING POWER STRUGGLES

Power struggles are best understood as counterefforts by patients and therapists to maintain control over therapy content or process. The following are some examples of power struggles between therapists and patients:

- Jim enters therapy for help with an alcohol problem and his therapist asks about his childhood, in order to determine risk factors for alcohol use disorder. Jim says he sees no reason to talk about his past or "play the blame game." Jim's therapist insists that he needs this information to help Jim, but Jim holds his ground.

- Sherry has been seeing a therapist for gambling disorder. Sherry is in serious financial trouble as a result of her frequent visits to a nearby casino. Sherry says therapy is helpful, and her goal is to limit her casino spending to $20 per visit, no more often than three times per week. Sherry's therapist insists that Sherry completely stop going to the casino, but Sherry says it's the only fun thing she does. At each visit, Sherry's therapist insists that Sherry stay away from the casino. Sherry holds her ground.

- Phil has worked closely with his therapist to reduce the amount of prescription pain medication he takes. He tells his therapist he has reached a plateau and wants to check into medication-assisted treatment (MAT). His therapist responds by telling Phil that he has done well in therapy and turning to MAT now would reinforce Phil's helpless thoughts. Phil disagrees and holds his ground.

Most human beings want to control their own lives, but most who enter therapy for addictions have had difficulty controlling their lives. As a result, they are likely to enter therapy feeling ambivalent. In fact, most people with addictions vacillate between wanting to change and wanting to maintain their addictive behaviors. So even when patients and therapists agree on goals for therapy, it is possible for them to enter into power struggles, where patients move in and out of readiness to change, while therapists remain steadfast in their wish to see patients change.

Cognitive-behavioral therapists may unwittingly enter into power struggles with patients as a result of the goal-oriented nature of CBT. Therapists need to remain aware of this risk and continually remember that *collaboration in CBT is more important than goal achievement.* As a reminder, collaboration is defined as engaging cooperatively, *as a partnership,* to establish and accomplish goals. Power struggles occur when therapists and patients no longer agree on goals. From the examples above, Jay's goal is to change his drinking without consideration of family history, Sherry's goal is to spend up to $20 per day at the casino, and Phil's goal is to learn more about MAT. As long as their therapists do not share these goals, they are at risk for entering into power struggles. In each case, these therapists should be clear about the injunction above: *Collaboration in CBT is more important than goal achievement.*

We offer therapists the follow recommendations for avoiding power struggles:

- Recognize circumstances that might develop into power struggles before they actually develop (e.g., when a patient says, "I haven't done the homework we talked about.")
- Regularly ask patients for feedback regarding the therapy process (as we will discuss in the next chapter). For example, "What are your thoughts about our session today? To what extent is this session meeting your needs?"
- Identify and resolve therapeutic ruptures as soon as they occur, so they don't turn into power struggles.
- Pay attention to your own internal thoughts and feelings, and especially feelings of pressure, tension, frustration and irritation. Resolve these feelings by minimizing negative thoughts and maximizing empathy for the patient.
- Remind yourself to be patient and compassionate with patients. Most come to therapy feeling frustrated and inadequate, and power struggles may heighten their discomfort and contribute to treatment failure.

Another way to avoid power struggles is to stay focused on patients' strengths. Power struggles in therapy are sometimes activated by therapists' negative biases. For example, therapists may feel tension toward patients as a result of over-focusing on patients' problematic thoughts and behaviors, while neglecting to think about their strengths. In such instances, therapists need to identify their own problematic thoughts such as:

"This patient *never* does what he says."
"I'm ready to give up on this patient."
"I really can't believe *anything* this patient says."
"She is trying to manipulate me like she manipulates everyone else."
"This patient doesn't have the capacity to change."

Clearly, such automatic thoughts are counterproductive. In direct response to these thoughts, therapists can deliberately generate the following alternative thoughts:

"This patient meets an important commitment by attending all of our scheduled therapy sessions in a timely manner."
"It takes courage to come to therapy, so of course I won't give up on this patient."
"This patient has told me things he's never told anyone else, which takes guts."

"Rather than labeling this patient as manipulative, I acknowledge that she has had to work hard for everything she has in the world."

"This patient has made substantial improvements in several areas of her life. I'm allowing my unrelenting standards to get in the way of seeing her accomplishments."

By monitoring and modifying their own thoughts, feelings, and behaviors, therapists are able to avoid power struggles. The negative thoughts listed above are similar to those held by a society that stigmatizes people with addictions. By activating new, more positive thoughts about patients with addictions, and working hard to reduce their cognitive biases and resolve them, therapists facilitate their own personal growth.

SUMMARY

This chapter has emphasized the vital challenges of establishing a positive therapeutic relationship with patients who struggle with addictions. We have illustrated ways therapists can engender a sense of rapport, trust, and collaboration with such patients, while minimizing the risk of inadvertently propagating patients' maladaptive behaviors and beliefs. We have also described ways to reduce the risk of becoming adversarial in treatment, and therefore maintain the collaborative spirit that is central to CBT.

CHAPTER 5

INDIVIDUAL SESSION
STRUCTURE

The structure of an individual CBT session is among its most conspicuous and essential characteristics. Well-structured sessions make the best use of available time, rather than drifting aimlessly from topic to topic and problem to problem. This is vitally important, since patients with addictions are likely to suffer a wide range of chronic and acute problems that need to be resolved. Also, a well-structured session contributes to collaboration between patient and therapist, as they work together to identify and address problems. Structure enables therapists and their patients to prioritize and focus on the most essential problems. Structuring the session sets the tone for a working atmosphere, necessary for learning new skills and problem solving. Furthermore, structured sessions decrease the likelihood of session drift (i.e., meandering around from topic to topic), resulting in a loss of continuity. Knowing the elements of a structured CBT session facilitates adherence to the cognitive-behavioral model and minimizes the chances that drift will occur.

Various CBT approaches (e.g., behavioral activation, acceptance and commitment therapy, rational emotive behavior therapy, and dialectical behavioral therapy, among others) differ in how they structure sessions. This chapter focuses on eight elements we consider important during individual therapy sessions:

1. Setting the agenda (including urges to engage in addictive behaviors, actual addictive behaviors, or high-risk situations)
2. Checking mood (e.g., sadness, anxiety, restlessness, boredom, anger, frustration)
3. Bridging from prior sessions (including any homework assigned, problems encountered, addictive behaviors, major life changes, problematic moods, etc.)

4. Prioritizing and addressing agenda items (through guided discovery and the application of structured techniques)
5. Providing capsule summaries throughout
6. Assigning homework as needed
7. Exchanging feedback
8. Closing and planning for follow-up

In the following sections we describe these elements in detail and provide instructive examples.

SETTING THE AGENDA

Time is precious. Setting the agenda facilitates efficient use of time and provides a focus for the therapy session. It also teaches patients to set priorities—a skill sometimes lacking in people with addictions. Because people with addictions spend considerable time seeking, using, or recovering from their addictive behaviors, they are at risk for spending insufficient time addressing important life challenges.

Effectively setting the agenda can deepen the therapeutic relationship. It can reinforce the spirit of collaboration, as both patient and therapist have an opportunity to contribute to each encounter. Setting the agenda allows patient and therapist to target specific goals and discuss the appropriateness of focusing on specific topics. It also sets the stage for potential conflict resolution when a patient's concern seems incompatible with the therapist's concern for the patient. Consider circumstances in which the patient says, "I need to tell you the whole story to get it off my chest. It makes me feel better to talk about it." For the sake of collaboration the therapist might agree that a certain portion of the session can be used to tell the whole story but also suggest that time is needed to address other potential problems, such as ambivalence about abstinence, continued addictive behaviors, triggers, urges to use, and so forth.

Many patients do not want to feel vulnerable, so they avoid placing sensitive topics on the agenda. As a result, therapists often find they have to recommend topics for the agenda. For example, when a patient who perpetually relapses does not place relapse on the agenda, the therapist might say, "In addition to the items you have already put on our agenda I'd like to suggest that we add relapse prevention." In doing so it is helpful to provide a rationale, for example: "Whether or not you've had a recent relapse, it's going to be a topic worth reflecting on for some time." Therapists also make good, collaborative use of the agenda by demonstrating empathy for their patients' reluctance to discuss sensitive topics such as relapse.

Therapists' efforts to set the agenda should not be thwarted when patients say, "I don't know what to put on the agenda." In fact, we believe good cognitive-behavioral therapists almost never take "I don't know" for an answer. They persist gently, find alternative ways to ask the question, or ask the patient to reflect on possible agenda items while the therapist silently, patiently waits. When encountering patients who say, "I can't think of anything to work on," the therapist might explain that one of the patient's responsibilities in therapy is to come to sessions prepared to work on matters that concern them. At first, the therapist may assist the patient by suggesting some agenda items, asking, "Which of these is most important to you?" The therapist might also ask, "What's been on your mind since our last visit? What's on your mind right now?" Later, if the patient continues to seem unable or unwilling to generate topics for discussion, this problem can itself become an agenda item. For example, the therapist may say, "Let's discuss your difficulty in thinking of things to talk about in session," or "Let's try to understand your difficulty setting an agenda, and how I might help you overcome it." In doing so, the therapist avoids accepting the patient's helplessness or hesitancy as an unmanageable fact. In addition, the patient learns that saying "I don't know" will not be reinforced, and will fail as a means of escape from the work of therapy.

Therapists often need to be flexible in setting the agenda. Patients may come to a session in crisis, for example after being fired from a job, getting arrested, or being evicted from their home. These types of problems may require immediate attention, superseding ongoing issues. Likewise, a lapse should be addressed immediately because patients who have a slip or lapse often feel discouraged about their ability to stay on course, and thus are at increased risk for a full relapse—which often leads to feeling hopeless about therapy and may precipitate dropout.

Therapists should avoid being rigid or authoritarian in setting and following agendas. For example, when it becomes clear that a high-priority agenda item will require most of the session, the therapist should be willing to delay less important topics until a future session. Also, therapists might decide to revise an agenda midway through a session to accommodate the amount of time left in a session. If there is insufficient time, patient and therapist may collaboratively decide which items might be addressed and which might be postponed.

The following is a transcript of the beginning of a therapy session. In reading this transcript, keep in mind that the therapist is working with the patient to set an appropriate agenda with a specific target problem, to keep the agenda suitable for the amount of time available in the therapy session, and to prioritize the topics:

THERAPIST: What would you like to work on today?

PATIENT: Some things, but you know . . . my big problem now . . . the thing is . . . [*pause*] . . . I really need a job.

THERAPIST: A job. That makes good sense. Let's put it on the agenda. Are there other things we need to talk about, like any recent slips or lapses?

PATIENT: No, I'm doing alright as far as my addiction is concerned.

THERAPIST: Have you gotten high at all since I last saw you?

PATIENT: Not at all.

THERAPIST: Not once?

PATIENT: Not once. I go to my meetings now.

THERAPIST: No drinking? No alcohol?

PATIENT: Nothing.

THERAPIST: Urges or cravings?

PATIENT: No, none.

THERAPIST: How do you feel about that?

PATIENT: Pretty good.

THERAPIST: I'm glad to hear that. Congratulations on another week of success. Is there anything coming up that might put you at risk for relapsing?

PATIENT: No, I don't seem to crave anymore. Now my challenge is finding the energy to get out of bed in the morning. I need to get up, get out, and find a job. That's the real problem: I lack motivation.

THERAPIST: Okay, I'm making a list of things we need to cover like I always do. But I understand that getting a job is your greatest concern. As you well know, we might not get to everything today. So finding a job is first on the agenda. It sounds like difficulty getting up in the morning is another potential agenda item. The next thing I can put on the agenda is your success at not getting high this week so we can figure out what you need to keep thinking and doing as relapse prevention. Oh, and we can go over the homework from last week.

PATIENT: Finding a job is the most important thing.

THERAPIST: Okay, let's start with that.

As this brief transcript illustrates, the agenda sets the stage for focusing on multiple potential topics: finding a job, difficulty getting motivated, possibly depression, and relapse prevention. In the exchange above, the therapist also raised three questions that are important to ask at every session: (1) "Have you used since the last session?" (2) "Have you had any urges/cravings to use?" and (3) "Are there any situations coming up before our next session where you might be at risk to use?"

CHECKING MOOD

Since negative emotions (e.g., boredom, restlessness, despair, anxiety, anger) are internal triggers that may activate continued use or relapse, it is important to monitor emotional states (i.e., moods) at every visit. In addition to their potential impact on relapse, intense negative emotions have the potential for putting patients at risk for suicide. Therapists should pay special attention to feelings of despair associated with hopelessness, as it has been shown that a chronic, marked negative view of the future is a reliable predictor of suicide (Beck, Steer, Kovacs & Garrison, 1985).

It is helpful to have the patient complete brief screening instruments on a regular basis, or even at every session. Such instruments might include the Beck Depression Inventory (BDI; Beck, Steer, & Brown, 1996), Beck Anxiety Inventory (BAI; Beck & Steer, 1993), Patient Health Questionnaire (PHQ-9; Kroenke, Spitzer, & Williams, 2001), General Anxiety Inventory (GAD-7; Spitzer, Kroenke, Williams, & Lowe, 2006), and the Columbia Suicide Severity Rating Scale (C-SSRS; Posner et al., 2011). Scores and their meanings should be discussed with the patient, especially if there are substantial changes in scores from one session to the next. Sometimes there are changes in mood that are not within the patient's awareness, but they become apparent by reflecting on these instruments. The therapist might say, "Your score on the BDI/PHQ-9 is higher this week, which may indicate that you have been feeling more depressed. Do you agree with that?"

Because therapists regularly discuss emotions in their daily lives, they may overestimate patients' knowledge about them. Many people grow up in families that never talk about feelings. Some are taught directly to refrain from having vulnerable feelings (e.g., "Big boys and girls don't cry," or "If you don't stop crying, I'll give you something to cry about"). And others have had strong painful feelings in the past but learned to numb them with addictive behaviors. In these cases the therapist needs to be aware and ready to help patients identify and label their feelings, the triggers that activate them, and the most effective strategies available to master feelings.

BRIDGING FROM PRIOR SESSIONS

Many people with addictions live chaotic lives, and therefore therapists may find that some jump from topic to topic in a disjointed fashion—both within and across sessions. Hence, therapists should be determined to stay focused and maintain continuity across therapy sessions by asking themselves, "How do today's agenda items relate to what we discussed in previous sessions, and how do these items relate to the overall goals of therapy?"

As an extension of bridging, therapists should reflect on any patient feedback from previous sessions. For example, the therapist might ask for any unfinished business from the most recent session, including any negative or positive thoughts or feelings. Further, the therapist might reflect on chart notes from prior sessions. Usually this is a brief process; however, some responses might require considerably more attention and time to address. For example, consider the patient who says that he did not expect to make any progress in the last session, that he did not in fact make any progress, and that he did not expect to make progress in future sessions. The therapist should recognize that this feedback reflects negative and possibly even hopeless views about therapy that need to be discussed in the current session.

Regular bridging provides a convenient backdrop for checking on homework (see Chapter 7), as well the status of an individual's addiction. For example, a therapist might say something like, "When we talked about homework last week, you especially liked the idea of *urge surfing*, by taking a short walk any time urges and craving seem unbearable. How did that work out? Did you take any walks this week or even have cravings that might precipitate an urge surfing walk?"

And finally, to get a sense of the patient's world, it is sometimes helpful to focus on the general quality of a patient's life from session to session. Therapists might consider using structured self-monitoring strategies (e.g., activity schedules) to facilitate this process, focusing on the most relevant events and circumstances (see Form 7.2 in Chapter 7). A less structured approach might be to simply recommend journaling. These activities sometimes make it easier for some patients to bridge from prior sessions and generate new agenda items.

PRIORITIZING AND ADDRESSING AGENDA ITEMS

In reality, some patients come to therapy with no agenda items, some come with a few items, and some come with too many items to cover in a 50-minute session. When patients come with no items, therapists might say, "Let's just discuss what's concerned you most this week." Regardless of how agenda items are generated, prioritizing them is vital. This process may be simple, requiring only the question, "Where do you want to begin?" or it might require more careful probing and asking the patient to choose each item carefully. When too many items are introduced at the beginning of a session it might be necessary to delay some until a future session. By deliberately prioritizing agenda items, therapists can avert problems such as learning about a crisis with only minutes left at the end of a session.

Therapists must be alert to patients' tendencies to stray from agenda items and go off on tangents. A polite but prompt statement is usually sufficient, such as, "I prefer not to interrupt you, but I think we should refocus on the topic we began talking about." At times, when patients seem to stray to even more important issues (e.g., a discussion of the patient's pending divorce leads to hints that the patient is contemplating suicide), it is advisable to reprioritize the agenda in order to address these important topics. In general, topics such as the patient's active drug use, suicidality, or problems with therapy will supersede most other agenda items.

Therapists need to be conscious of time so topics presented are addressed in sufficient breadth and depth, and transitions can be made in a timely manner. At times, therapists may interject with a question in order to facilitate this process, for example: "We're about halfway through the session. Should we keep talking about this topic or would it make sense to wrap this up and move to our next agenda item?" This is a collaborative, flexible way to stay focused on meaningful therapeutic material, and to be as efficient as possible in making the best use of valuable therapy time.

Guided Discovery

Agenda items are addressed by means of a systematic process known as *guided discovery*. Guided discovery involves asking questions of patients to facilitate their own contemplation, evaluation, and synthesis of diverse information. Guided discovery should be continuous throughout entire sessions. Typical guided discovery questions might include:

> "How did you make that choice?"
> "What were you feeling when you made that choice?"
> "What were you thinking when you made that choice?"
> "What else could you have done in that situation?"
> "How accurate or helpful are those thoughts/beliefs?"
> "What is the consequence of thinking that way?"
> "How else could you have reacted to that issue/problem?"
> "What are the advantages and disadvantages of thinking and acting that way?"
> "What are your most deeply held values?"
> "What future behaviors will be most consistent with your values?"

In contrast to questions meant to gather information regarding the frequency, intensity, and duration of problems, guided discovery is used to bring information and solutions into the awareness of the patient. Guided discovery aims to promote insight and effective decision making. Questions should be formulated to stimulate thought and increase awareness, rather than requiring a correct answer. The proper choice, phrasing, and ordering of questions has a strong impact on patients' thinking patterns and content. Over the years we have learned that most patients respond more favorably to exploratory questioning and listening than lecturing. In fact, guided discovery, like motivational interviewing, is based on the principles and techniques of active listening.

Guided discovery is a powerful technique for addressing agenda items. Through the process of guided discovery, patients are helped to examine their thinking, reflect on self-defeating behaviors, and generate more effective approaches to living. This often leads to patients' questioning their own thoughts, motives, and behaviors *even after they have left therapy sessions*. Also, guided discovery establishes a nonjudgmental atmosphere and thus facilitates collaboration between patients and therapists. This kind of atmosphere can help patients come to their own conclusions about the seriousness of their addictive behaviors.

Therapists should start utilizing guided discovery from the outset of therapy so that patients become oriented to an active, reflective problem-solving mode. Occasionally, therapists will find that patients struggle with guided discovery. When this occurs therapists may choose to be more direct by frankly identifying inconsistencies and discrepancies, followed by asking if the patient agrees. For example, instead of asking, "What were you thinking when you did that?" a therapist might state, "You must have had *some* angry thoughts when you chose to hit that guy," and then ask, "Do you agree?"

While it is important to use questioning to explore problems and to help patients draw their own conclusions, there should be a balance between questioning and other more direct modes of intervention, such as reflection, clarification, giving feedback, and educating the patient. The following dialogue illustrates such a balance, with the therapist starting with some basic assessment questions:

THERAPIST: Sarah, what happened to your arm?

PATIENT: Oh nothing, those are just old bruises.

THERAPIST: Why do you think I asked that question?

PATIENT: Because you think I've been shooting up again.

THERAPIST: How do you feel about me asking that question?

PATIENT: I don't like it.

THERAPIST: What bothers you about my question?

PATIENT: Nobody trusts me. Everyone thinks I'm still a junkie.

THERAPIST: That thought must really hurt.

PATIENT: Yeah it hurts, especially since I've been clean and sober for six months now.

THERAPIST: Six months. That's a huge success.

PATIENT: Not to the people in *my* world.

THERAPIST: Sarah, how long do you think it should take for people to trust you?

PATIENT: I don't know. Maybe it's still too early.

THERAPIST: Maybe. More importantly, are you starting to trust yourself to stay clean and sober?

PATIENT: Well, it gets easier every day.

THERAPIST: Maybe it will get easier for others to trust you over time.

PATIENT: Yeah, I guess.

Note that the therapist acts as a role-model who demonstrates inquisitiveness, partly to help the patient become more *self-inquisitive*. In other words, *the therapist guides discovery so the patient will learn to guide their own self-discovery.* The fact that the patient is upset at times during guided discovery should not deter the therapist. Instead, the therapist should identify tactful, collaborative strategies to encourage each patient to exert more cognitive effort, facilitated by guided discovery.

Psychoeducation and Structured Techniques

In Chapter 1 we presented the five components of CBT: structure, collaboration, case conceptualization, psychoeducation, and structured techniques. It is while prioritizing and addressing agenda items that the therapist provides the majority of psychoeducation and structured techniques—in addition to engaging in guided discovery. Psychoeducation can involve many topics, including:

- An overview of the CBT model of addictions (the "ABC" model)
- Strategies for dealing with urges and craving
- Relapse prevention
- Behavioral activation strategies
- Emotion regulation strategies
- Interpersonal skills
- Problem-solving skills
- Mindfulness and meditation techniques
- The role of acceptance and commitment in recovery
- Basic addiction facts and principles (causes and consequences of addictions, treatment efficacy, etc.)

The timing of psychoeducation during a CBT session is vital. Novice CBT therapists are at risk for teaching patients without adequately conceptualizing them or establishing a collaborative therapeutic relationship. For example, some therapists (in their great enthusiasm for CBT) will immediately start describing the CBT model, structure of therapy, and techniques—right at the start of therapy. The problem with doing so is that patients may not be ready to focus on this information, they may not be ready to make changes, the therapist may not fully understand the problem to be treated, and the therapeutic relationship has not been well established. Alternatively, the therapist should first collect information about the patient's background, occasionally asking questions like, "Would you like more information about how CBT works?" or "Would you like to know more about the likely cause or consequence of the behavior you're describing?"

Numerous structured CBT techniques have been developed for addressing addictive behaviors, and as described above, these techniques should not be administered until the therapist has collected enough information to understand the needs of the patient. The following are just some of the CBT techniques available for help patients with addictions:

- Targeting problematic beliefs
- Rational responding
- Stimulus control
- Daily thought recording
- Activity monitoring and scheduling
- Delaying and distracting
- Urge surfing
- Role playing
- Advantages–disadvantages analyses
- Prolonged exposure
- Mindfulness and meditation techniques

Most of these techniques are described in Chapter 7. For these techniques to be effective, they need to be effectively explained, learned during the session, and practiced as homework.

PROVIDING CAPSULE SUMMARIES THROUGHOUT

It is essential to the learning process that therapists and patients summarize their discussion at various times throughout each session. Capsule summaries provide opportunities to adjust agendas and to maintain the focus of therapy sessions. Cognitive-behavioral therapists should strive to provide no less than three capsule summaries each session. For example, an early capsule summary might occur right after the agenda has been set, others might occur during the therapy session, and yet others might occur toward the end of the therapy session.

A capsule summary provided early in a session might link the current agenda to the patient's long-term goals. The following reflects such a capsule summary:

THERAPIST: Okay, let's summarize today's agenda: The first agenda item was your strong urge to purchase a pack of cigarettes this morning. The second agenda item has to do with a crisis at work. And your third involves your ongoing anxiety about your marriage. Have I missed anything?

PATIENT: No, that's it.

THERAPIST: It seems to me that all three agenda items fit well with your long-term values. You've repeatedly said that you want to be in better physical health, and you've often said that you value your family and want to provide for them.

PATIENT: Yeah, that's true.

A capsule summary provided later in the session might help the therapist reflect, decide what to do next (such as advancing to the next item on the agenda), convey understanding, correct any misunderstanding, and make therapy more understandable to the patient.

Every CBT session should conclude with final summaries provided by both therapist and patient. When patients are encouraged to summarize, they are reminded that they have a responsibility for processing the session. Patients' summaries enable therapists to check on patients' understanding of what occurred in the session. Further, patients improve their retention for the contents of the session when they actively review what has been discussed.

ASSIGNING HOMEWORK AS NEEDED

The assignment of homework is a collaborative enterprise generated and agreed upon by the therapist and patient as a team. Its two main functions are to serve as a bridge between sessions, ensuring that patients continue to work on their problems, and to provide an opportunity for patients to collect information to test personal beliefs and to try new behaviors. Patients are encouraged to view homework as an integral and vital component of CBT. Since the therapy session is time-limited, homework assignments become extremely important as opportunities to practice new skills between sessions.

It is best to assign homework that draws from the therapy session, as a logical extension of the therapy session. This can be done by reviewing insights from the session and how these can be continued and reinforced outside treatment. Ideally, such assignments lead to continued use of new skills even after the termination of formal treatment.

It is generally advisable to review the previous week's homework as an early agenda item in each therapy session (i.e., after bridging from prior sessions). By doing so, therapists convey to patients that homework is an important part of the therapy process. Also, by reviewing homework from previous sessions, therapists can correct patients' mistakes early in treatment—for example, in completing automatic thought records (see Chapter 7). By making sure that the homework assignment is reviewed, therapists can make certain that patients are effectively practicing new cognitive and behavioral skills.

Therapists who do not review homework might inadvertently contribute to three problems. First, their patients might conclude that homework assignments are actually not important. Second, their patients might miss opportunities to identify and correct misconceptions about assignments or new skills. And third, their patients might miss opportunities to draw helpful lessons from homework and reinforce these lessons.

Therapists can minimize homework failures by explaining the rationale for assignments and discussing any possible or expected difficulties. For example, the therapist might ask: "How might you benefit from doing this homework?" "What are the odds of your completing this assignment?" or "What could get in the way of completing this homework assignment?" In addition, when therapists doubt patients' understanding of homework, they should rehearse the assignment before the patient leaves the session.

When homework assignments are not completed, therapists should ask about the barriers that may have interfered with homework completion. In our experience, some of the most common barriers cited by patients are:

"I was too busy. I didn't have enough time."
"I forgot about the homework."
"I kind of did the homework. I just didn't do it the way we talked about it."
"I tried to do what we talked about, but it didn't help."
"It was a good week, so I didn't need to do the homework."
"I was too depressed to do anything this week."
"I didn't think it would really help me."
"Nothing can help me so there is no point in trying."

Each of these thoughts has the potential to be transformed into an agenda item. For example, the response, "I was too busy," might lead to a discussion of time management. The response, "I forgot about the homework," might lead to a discussion about the hard work required for making complex personal changes. The response, "I didn't think it would really help me," might lead to a discussion about helplessness, or even the value of therapy.

In summary, homework functions as a bridge between therapy sessions and provides an opportunity to test beliefs and practice skills learned in the session. Actual assignments should serve as logical extensions of sessions and be relevant to the goals of therapy. Therapists can reduce noncompliance by giving a rationale for each assignment and addressing possible difficulties that might arise. To facilitate patients' understanding, homework assignments should be rehearsed in session. Therapists should explain the importance of homework and review assignments at each session. Incomplete assignments should be discussed as agenda items in the session. Reasons for not doing homework should be ascertained and addressed.

EXCHANGING FEEDBACK

Therapists and patients should regularly exchange feedback during therapy sessions. During all sessions, therapists should determine whether patients understand both the session content and the process. For example, the therapist might ask, "Can you tell me what point I'm trying to make with these questions?" Sometimes patients misunderstand what therapists are trying to accomplish. Asking questions provides patient and therapist opportunities to discover any miscommunications in the therapy session. At the end of each session, therapists should elicit feedback from patients regarding (1) what was learned in the session, (2) how the patient felt during the therapy session, and (3) how the patient feels about the therapy in general.

For example, the therapist might ask: "What did you get out of today's session?" "Was there anything I said or did that was particularly troubling?" or "What do you think we accomplished?"

Other ways of eliciting feedback include responding to nonverbal behavior in the therapy session. For example, if the therapist notices that the patient is frowning, the therapist might say, "I noticed you just had a frown on your face. What thoughts were going through your mind right then?" This will often result in eliciting valuable feedback.

Key points to remember are that therapists should be adept at eliciting and responding to verbal and nonverbal feedback throughout the therapy session, they should regularly check for patients' understanding, and they should provide summaries periodically throughout the session. These actions, in turn, help to build a strong collaborative relationship.

CLOSING AND PLANNING FOR FOLLOW-UP

In movies portraying psychotherapy it is not unusual for session endings to occur suddenly and sound something like this: "Okay, time is up. I will see you back in one week." In reality, human beings rarely get up suddenly and walk away from social encounters. In the course of conventional interpersonal discourse, time together ends with at least a semiformal conclusion. The same should be true in psychotherapy.

We suggest therapists take at least a few minutes at the end of every session to get closure. For example, if a session is 50 minutes in length, the therapist might (at 45 minutes) say something like, "We only have about five minutes left. Let's make sure we discuss what you got out of this session, and if you agree with the homework. We can also schedule another appointment if you like." Statements like these prepare patient and therapist for the patient's departure. In doing so, the collaborative atmosphere that began during agenda setting is maintained right up to the end of the session.

SUMMARY

In this chapter we discussed the importance of session structure and its eight components. Setting an agenda helps to make optimal use of time, keeps the session focused, sets the tone for a working atmosphere, and counters session drift.

Repeated mood checks identify changes in mood that might detract from the session or lead to relapse. Bridging sessions provides continuity across sessions and keeps therapy focused on treatment goals. While addressing the list of agenda items, therapists help patients prioritize, stay focused on important material, make the most efficient use of time, and contribute actively to the discussion. Guided discovery helps patients draw their own conclusions and make their own decisions. Capsule summaries help to reinforce learning. Homework must be understood by patients, and appropriate steps for minimizing barriers should be taken. Therapists should continually provide and elicit feedback to clear up possible misunderstanding or misinterpretation of what is happening in each session.

CHAPTER 6

GUIDED DISCOVERY, MOTIVATIONAL INTERVIEWING, AND FUNCTIONAL ANALYSIS

Guided discovery is an essential CBT process involving careful, deliberate, systematic exploration of patients' thoughts, feelings, and behaviors, with emphasis on how these all impact each other. When effectively practiced, guided discovery helps patients recognize cognitive, behavioral, and affective patterns, and learn that some patterns are more adaptive than others. As patients learn to recognize patterns, they are better equipped to manage them. We consider guided discovery essential: Cognitive-behavioral therapists, throughout each session, aim to *guide* their patients to *discover* adaptive strategies for effectively coping with life challenges. As an exploratory process, guided discovery aims to answer such questions as:

- What are your thoughts about ... [past, present, or future concerns]?
- What are your beliefs about ... [past, present, or future concerns]?
- How do you feel about ... [past, present, or future concerns]?
- How do you behave when confronted with ... [past, present, or future concerns]?
- What thoughts or beliefs typically precede your ... [particular feelings or behaviors]?
- What are the likely consequences of ... [past, present, or future behaviors]?
- How closely do your ... [past, present, or future behaviors] ... align with your values?
- In the future, what behaviors might you choose in response to ... [past, present, or future challenges]?

94

It is a mistake to assume that answers to these questions come easily to patients. If such answers came easy, many more people would likely solve their own problems. Many patients have never before been asked questions like these, and therefore the questions themselves have the potential to facilitate learning. It is important to remember that there are two primary aims of guided discovery: (1) to help the *therapist* understand the *patient's* personal world, and (2) to help the *patient* understand the *patient's* own personal world.

Standardized techniques, like those described in the next chapter, tend to be highly *structured* and *focused*. Structure involves distinct steps, while focus involves continuous attention and responsiveness to therapeutic content—in order to avoid meandering, or drift from topic to topic. Guided discovery is necessarily focused (avoiding drift), but it is not necessarily highly structured, since each guided discovery question and response is influenced by the often-unpredictable patient content that precedes it.

GUIDED DISCOVERY AND MOTIVATIONAL INTERVIEWING

Clinicians are often surprised to learn about the similarity between guided discovery and motivational interviewing (MI; Miller & Rollnick, 2013). Both are sophisticated approaches aimed at helping patients reflect on their own thoughts, beliefs, feelings, and behaviors, in order to intentionally evaluate them. Both guided discovery and MI are based on the assumption that people will act in their own best interests when they are helped to acknowledge, understand, and realize their own best interests.

Some specific similarities between guided discovery and MI include:

- Asking patients how they have made certain decisions, and then helping them consider additional or alternative decisions.
- Appealing to patients' best interests in considering changes, rather than focusing on what is right or wrong by normative standards.
- Utilizing and validating patients' own words as leverage in making a related therapeutic point. This increases the chances that patients will be more agreeable with therapists' comments and decreases the chances that patients will view therapists' comments as being contrary, judgmental, or adversarial.
- Summarizing patients' comments in a positive (though strategic) manner, with the purpose of enabling them to hear their own words. This sometimes leads to reconsideration of what they have said and may open the door to changing the way they think, feel, or act.

- Making seemingly casual comments that are actually important therapeutic messages. This enables patients to hear a therapeutic message that might ordinarily run counter to their beliefs, without necessarily viewing it as a challenge. The result is that patients may consider or adopt the therapeutic message while still saving face.
- Not expecting that patients will accept therapists' messages during the present session, but rather being content to *plant the seed* for further consideration later.

The following dialogue illustrates a therapist engaging her patient, Jennifer, in guided discovery. This interaction between Jennifer and her therapist was chosen to highlight the similarities between guided discovery and MI:

JENNIFER: I'm not one of those people who drinks to get drunk. I might have just one or two glasses of wine to relax over the course of an evening and on weekends. I always take my time when I'm drinking. Believe me, I have seen other people drink much more than me, and they're not alcoholics . . . so I know I'm okay. Never mind what my husband thinks or says.

THERAPIST: So, Jennifer, you see yourself as a leisurely drinker, and not someone who drinks to get drunk. You feel secure in knowing that other people are much heavier drinkers, so you feel pretty safe by comparison.

JENNIFER: Right. I'm not one of those falling down or passing out drunks. I just want to enjoy some wine . . . or a few cocktails.

THERAPIST: Based on what you just said, would it be fair to say that the actual problem is that your husband is worried about you?

JENNIFER: You could say that . . . plus the expense. [*Laughs nervously.*]

THERAPIST: The expense? So, you're concerned about how much you spend on alcohol.

JENNIFER: It's more than I want to admit, but I've gotten pretty sick from drinking the cheap stuff.

THERAPIST: So, you're worried about two costs of drinking: one to your marriage and the other to your bank account.

JENNIFER: [*Brief silence.*] I just want to relax. That's all. I have a stressful job. Is it a crime to relax?

THERAPIST: Of course not. You've mentioned several times that you have a stressful job. Does it seem like some people are saying your drinking is a *crime*? Does it come across as that sort of accusation?

JENNIFER: It sure feels that way. I'm tired of defending myself. [*Begins to tear up.*]

THERAPIST: I hope I don't sound accusatory. That's not my intention. I was just trying to figure out if you had ideas about why your husband might be worried about you, even though you're not worried about yourself.

JENNIFER: I worry sometimes too. I'm not oblivious. I'm not in total denial. I just want people to trust my judgment and not jump to all the wrong conclusions about me. [*Long pause.*] I have no intention of turning out like my mother. [*Starts to cry.*]

THERAPIST: [*Gently pushes a tissue box on the table toward the patient.*] Do you mind telling me what you're thinking right now?

JENNIFER: I don't want to turn into my mother, I don't want my husband to lose respect for me, and I don't want you to think I'm not interested in considering some changes. But I need a way to relax. What am I supposed to do? I take precautions when I drink: I never drink and drive, I never mix drugs and alcohol, and I never drink in the morning.

THERAPIST: You've just said so many important things. Is it okay if I summarize? [*Jennifer nods "yes."*]. On the one hand, you are doing everything you can to keep your drinking in what you believe is a safe zone. On the other hand, the drinking has become very important to you as your main way of relaxing, to the point where it's hard for you to imagine stress relief without it. You feel frustrated with your husband's worrying about your drinking, but you also realize that marital strain is one of the costs of your drinking, along with the financial expense. And then there's that thing you just said about not being oblivious and not being in denial, because you're very aware of your family history. I hadn't mentioned your mother, but you suddenly mentioned her because you connected the dots yourself—without any help from me. Jennifer, can you tell me more about your concerns?

JENNIFER: This is hard. [*Pauses.*] I *know* I have to be careful with my drinking. I *know* that, okay? I'm not stupid.

In this exchange, Jennifer's therapist never said her thoughts were wrong or dysfunctional, never instructed her on what she *ought* to do or think, and never got into a power struggle. Instead, her therapist used guided discovery, like MI, to highlight certain cognitive, behavioral, and affective patterns. Note that by the end of the dialogue, Jennifer began to shift from minimizing her drinking to saying she worried about it too, and knew she had to be careful. This disclosure allowed the therapist to use Jennifer's own words in future sessions to discuss her alcohol consumption. By paying attention to Jennifer's comments about her mother's drinking, her therapist further develops her case conceptualization by establishing historical and developmental antecedents to Jennifer's pattern of alcohol consumption. This brief dialogue illustrates the interplay between guided discovery, case conceptualization, and collaboration. In the sections that follow we introduce and describe functional analysis and demonstrate how it is facilitated by guided discovery

GUIDED DISCOVERY FOR LINKING THOUGHTS, FEELINGS, AND BEHAVIORS

Patients new to CBT typically underestimate the role thoughts and beliefs play in the development and maintenance of their addictive behaviors. Many view addictive behaviors as directly caused by external events (e.g., situations and circumstances) or internal feelings (e.g., craving, restlessness, anxiety, depression, physical pain) and therefore view addictive behaviors as being out of their control. They may not realize the impact of their own thoughts or beliefs, and they may not believe that changing these will help them change problematic behaviors.

Therapists help patients by focusing on the role of thoughts and beliefs in the development and maintenance of addictive behaviors. They assist patients by continually eliciting addiction-related thoughts and beliefs, and helping patients link these to addictive behaviors. The real work in CBT begins as patients are taught, through guided discovery, to understand the link between their addictive behaviors and such thoughts and beliefs as:

"I can't stand the way I feel."
"I just want some relief."
"I need to feel better."
"I'll have just a couple of drinks."
"I just want to get buzzed."
"Life is boring without getting high."
"I've always been a drinker and smoker. It's just who I am."
"I always have a good time when I'm partying with friends."
"Gambling is the only thing I do that's fun."

Thoughts and beliefs like these all have the potential to trigger addictive behaviors. Therapists who elicit such thoughts and link them to addictive behaviors provide a valuable resource to their patients. This process requires considerable patience. It is tempting for therapists to prematurely challenge thoughts and beliefs that activate addictive behaviors. However, doing so runs the risk of alienating patients and putting them on the defensive. Alternatively, therapists who patiently elicit thoughts and beliefs without prejudging them assist patients in learning about the link between thoughts, beliefs, and addictive behaviors. The following exchange between Jill and her therapist demonstrates this guided discovery process:

JILL: I messed up.

THERAPIST: What do you mean by "messed up"?

JILL: I smoked a cigarette this weekend.

THERAPIST: Tell me what happened.

JILL: I ate dinner with some friends at a restaurant and afterward I smoked a cigarette.

THERAPIST: Tell me more.

JILL: My friends lit up after we left the restaurant. We were just standing around in the parking lot, talking.

THERAPIST: What went through your mind when you saw them light up?

JILL: What do you mean?

THERAPIST: Try to remember what you were thinking.

JILL: I remember thinking, "Damn, I wish I could smoke just one."

THERAPIST: And then what happened?

JILL: My friends saw me just standing there, looking like a fool, and one of them offered me a cigarette. Of course, I took it.

THERAPIST: Jill, can you remember what you were thinking right before you took the cigarette?

JILL: Yeah, I was thinking lots of things. I was thinking I really wanted a smoke. I was thinking I couldn't say no to my friend. I remember . . . [*pauses for a moment*] . . . it was like one little voice in my head said, "Don't do it." But then another louder voice said, "Just this one."

THERAPIST: So, there were several thoughts that were directly linked to your smoking. One thought was, "Damn, I wish I could smoke just one." Another thought was, "I looked like a fool just standing there." Another was, "Of course I'm going to take a cigarette if a friend offers it to me. I can't say no to a friend." Other thoughts were, "I really want a smoke. Just this one."

JILL: Yeah, that about sums it up.

THERAPIST: Jill, it's important to recognize that your thoughts and beliefs are directly linked to your decision to smoke. We just identified half a dozen thoughts that all occurred within seconds of each other. I'd like to help you get into the habit of recognizing the thoughts that are so often linked to your smoking.

JILL: How will that help?

THERAPIST: Eventually you will be able to catch these thoughts and challenge them. This will become one of your new skills as a nonsmoker.

JILL: Now that you explain it, I realize that I've been doing just that for months now to stay away from smoking. When I think it would be great to have a smoke, I remind myself how good I feel about quitting.

As Jill explained, she has been able to stop smoking by reminding herself that it feels good to be a nonsmoker. She *implicitly* understands that both smoking and quitting are linked to various thoughts. Hence, a major role of the cognitive-behavioral therapist is to make this link *explicit* through guided discovery, so patients can be more deliberate and intentional in their own efforts to control these thoughts and abstain from addictive behaviors.

Most people (including therapists and patients) do not appreciate the subtle differences between thoughts and beliefs. Therapists who teach patients to distinguish between their thoughts and beliefs play a helpful role in their patients' recovery. Doing so helps patients target each thought and belief for change. One way to differentiate between the two is to understand that thoughts are generally *sudden, spontaneous, and fleeting*—and they grow out of more *deeply held* beliefs. Based on these differences, we tend to think of thoughts as *automatic* and beliefs as *basic* or *underlying* processes.

For example, as a young child Jay developed the basic belief, "I am inherently shy and quiet." In middle school he discovered the disinhibiting effects of alcohol. Over several years of ongoing alcohol consumption, Jay naturally developed the new belief, "I am less shy and more sociable when I drink alcohol." At the same time, he developed the automatic thoughts, *"Drinking is fun!"* and *"More drinking is more fun!"* These automatic thoughts and many more like them tended to permeate Jay's heaviest drinking episodes. It is helpful, especially early in therapy, to teach patients like Jay that they will be more effective at controlling emotions and behaviors when they understand the direct links between their beliefs, automatic thoughts, and addictive behaviors. Jay appreciated learning that his drinking was precipitated by proximal thoughts like "Drinking is fun," but also by more deeply held beliefs like, "I don't want to be quiet or shy anymore."

Most experienced therapists have heard patients say, "Just changing my thoughts isn't going to make me stop using drugs" (or other addictive behaviors). These patients are correct. Patients who struggle with addictions typically need to learn numerous skills, and learning these skills takes time and practice. The ability to identify and label thoughts and beliefs provides the foundation for linking them to complex addictive behaviors. Eventually, identifying and labeling thoughts and beliefs makes it possible to change them, and the complex behaviors they prompt.

We find it helpful to begin therapy by assessing the degree to which patients are able to identify thoughts, beliefs, and feelings. Most patients do not clearly differentiate between these three processes. In fact, many people when asked how they feel about something will respond with a statement like, "I feel *that* . . ." In doing so, they express what they *think* or *believe*, rather than what they *feel*. A patient who says, "I *feel like* I'll always be addicted," is really saying, "I *believe* I'll always be addicted." A patient who says, "I *feel like* he is wrong," is really thinking, "I *think* he is wrong."

Categories of Thoughts and Beliefs

There are likely as many addiction-related thoughts and beliefs as there are human fingerprints. We find it helpful to place addiction-related thoughts and beliefs into various categories:

- Thoughts and beliefs about the *nature* of specific addictive substances and behaviors
- Thoughts and beliefs about the *benefits* of addictive substances or behaviors
- Thoughts and beliefs about urges and cravings
- Permission-giving thoughts and beliefs

Thoughts and Beliefs about the Nature of Specific Addictive Substances and Behaviors

Addictive substances and behaviors are complex and misunderstood by most people. For example, most people believe tobacco use is safer than other drug use, when in fact more deaths are caused by tobacco than any other drug. Many people believe alcohol helps them get a good night's sleep, when in fact alcohol interferes with good sleep. Most people with gambling disorder believe they will eventually recover their losses by continued gambling when in fact the more they gamble, the more money they are likely to lose. The following are examples of other common misconceptions about addictive substances and behaviors:

"I don't have a drinking problem as long as I only drink beer."
"Prescription drugs must be safe, since they're prescribed by physicians."
"Marijuana is harmless, or it wouldn't be legal in so many states."
"Spending money on gambling is no different than spending on any other form of entertainment."
"Online gaming can't possibly be a problem; they're just games."

When patients maintain thoughts and beliefs such as these, therapists can identify them, invite patients to examine them carefully, and eventually help them better understand how such beliefs may lead to lapses and relapses, despite patients' strong desires to change. It should be apparent that the eventual long-term goal of such interventions is to help individuals make healthy decisions by resolving their misconceptions about addictive substances and behaviors. In order to learn about patients' erroneous thoughts and beliefs about addictive chemicals and behaviors, a therapist might ask:

"What is your understanding of safe drinking limits?"
"How does cigarette smoking impact a person's physical health?"
"What does it mean to become tolerant to pain medication?"
"To what extent might marijuana be addictive?"
"How likely is it that a person will win back their gambling losses?"
"What are some potential risks associated with online gaming?"

It is important for therapists to learn as much as possible, through guided discovery, about patients' beliefs prior to challenging them. As previously mentioned, premature challenges are likely to put patients on the defensive. It should be apparent that the questions above are asked in a general, rather than personal, manner. This is done to minimize the likelihood that a patient will feel accused of doing something wrong by the personal nature of questioning. Fortunately, many patients respond to questions like these by reexamining their own beliefs. As a result, they may ask for factual information about addictive substances and behaviors. When this occurs, it is certainly acceptable to provide evidence-based resources that provide answers to their questions (e.g., *www.niaaa.nih.gov, www.drugabuse.gov, www.samhsa.gov*).

Thoughts and Beliefs about the Benefits of Addictive Substances or Behaviors

It is well understood that people engage in addictive behaviors for their reinforcing properties. But what does this mean? It means different things to different people, and therefore it is essential to conceptualize the benefits each patient associates with their own addictive behavior. For example, some people believe they can only stop feeling anxious by drinking alcohol. Some people believe they can only have fun at parties where everyone is getting high. Some people believe that the only way they can get motivated to do anything is by taking narcotic pain medication. Some people believe that their only reward in life is food, which leads them to binge eat. Some lonely people believe they can only find relief from loneliness by visiting a casino. In other words, for some people the benefits of addictive substances and behaviors are that they provide relief from suffering. For others, addictive substances and behaviors are needed for making a good or neutral mood even better.

Many patients use addictive substances and behaviors to self-medicate co-occurring conditions such as depression, anxiety, personality disorders, and other psychiatric problems. When this is the case, CBT is used as a *dual treatment* for patients with *dual diagnoses*. The aim of this dual treatment is to help patients with their addictive behaviors, but also with the mental health problems they seek to medicate with addictive behaviors. This work is best done in an integrated fashion, rather than separately (SAMHSA, 2009). The message sent to patients is that their depression, anxiety, personality, and other mental health problems are associated with problematic thoughts and beliefs, just as their addictive behaviors are.

For patients who use addictive substances to celebrate (i.e., make a good mood even better) or maintain emotional status quo, it is just as important to identify thoughts and beliefs regarding perceived benefits of continued addictive behaviors. Eventually, these thoughts and beliefs may be challenged by therapists, but early in therapy it is important to simply encourage patients to recognize thoughts and beliefs associated with addictive behaviors.

Thoughts and Beliefs about Urges and Cravings

Urges and craving are psychological and physiological sensations that create an uncomfortable, unsettling sense of "hunger" or "drive" to alter one's state through the use of psychoactive chemicals or nonchemical addictive behaviors. The following are examples of commonly encountered beliefs about urges and craving:

"Urges and cravings are intolerable."
"The only way to stop craving is to give in to it. Otherwise, it just gets worse."
"Unsatisfied urges or craving will drive me crazy."
"I can't think about or do anything else when I'm having urges or craving."

As one may infer from the above, many patients have a linear view of urges and craving, anticipating that these feelings will take an ever-ascending course that is unalterable and unmitigated unless satisfied by engaging in addictive behavior. In some respect this faulty notion is analogous to an avoidant patients' view of anxiety, in which it is believed that anxiety will keep increasing until it makes the person crazy or kills them, and the only way to stop feeling anxious is to avoid the anxiety-provoking situation. In both cases—with addicted patients and avoidant individuals—there is a failure to understand that discomfort is time-limited and will eventually subside.

As we will see in a later section on challenging addiction-related thoughts and beliefs, therapists can help patients examine concrete evidence from prior experiences in which they had craving or urges that subsided on their own. For most patients, in most situations, urges and craving decrease over time when not accommodated. Many patients are incredulous when told they can *ride out the wave* of discomfort associated with urges and craving, but their own personal histories usually provide evidence that they have done so before and can do so again. When they combine this knowledge with other strategies and social support (e.g., mutual help groups, therapists, counselors, friends, loved ones), patients can eventually allow their urges and craving to peak and decline. Success in this endeavor is a victory both of self-realization and self-help. In the next chapter we describe the *delay and distract* technique, in which patients lengthen the time they are willing to endure urges and craving.

Permission-Giving Thoughts and Beliefs

Permission-giving thoughts are sometimes referred to as rationalizations, excuses, or justifications for engaging in addictive behaviors. Therapists are alerted to patients' permission-giving thoughts when patients imply that they had *good reasons* to engage in their addictive behaviors or *it's okay this time*. Examples of permission-giving thoughts include:

> "Just this one time."
> "Just a small amount."
> "This is a special occasion."
> "No one will know."
> "I'm not hurting anyone but myself."
> "My life can't get any worse."
> "I've been sober long enough."
> "It's not fair that everyone else gets to do it."

We have observed that permission-giving thoughts tend to be activated at key moments when patients feel ambivalent about giving in to a temptation, as they wrestle with the question, "*Should I?*"

During guided discovery, therapists listen for permission-giving thoughts, identify them as such, and invite patients to consider them carefully. In the interest of maintaining a strong therapeutic relationship, therapists should express concern that such thoughts put patients at risk, without sounding judgmental. Given that patients will often experience ambivalence when considering use, it is imperative that they learn to identify their permission-giving beliefs and understand their potential effects on decision making (Newman, 2008).

Patients need to develop well-rehearsed adaptive responses to counteract permission-giving thoughts. They should be encouraged to generate some adaptive responses with their therapists in session and then generate more adaptive responses as homework. As we will discuss in the next chapter, therapists can engage patients in role playing in order to practice adaptive responses to permission-giving thoughts. Examples of some adaptive responses include, "There's no such thing as *only* one drink; one drink generally leads to many drinks," "The best way to pass the test is to not test myself in the first place," and "I'm determined to keep my sobriety streak alive." Additionally, patients are taught to notice when they use words such as *only, just,* and *a little bit* in their self-statements, as these are clues that they might be engaging in permission-giving. Patients are instructed to repeat their comments *without* those words and listen for the qualitative difference. For example, "I *only* want one drink," becomes "I want a drink," and "I *just* want to use *a little bit,*" becomes "I want to use." This exercise drives home the stark reality of what patients are proposing to do when they engage in permission-giving.

FUNCTIONAL ANALYSIS

Perhaps the simplest and most important processes for identifying and linking thoughts, beliefs, and feelings is the *functional analysis* (also referred to as a *chain analysis*). *Functional analysis,* as the name implies, helps patients to analyze the chain of triggers, thoughts, feelings, and behaviors associated with the functioning of addictive behaviors (Budney & Higgins, 1998; Magidson, Young, & Lejuez, 2014). Liese and Esterline (2015) explain how functional analysis can be facilitated by employing concept maps (i.e., diagrams that represent causal relationships between triggers, thoughts, feelings, and behaviors). The simplest example of a functional analysis is presented in Figure 6.1. Many cognitive-behavioral therapists recognize this simple ABC model, where A represents *A*ntecedents, B represents *B*eliefs or thoughts, and C represents the emotional and behavioral *C*onsequences associated with thoughts and beliefs.

We often refer to antecedents as "triggers" or "activating events" because they activate thoughts and beliefs that in turn activate addictive behaviors. Triggers may be internal and experienced emotionally or physically, or they may be external

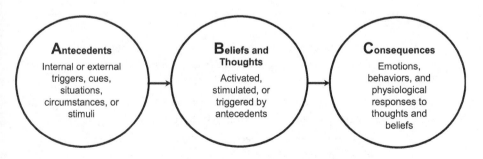

FIGURE 6.1.   The ABC model.

and encountered in the environment. Examples of internal triggers include emotions like sadness, loneliness, restlessness, boredom, anxiety, anger, and frustration. Internal triggers might also be experienced as pain, craving, tension, or pressure. Examples of external triggers might include others who are engaging in addictive behaviors, the availability of addictive substances or activities, or situations in which addictive behaviors took place in the past. It is important to remember that triggers may involve negative, neutral, or positive circumstances. They may trigger thoughts about celebrating happy circumstances or self-medicating unhappy circumstances. They may involve relationship conflicts or celebrations, failure or success at achieving desired goals.

While conducting a functional analysis, Ben's therapist learned that he "found it impossible to walk past a panhandler on the corner of a busy street without getting triggered." When asked to elaborate, Ben explained, "Just seeing someone begging for money on a street corner makes me think of times when I begged for money on street corners to support my heroin addiction." He further explained that this visual trigger would lead to thoughts about using heroin, which would lead to strong urges to use, which would lead to permissive thoughts, which would lead to panhandling, which would lead to purchasing heroin, which would inevitably lead to heroin use. In just a few sentences, Ben provided his therapist with a relatively detailed functional analysis.

We recommend a two-step process in formulating a thorough functional analysis. In step one, therapists help their patients identify the most salient processes (e.g., triggers, circumstances, thoughts, beliefs, feelings, and behaviors) associated with their addictive behaviors. These are organized into a list. In step two, therapists help patients draw a flowchart that reflects causal relationships between these processes. For example, Margaret comes to a therapy session and explains that she feels guilty and ashamed about a recent cocaine relapse. Margaret's therapist asks her to explain, via guided discovery, what happened. The following dialogue proceeds:

THERAPIST: Margaret, you seem terribly upset with yourself.

MARGARET: Well shouldn't I be? I've been clean for half a year, and then I go and screw it all up.

THERAPIST: Margaret, it's normal to feel disappointed about your lapse, but it isn't helpful to beat yourself up. Instead, let's figure out exactly what happened. Tell me the story.

MARGARET: I'm not quite sure how it happened. One minute I'm doing okay and the next minute I'm sucking that shit up my nose.

THERAPIST: Let's be deliberate here. What time of day was it? What were you doing before, during, and after you used? What were you feeling?

MARGARET: It was Saturday afternoon and I didn't have anything going on. I was just kind of hanging around the apartment, mostly watching TV. Is that what you mean by "What was I doing?"

THERAPIST: Exactly. Tell me more. And be sure to tell me how you felt along the way.

MARGARET: Well, I can tell you that I was sick of watching TV. I was probably bored and restless. Those feelings have always been big triggers for me.

THERAPIST: Go on.

MARGARET: The phone rang, and it was my friend Fran. I hadn't talked to Fran in around six months, since I stopped using. She's one of those people I needed to avoid if I was going to keep to my program. She was always ready to party, but she said she called because she missed me. She asked if I wanted to go to lunch. I hadn't eaten and it seemed innocent enough.

THERAPIST: And then what happened?

MARGARET: I hung up and got ready to meet her. That's when the old feelings started to come back.

THERAPIST: What old feelings?

MARGARET: I started to feel excited, like something great was going to happen.

THERAPIST: And by great, you mean . . .

MARGARET: Like I almost felt high again. Just thinking about meeting Fran gave me a rush. I started to imagine those feelings again.

THERAPIST: The rush of getting high?

MARGARET: Yeah, and my mind kept racing back and forth. First it was like, "No, I can't do this!" And then, almost like hearing another voice I thought, "Yes, I can . . . I can use with her just this one time." And then I thought, "You've been clean for six months. Call her back and tell her you can't make it." But I didn't.

THERAPIST: So the permissive thought won the battle? You decided you could see her and maybe use again?

MARGARET: Yup, that's exactly right.

THERAPIST: And then you had lunch with her?

MARGARET: No, of course not. I parked my car at the restaurant and started walking through the parking lot, when I heard Fran call to me from her parked car. She told me to hop in for just a second before lunch, and sure enough she had laid down a few lines for us. What was I going to do? I couldn't say no. Again I thought to myself, "Just this time."

THERAPIST: I've been listing all the circumstances, thoughts, and feelings you've described. Tell me if this is right: You were at home on a Saturday afternoon with nothing to do. You were feeling bored. Fran called and you knew you were at risk. You said to yourself, "Don't go with her." She has always been a trigger for you. You thought about that, but then changed your thoughts and told yourself that it would be a nice, pleasant lunch, and that's all. But then another thought popped up. You thought you might be able to use just a little. And as a result of that thought, you felt excited. And then you had a competing thought, "I shouldn't do this." You then got into your car and drove to the restaurant, thinking you might just get lunch . . . or something else. And in her car, faced with a few lines of coke, you had the thought, "Just this time" or something like that.

MARGARET: Exactly.

THERAPIST: Let's draw this out. [*Proceeds to do so.*]

The dialogue presented above enabled Margaret's therapist to sketch out her functional analysis (see Figure 6.2). As is often the case when patients actually visualize their thoughts, feelings, and behaviors organized as a functional analysis, Margaret responded with surprise and exclaimed: "That makes sense. It helps to draw it out like that. I guess I could have done something different at each of those points."

In conducting a functional analysis, it is important to point out that most circles represent *decision* or *choice points,* where patients can decide between more or less beneficial thoughts or behaviors. Of these choices, some are more and some are less likely to result in addictive behaviors. The primary aim of the functional analysis is to encourage conscious, deliberate decision making, in order to decrease the risk of lapses and relapses.

Regardless of the technique chosen by a therapist, it is vital that the underlying guided discovery process is collaborative. The process of change is difficult, and most people with addictions are at least ambivalent about changing. Hence, techniques should be presented in such a way that patients understand it is their choice to submit to various techniques. Most people have engaged in a process of *white knuckling* their way through urges and craving. This term is meant to reflect the forceful, often painful, process of avoiding addictive behaviors. Alternatively, we encourage patients to take an active role in reducing their urges and craving by challenging their addiction-related thoughts and beliefs. When this process is successful, we enable people to engage in more adaptive responding.

Adaptive responding is the term given to the process of establishing new, effective ways of thinking that serve to counteract addiction-related thoughts and

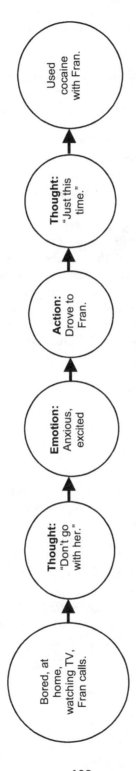

FIGURE 6.2. Functional analysis of Margaret's cocaine lapse.

beliefs. An example of this process was introduced at the end of the last section, where we described how therapists might identify *decision* or *choice points*. The term *adaptive* has been chosen deliberately, to emphasize that CBT aims to help patients recognize and choose thoughts and beliefs that make life better, instead of worse or more difficult. Patients who learn how to produce adaptive responses generally feel an improved sense of self-efficacy, satisfaction, and hope.

When patients experience emotions and physiological triggers associated with addictive behaviors (anger, anxiety, restlessness, loneliness, boredom, tension, urges, craving, pain, etc.), they are encouraged to ask themselves, "What's going through my mind right now that might be contributing to these feelings?" The goal is to teach patients, through guided discovery, the skills of identifying their *automatic thoughts* under specific circumstances, evaluating these thoughts, testing their validity, and modifying them so they are more adaptive. Recognizing their thinking patterns is certainly a prerequisite to addressing or changing their thinking patterns. With practice, patients can learn to recognize and challenge thoughts that otherwise would maintain or exacerbate their addictive behaviors. Patients are encouraged to use questions to help themselves reconsider the validity or utility of their thoughts. Such questions may include:

"How else can I look at this situation?"
"What concrete evidence supports or refutes my thoughts or beliefs?"
"What constructive action can I take to deal with this situation?"
"What advice would I give to a good friend in the same situation?"
"What is the worst-case scenario in this situation? What is the best-case scenario?"
"Considering all options, what is the most adaptive choice I can make?"
"What are the pros and cons of continuing to believe my current thoughts?"
"What are the pros and cons of changing my thoughts?"

Although the above questions can be used to test and modify problematic thinking, it is not necessary to ask all of these questions, for all thoughts, in all cases. These questions serve as prompts, and when patients become adept at using them, they improve their ability to reflect on their thoughts, feelings (including cravings), and actions, rather than acting reflexively. A few good, all-purpose adaptive responses are, "Be reflective, not reflexive," "Be responsive, not reactive," and "My first thought may not be my best thought."

SUMMARY

In this chapter we focused on guided discovery, the process that underlies most standardized cognitive and behavioral techniques. In early sessions, therapists use guided discovery to facilitate awareness and changes in thoughts, feelings, and behaviors. And then eventually, patients find themselves asking themselves questions about their own thoughts, feelings, and behaviors. In other words, they start doing their own self-guided guided discovery—until more adaptive responding becomes natural and automatic.

Cognitive and behavioral techniques are methods, procedures, and activities aimed at helping patients make desired cognitive, behavioral, and emotional changes. Hence, problematic thoughts, feelings, and behaviors are *what* need to be changed. Techniques are *how* change is facilitated. In the next chapter we present specific standardized cognitive-behavioral techniques that target addictive behaviors.

CHAPTER 7

STANDARDIZED CBT TECHNIQUES

A wide range of standardized CBT techniques are available for helping people with addictions. These techniques aim to accomplish specific targeted clinical goals. For example, delay and distract techniques help patients tolerate urges and craving, thereby reducing the likelihood of relapse. Activity monitor and scheduling helps patients effectively organize their time to accomplish important, healthy life goals. We have been applying these techniques to addictive behaviors since publishing *Cognitive Therapy of Substance Abuse,* and many cognitive-behavioral therapists have also found these techniques to be helpful in addressing other mental health problems (e.g., depression, anxiety, personality disorders). We present 12 standardized techniques here, acknowledging there are many more (perhaps hundreds) that could not be included due to space limitations. Techniques in this chapter include:

1. Stimulus management
2. Delay and distract
3. Advantages–disadvantages analysis
4. Hierarchy of values
5. Activity monitoring and scheduling
6. Behavioral activation
7. Automatic thought records
8. Acceptance and commitment
9. Relaxation training
10. Mindfulness and meditation training
11. Contingency management
12. Role playing

Before describing these 12 standardized techniques we want to reemphasize the importance of formulating an accurate case conceptualization prior to choosing any one technique over another. We explained earlier that addictive behaviors are often engaged to compensate for skills deficits (i.e., as compensatory strategies). In other words, addictive behaviors are often initiated when individuals lack skills for addressing persistent problems. Each of the targeted techniques described below aims to facilitate skill development and thus reduce the client's need for compensatory strategies.

STIMULUS MANAGEMENT

An important aim of CBT for addictions is the management of stimuli that activate urges, craving, and opportunities to engage in addictive behaviors. Many different terms have been used to identify such stimuli, for example: *triggers, cues, high-risk situations, proximal antecedents,* and so forth. We refer to these mostly as *triggers,* as patients readily relate to this term.

We have found it helpful to organize *stimulus management* into four steps. Step 1 involves asking patients to list and describe triggers that have been problematic over the course of their addictions. In Step 2 therapists and patients discuss past successful and unsuccessful strategies for managing these triggers. In Step 3, patients are asked to identify the triggers of greatest concern presently (i.e., those most likely to trigger relapse). And in Step 4, therapists and patients brainstorm how these triggers might best be managed, given patients' current challenges, skills, and circumstances. It is understood from the start that some stimuli are best avoided, and other (often unavoidable) triggers require other self-management strategies.

While it is impossible to avoid all triggers, patients can learn to *plan* their activities in such a way that they reduce the *likelihood* of being exposed to triggers. This requires motivation and a high degree of vigilance. Most people who struggle with addictions are surrounded by triggers, and their lives are typically intricately entangled with people, places, and things associated with addictive behaviors. Consider for example, that people with addictions typically have friends and family members with addictions. They typically frequent places where their addictions are perpetuated (e.g., bars, casinos, homes of people who use). Rather than making the naïve assumption that all triggers can be avoided, patients are encouraged to list triggers that can and cannot be avoided—and then avoid the most obvious triggers. For example, people with marijuana use disorder certainly can *and probably should* remove all bongs, pipes, and other drug paraphernalia from their homes. Individuals trying to quit drinking certainly can and probably should remove favorite alcoholic beverages from their homes and avoid visiting favorite drinking establishments—at least early in recovery. They cannot change the fact that bars, liquor stores, and liquor ads exist all around them, but they can distance themselves from these triggers.

The identification of triggers should be a standard feature of the case conceptualization process. As we discussed in Chapter 3, lapses and relapses are often preceded by proximal antecedents (i.e., triggers) that may be internal or external. During the case conceptualization it is important to characterize triggers as more or less avoidable (per above), so that avoidable triggers are avoided while unavoidable triggers are managed with coping skills. For example, both good and bad moods are unavoidable, and both have potential for triggering addictive behaviors. Patients at high risk for relapsing when in good *or* bad moods should certainly learn and practice relapse prevention skills in therapy that involve emotion regulation. Patients with alcohol use disorder who dine in restaurants featuring alcohol drinks should practice saying, "No, thank you," when asked before a meal if they would like to try one of these drinks. Similarly, patients with binge eating disorder should practice saying, "No, thank you," when eating dinner at friends' houses, where they are likely to be offered second and third food helpings. In addition to learning and practicing these behavioral refusal skills, it is essential for patients to learn and practice cognitive and behavioral skills for reducing the internal urges and craving that corresponds with these triggers. In the section that follows, describing delay and distract techniques, we discuss specific strategies for accomplishing this objective.

DELAY AND DISTRACT

Patients who suffer from addictions often act on impulse when they experience an urge or craving. They become accustomed to reacting reflexively when temptations emerge, and they succumb to these temptations without deliberate consideration. In doing so, they reinforce their belief that there is no other way to cope and there is no point in trying. To counter this belief, therapists explain that creating time and distance between an impulse and actual behavior is a skill vital to recovery and impulse control.

Delay and distract (D&D) techniques help with impulse control by teaching patients to refocus their attention away from, rather than toward, addictive behaviors. Patients are encouraged to pause and consciously choose constructive alternative actions, with the goal of improving their endurance in coping with urges and craving. By postponing addictive behaviors, they learn that urges eventually subside on their own. Those striving for abstinence can learn to tolerate a discrete period of elevated urges while they seek more meaningful activities (e.g., time with friends or loved ones, exercise, reading, healthy hobbies). This method should also be helpful to patients who have not yet fully committed to abstinence, but who are open to the idea of learning better self-control.

As an important component of D&D, patients are encouraged to generate a list of as many positive activities they can think of—both cognitive and behavioral. Therapists and patients work together to brainstorm this list, and patients are encouraged to add activities to the list as an ongoing homework assignment. Many patients choose to write this list in their smart phones for easy reference. A nonexhaustive sample of such D&D activities, taken from actual cases, is provided below, preceded by instructions:

Before I act on my urge, I will do some of the following things for as long as I can. If these distraction methods help me refrain from acting on my addiction, that's a victory. If I wind up doing the addictive behavior, it is still a partial victory if I build endurance and learn not to act on impulses. My D&D options include:

1. Returning phone calls, text messages, or e-mails
2. Reading something interesting, such as a newspaper, magazine, book, or my own writings from previous CBT homework assignments
3. Mentally picturing the faces of the people who are counting on me to make positive changes and cheering me on
4. Watching something entertaining on television or my computer
5. Doing sit-ups or push-ups
6. Eating healthy, nutritious foods or snacks
7. Brushing my teeth, taking a shower, or otherwise practicing good hygiene
8. Getting on the exercise bike
9. Going for a walk
10. Going grocery shopping
11. Reading a prayer book
12. Working on a crossword puzzle
13. Playing Solitaire
14. Playing a musical instrument
15. Writing in my journal, explaining how I feel and what I'm thinking
16. Listening to music while resting
17. Attending a mutual-help group meeting (e.g., 12-step or SMART Recovery)
18. Imagining the benefits of being abstinent from addictive behaviors
19. Practicing breathing control, yoga, or doing other mindfulness activities
20. Cleaning or otherwise maintaining my car or home

This list can continue to grow and is limited only by patients' energy and imagination; the more options the better. When patients succeed at practicing D&D on a regular basis, they achieve dual benefits: They experience satisfaction when they have fully resisted urges, and they experience a sense of accomplishment when they complete important tasks as distractions.

The D&D technique is used to avoid, abort, interrupt, or otherwise counteract the progression of addiction rituals. When an addiction is substance-based, a common strategy is to make acquisition and use of substances as inconvenient as possible, which facilitates the delay in acting on the subjective temptation (Newman, 2008). This may involve removing alcohol, drugs, and paraphernalia from surroundings, as well as structuring daily activities so time is spent with people who are not substance users. For example, patients who have had a habit of stopping at a local tavern on the way home from work might instead stop at a mutual-help group meeting or go to a gym. When patients break their addiction routines, they buy time to implement self-help skills and seek appropriate social support. Any delay caused by interrupting addiction rituals increases patients' chances of finding ways to cope and remain abstinent in situations that might otherwise lead to relapse.

Patients also have opportunities to use D&D techniques in live CBT sessions, as they experience urges or craving while discussing their addictive behaviors. Because in-session urges and craving are common, it is important for therapists to determine whether discussions regarding addictive behaviors are triggering urges or craving. When patients do experience urges or craving in session, therapists can frame this situation as an in vivo opportunity to practice coping skills, including D&D.

It is important to acknowledge the groundbreaking work of Alan Marlatt here. Marlatt and his colleagues (Marlatt & Gordon, 1985; Marlatt & Witkiewitz, 2005) originally coined the term *urge surfing*. They described urge surfing as the D&D process of *riding the waves of urges and craving*, rather than allowing them to prevail (Marlatt & Kristeller, 1999). They reported that this metaphor was conceived in a session with a surfer who described how he learned to keep his balance on the waves until they "gradually crested and subsided" (p. 78).

D&D strategies are appropriate for patients trying to control or abstain from addictive behaviors and any other undesired behaviors, especially those in the action stage of change. These patients want to make changes and are willing to consider ways to avoid addictive behaviors. As stated earlier, the decision to use this and other techniques should result from a well-formulated case conceptualization. Patients who already describe good impulse control may be less likely to benefit from D&D strategies. Hence, efforts to impose these strategies on such patients are likely to be viewed as unhelpful or even invalidating.

ADVANTAGES–DISADVANTAGES ANALYSIS

People with addictions usually magnify the advantages and minimize the disadvantages of their addictive behaviors. For example, people who regularly gamble believe that gambling is fun, exhilarating, and a potential source of financial gain.

Similarly, people who heavily use marijuana generally believe that marijuana is safe, natural, and a great way to mellow out. Like those with other addictions, such individuals tend to overlook or dismiss the disadvantages of engaging in addictive behaviors as they initiate these behaviors.

An *advantages–disadvantages analysis* (ADA) highlights the advantages and disadvantages of engaging versus not engaging in addictive behaviors. In order to conduct an ADA, therapists can use the four-cell, advantages–disadvantages analysis matrix (Figure 7.1; a blank version of this figure is available in Form 7.1, at the end of this chapter, for use with clients). In this matrix, one axis is represented by "advantages" and "disadvantages," and the other axis is represented by "using" and "not using" addictive behaviors. Therapists and patients work together to brainstorm items for each of the four cells, until each cell is well-represented.

A therapist might introduce the ADA by stating: "I would like to understand your thoughts about gambling. It seems that you have thoughts both for and against gambling. If it's okay with you, I'd like to use this form (Form 7.1), where we can enter your thoughts about the advantages and disadvantages of continuing to gamble and quitting. As you tell me your thoughts, I'll fill in each of these four cells."

It is often a good idea to begin by generating items in the "advantages of using" cell, as patients are typically more focused on the advantages of their addictive behavior, and this provides therapists with useful data regarding patients' reasons for engaging in addictive behaviors. Further, focusing on this cell demonstrates therapists' willingness to understand patients' reasons for using, which may ultimately gain patients' trust, especially as they discuss thoughts and beliefs pertinent to the other cells in the ADA. Patients' responses in this cell also often provide the therapist with examples of their problematic beliefs. For example, one patient offered that an advantage of using cocaine was that "It gives me self-confidence."

	Advantages	Disadvantages
Using Tobacco	1. "Smoking reduces my appetite and helps keep my weight down" 2. "Smoking relaxes me"	1. "Bothersome little cough" 2. "More serious medical problems" 3. "People stereotype me" 4. "My clothes and my car smell like smoke"
Not Using Tobacco	1. "I'll save money" 2. "I'll breathe better" 3. "Maybe I'll start exercising" 4. "More men might date me" 5. "It will make my mother happy"	1. "Withdrawal symptoms" 2. "Irritability, anger" 3. "Depression, despair" 4. "Likely to eat more, gain weight"

FIGURE 7.1.   Julie's advantages–disadvantages analysis matrix.

There is no need to calculate the ratio of advantages and disadvantages or generate conclusions about which side of the argument has "won." It is sufficient to spell out patients' thoughts and generate even more thoughts, to raise patients' awareness about the consequences of their addictive behaviors. As mentioned above, the ADA has the added benefit of highlighting the patient's reasoning processes, thus bringing to the fore some of their problematic beliefs that may be reevaluated (such as the patient writing that a disadvantage of not using drugs is that "I will just get more and more depressed if I can't get high").

Figure 7.1 illustrates an ADA in which Julie and her therapist have evaluated her tobacco use. We can see that one of Julie's associated concerns is weight gain; she views smoking as offering the advantage of controlling her weight. The entire ADA helps the therapist understand that Julie's difficulties go well beyond nicotine cravings. The four cells pave the way for a more complete set of therapy focal points (e.g., improved nutrition, increased exercise, emotion regulation). Additionally, Julie's *disadvantages of not smoking* show her therapist that she is fearful of the effects of withdrawal, including increased irritability, anger, depression, despair, and food consumption. Such information helps the therapist be even more empathetic and able to address important clinical problems.

A related way to use the ADA is to ask the patient to generate a list of advantages and disadvantages of their addictive behaviors *as those behaviors affect their loved ones.* This can be especially useful when patients profess not to care about themselves, and therefore they are not moved by the evidence that their addictive behaviors are harmful to them. By reflecting on the impact of their addictions on the lives of people close to them, patients may gain more compelling reasons for change. For example, it is often the case that patients cannot think of advantages for their addictive behaviors related to their loved ones in the way that they think of advantages for themselves. Likewise, focusing on the disadvantages of their addictive behaviors on the important people in their lives may encourage patients to pay attention to drawbacks that they previously had been minimizing or ignoring.

The ADA is most appropriate for patients interested in controlling or abstaining from addictive behaviors. Such individuals might be categorized as being in the contemplation or preparation stages of change. Therapists who try to introduce the ADA to patients who do not perceive themselves to have addiction problems run the risk of being perceived as pushy or out of touch with the patients' needs.

As illustrated in Julie's case, an additional benefit of the ADA is that it sometimes uncovers problems that may have been previously unknown to the therapist (or even the patient). This is especially apparent when cessation of an addictive behavior precipitates a coexisting mental health problem. In the example above, as Julie discusses the disadvantages of not smoking, it becomes apparent that she smokes to avoid symptoms of major depression. Hence, the ADA may effectively serve as both a therapeutic technique and a means of collecting case conceptualization data. When working with patients who do not perceive themselves as having addictions, it is important to explain that the ADA is often used to *understand* behaviors and does not necessarily imply that patients have addictions.

HIERARCHY OF VALUES

Values are deeply held core beliefs (e.g., principles, standards, morals, ethics) that ideally guide desired behaviors. When asked about their values, most people list relationships with family, friends, and community as highly valued, as well as virtues such as dependability, honesty, commitment, consistency, wisdom, kindness, and compassion. Because human beings are fallible and imperfect by nature, most do not live up to all their values or standards. And when individuals develop addictions, their excessive focus on addictive behaviors makes it even more difficult to live up to their values. This causes a wide gap that creates the potential for people with addictions to lose sight of their most deeply held values. This problem may be understood as a result of overfocusing on acquiring, engaging in, and recovering from addictions, and it may be experienced as living a life that is out of balance.

Hierarchy of values (HoV) is among the techniques offered in the SMART Recovery mutual-help program (SMART Recovery, 2021). In the HoV technique, individuals are asked to list the values that they consider most important. After listing as many as they can imagine, they are instructed to reduce this list to their top-five values. For those who might find this exercise difficult, several examples are provided (e.g., close relationships, physical health, financial well-being, personal integrity). Upon completion of this list, therapists review the results with patients. In most cases, there is no mention of addictive behaviors. Patients are helped to see that their addictive behaviors likely conflict with, or even detract from, their most closely held values. Hence, a central aim of the HoV is to help people with addictions rediscover the principles and standards they value most deeply and then help them consider behaviors more in accordance with their values.

The HoV may be helpful to patients who are contemplating or preparing to change addictive behaviors. But the HoV might also be used with an individual in the precontemplation stage of change. For example, we have worked with individuals mandated to treatment for addictions, who at least find this to be an interesting activity. When offered without judgment, this technique has the potential to move patients from precontemplation to contemplation. Therapists conducting the HoV should be aware that any obvious efforts to induce change through the HoV are likely to stifle honest responding. Put simply, patients who feel pressured to change in accordance with their values may shut down and be less honest with therapists. Or worse, they may completely disengage from therapy.

ACTIVITY MONITORING AND SCHEDULING

Addictions have a major impact on how people spend their time. When in the throes of addictive behaviors, patients tend to spend disproportionate amounts of time obtaining, using, and recovering from their addictive behaviors. They also tend to give up or reduce important social, occupational, or recreational activities due to addictive behaviors. Additionally, patients may find that their sleep-wake cycles are significantly disturbed, which further impedes their ability to lead effective lives. *Activity monitoring and scheduling* is useful for discovering and addressing deficits in self-care, delineating patterns of addictive behavior, and identifying existing and potential new opportunities for healthy activities.

When introducing activity monitoring and scheduling, therapists usually state: "It will help us determine how you spend your time on a day-to-day basis," explaining that addictive behaviors grow and expand, ultimately taking up more and more valuable time that might be better spent doing things that make life more rewarding. By collecting data on patients' activities, therapists and patients can assess the impact of addictive behaviors, while also identifying strengths and resources in the patients' life that may be reinforced. One of the easiest ways to monitor and schedule activities is to use a blank grid (see Form 7.2 at the end of the chapter) called the *daily activity schedule* (DAS; Clark & Beck, 2010; Beck et al., 1979; see Figure 7.2 for a partially completed DAS). The grid comprises the seven days of the week divided into 5-hour blocks, on which patients are instructed to record their activities during this time. Further, they are asked to rate each activity on a scale from 0 (none) to 10 (complete), according to how much mastery or accomplishment they derived from this use of their time (designated by the letter *M*), as well as how much pleasure or enjoyment they felt (designated by the letter *P*). Mastery and pleasure, when recorded in this way, provide an indication of patients' levels of reward or satisfaction across various activities. Patients are also asked to indicate how long they sleep, and in which time slots they engage in addictive behaviors. (Please note that the size of cells in the DAS should be adjusted by patients to reflect their activity levels during any given hour.) Figure 7.2 shows a daily activity schedule for Julie.

When patients are hesitant to document addictive behaviors for fear that others will discover them, therapists might encourage the use of encoded words, so that others are not able to ascertain their meaning. Therapists also explain that gaps in the DAS will be explored in session, as these may represent areas where patients have lost track of time—itself a warning sign of addictive behavior—or simply felt too ashamed to write anything. No blocked item should ever say *nothing*, or be left blank, as one is always doing *something*.

In addition to the potential benefits listed above, the DAS is used for at least three specific purposes. First, it serves as a journal of patients' present activities and offers a baseline understanding of how patients use their time. Second, the DAS serves as a prospective guide for planning upcoming activities, such as those that are less conducive to or incompatible with addictive behaviors. Third, the DAS is used to evaluate the extent to which patients have successfully followed proposed schedules. Often, failure to follow through with planned activities results from engagement in addictive behaviors or associated impaired functioning. When this is the case it is important for therapists to remain hopeful, helping patients to understand that useful information has been obtained, and that goals can still be achieved in spite of setbacks. Such occurrences serve as a reminder about plans and experiences forfeited as a result of addictive behaviors. On the other hand, when patients begin to succeed in planning and completing productive, addiction-free activities that give them satisfaction and build self-efficacy, they begin to view themselves as less helpless and hopeless, more in control of themselves and their lives, and less dependent on the addictive behaviors or substances.

Activity monitoring and scheduling is appropriate for patients who have expressed a desire and are making efforts to maintain control or abstain from addictive behaviors. Such individuals might be categorized as being in the preparation or action stages of change. However, activity monitoring and scheduling also have potential for helping individuals address other mental health problems (e.g., anxiety, depression, chronic procrastination, and more). The process of activity monitoring and scheduling will be discussed further below as we discuss behavioral activation.

BEHAVIORAL ACTIVATION

Behavioral activation (Dimidjian et al., 2006; Lejuez, Hopko, Acierno, Daughters, & Pagoto, 2011; Lejuez, Hopko, & Hopko, 2001) is an evidence-based approach to treating depression that has also been shown to be effective in helping people with addictions. Behavioral activation is best understood as an approach to improving the quality of an individual's life by increasing positive behaviors consistent with their values. Behavioral activation follows naturally from activity monitoring and scheduling, in that initiated behaviors follow directly from the process of activity monitoring and scheduling and completion of the HoV, so that chosen behaviors are consistent with an individual's most deeply held values.

Lejeuz and colleagues (2011), provided a helpful and convenient summary of their approach to brief behavioral activation for depression (BATD). They listed various key program elements, including (1) daily monitoring, (2) identification of important life areas (e.g., relationships, education, career, recreation, spirituality, daily responsibilities), (3) review of values, and (4) activity planning. They suggested that the process of behavioral activation may be enhanced by seeking

	Monday	Tuesday	Wednesday	Thursday	Friday	Saturday	Sunday
Early morning 5:00 A.M.–9:00 A.M.	Woke up 6 A.M., showered, ate breakfast, walked dog (M=0; P=5) Watched TV news, dressed, drove to work (M=2; P=2)	Woke up late (7:15 A.M.), got dressed, was too late for breakfast, quickly walked the dog, drove to work (M=0; P=0)	Woke up on time and got to do all the normal things like shower, eat breakfast, watch TV—and no smoking for over a week! (M=10; P=10)				
Midmorning–early afternoon 9:00 A.M. – 1:00 P.M.	At work, completed overdue project (M=6; P=2)	At work, attended staff meeting, discussed new projects, began working on new project, noon lunch alone (M=0; P=2)					
Late afternoon 1:00–5:00 P.M.	Sat at my work desk, surfed the Web, checked social media (M=0; P=4) Texted friends (M=2; P=8)	Back at my desk, starting to enjoy this new project, continued to work on it until end of day, drove home (M=5; P=6)					

122

Evening 5:00 P.M.–9:00 P.M.	Drove to 6 P.M. therapist appointment, stuck in traffic (M=0; P=0) Came home, watched TV for two hours (M=0; P=6)	5:30—made dinner and ate while watching TV, read for a while, got ready for bed early—didn't want to oversleep again (M=4; P=6)			
Late night 9:00 P.M.–1:00 A.M.	Got ready for bed, watched some more TV, went to bed at 11:00 P.M. (M=0; P=4)	Went to bed at 10:00 A.M., slept until 6 A.M.			
Predawn 1:00 A.M.–5:00 A.M.	Sleeping (M=0; P=8)	Sleeping (M=0; P=8)			

FIGURE 7.2. Julie's daily activity schedule.

help from supportive others who might be willing to help or even hold patients accountable for their behaviors. We have found their work in depression to be closely aligned with our work in addictive behaviors, so it is certainly worth mentioning here. We also think it helpful to present a case example that illustrates how behavioral activation might be employed.

Martha entered therapy 3 months ago after struggling with depression for years. In her early sessions it became apparent that Martha's depression was exacerbated by her daily marijuana use. She was receptive to reducing her use, and eventually chose to abstain from marijuana completely. During their time together, Martha's therapist had her complete 2 weeks of daily activity monitoring. They also spent an entire session focusing on Martha's HoV. The following is a discussion between Martha and her therapist, as they review Martha's plans moving forward:

THERAPIST: Martha, let's review your understanding of behavioral activation and your plans for the program we've been discussing.

MARTHA: Okay. It was shocking to do that daily monitoring thing you had me do. It made me realize how much my life was consumed by smoking weed. I'd get high in the morning before work, take a few hits over lunch, come straight home after work, and smoke a joint while watching hours of television. I'd go to bed, wake up, and do it over and over again, every day. My whole life revolved around weed, sleep, television, and work.

THERAPIST: You and I also completed the hierarchy of values together and you seemed surprised at how far you had strayed from the values you hold most near and dear.

MARTHA: Yeah, I stopped talking to my family, I was too depressed to go out with friends, I went to work but stopped enjoying my job, and I totally stopped exercising. My life had become a vicious cycle of smoking weed, withdrawing from everything and everyone, getting depressed, smoking more weed, avoiding life, smoking more weed, and on and on. It's no wonder I was depressed.

THERAPIST: So, what's the plan moving forward?

MARTHA: I understand that I can't expect things to get better just because I've stopped smoking weed. I need to get back into life and start living again. And I also can't expect that these activities will make everything better right away.

THERAPIST: Exactly. So, you have offered to start slowly and gradually increase the activities that give your life meaning.

MARTHA: Yes, I have committed to scheduling at least two activities a day for starters. Instead of getting high before work in the morning I'll take at least a 20-minute walk. And after work I'll reach out to some friends . . .

nonsmokers of course! And if I don't have plans with friends, I'll read or look into taking a class—or something other than watching TV all night.

THERAPIST: That sounds great, Martha.

From this example it should be understood that behavioral activation is a gradual, cumulative process. It actually consists of several other processes (at the very least), that include the identification of values, activity monitoring, and activity scheduling. It should be immediately apparent that behavioral activation is among the many CBT techniques that simultaneously address multiple problems (e.g., depression and substance use disorder).

AUTOMATIC THOUGHT RECORDS

Automatic thought records (ATRs) are foundational for helping patients understand relationships among their automatic thoughts, beliefs, emotions, and behaviors. Figure 7.3 (a blank version of which is available in Form 7.3 at the end of the chapter) illustrates a completed ATR, including: (1) date, time, and location; (2) situations; (3) automatic thoughts or related beliefs; (4) emotions; (5) alternative beliefs or responses; and (6) outcomes.

This ATR illustrates the case of Billy, who persistently retained the permission-giving thought that he could succeed at limiting drug use to "only once a week, on Saturday nights." He insisted he could do so without negative consequences, and he appeared frustrated and even irritated by any notion to the contrary. He repeatedly expressed the belief that he deserves to "have fun at least once a week." However, after several weeks of failing to use only on Saturday nights, he was willing to reconsider. It is important to note that the ATR includes a rating of the degree to which patients believe what they think, as well as a rating of the intensity of their emotions, on a scale of 0 to 100. Billy's alternative responses (and related outcome) indicate that he continually struggles with giving up his drug use while also facing the uncomfortable physical consequences caused by his drug use.

Billy's therapist responds by giving him positive feedback for completing the ATR, discussing how Billy's alternative responses might impact future decisions, empathetically acknowledging that Billy may need to find new ways to have fun, and perhaps by beginning a process of problem solving. Well-construed alternative responses on the ATR serve to reinforce positive, healthy processes and identify areas of potential change. Successfully completed ATRs, such as the one in Figure 7.3, are just the beginning of a process of helping patients to make significant cognitive and behavioral changes. Many repetitions are required (as homework) over a period of time before patients become expert in spotting, evaluating, and changing their thinking as it relates to their addictive behaviors.

Date, time, location	Situations	Automatic thoughts or related beliefs (0–100% confidence)	Emotions (0–100 intensity)	Alternative beliefs or responses (0–100% confidence)	Outcomes
Wednesday June 3, 1:15 P.M., therapist's office	Discussing use of drugs only on Saturday nights, to enjoy the weekend and recover in time for work	"I know I can use only once a week." (100%) "I deserve to have fun at least once a week." (100%)	Frustration with therapist (50) Irritated that I can't party like everyone else (75)	"This therapist doesn't really know me." (90%) "I know what's best for me." (85%)	Make plans with friends to get high on Saturday night
Saturday, June 5, 11:00 A.M., home in bed with a nasty hangover	Didn't wait until Saturday night Partied too much last night Bad hangover Feel really sick	"I promised my friends that I'd party with them tonight." (100%) "I'll be okay by then." (75%)	Mad at myself for going out Friday and not waiting (80) Pissed off that I have this problem (90)	"Maybe I'll give it another chance." (85%) "I'll party less tonight." (85%) "I'll get home early." (50%)	Keep plans to go out on Saturday night Stop worrying about last night Go out and party again
Wednesday, June 10, 1:10 P.M., therapist's office	Feeling depressed, defeated, shame Admitting to therapist that I went out and got wasted on both Friday and Saturday nights	"I'm a total loser." (75%) "I really f**ked up." (100%) "I'm never going get right." (85%)	Disappointed and depressed (70) Angry at myself (85) Discouraged (90)	"At least I'm here." (100%) "Life could be worse." (60%) "I'm sick and tired of being sick and tired." (100%)	Relieved to be getting help Putting things in perspective Resigned to make bigger changes in my life

FIGURE 7.3. Billy's automatic thought record.

ATRs were introduced decades ago, to help patients understand and address problematic thoughts, feelings, and behaviors associated with depression (Beck et al., 1979) and anxiety (Beck et al., 1985). Hence, ATRs are appropriate for all therapy patients, regardless of readiness to change addictive behaviors. ATRs enable patients to identify and ultimately optimize the thoughts, feelings, and behaviors that are important to them. When patients are actively involved in changing addictive behaviors, ATRs enable them to manage emotions and behaviors that trigger addiction-related thoughts and beliefs. When patients are not willing, able, or interested in changing addictive behaviors, ATRs may can be helpful in emotion regulation and behavioral self-regulation. Like the process of activity monitoring, ATRs may be used both to facilitate change and to conceptualize patients' problems and processes.

ACCEPTANCE AND COMMITMENT

In the early 1940s, Alcoholics Anonymous (AA) adopted the ubiquitous serenity prayer:

> *Grant me the serenity to accept the things I cannot change,*
> *The courage to change the things I can,*
> *And the wisdom to know the difference.*

This prayer, originally written by Reinhold Niebuhr and then embraced as a cornerstone of AA (Shapiro, 2014), provides an excellent foundation for the CBT model of addiction treatment and recovery, with its grounding in both cognitive and behavioral processes. It states what perhaps should be obvious: It is important to *cognitively* distinguish between what can and cannot be changed, and *behaviorally* make personal changes, in order to maintain mental health and vitality.

We find it helpful to focus on acceptance and commitment as cognitive and behavioral processes. In fact, we have focused on these processes since the earliest formulation of cognitive therapy for addictions (Beck et al., 1993). Even earlier, when formulating cognitive therapy for depression, Dr. Beck and his colleagues (1979) focused on thoughts and behaviors that *can* be changed and encouraged acceptance of those that likely cannot (or even should not) be changed.

At least one CBT approach has focused principally on the concepts of acceptance and commitment and even identified its approach accordingly: *acceptance and commitment therapy* (ACT; Hayes et al., 2012). Like most other members of the CBT family, ACT has been effectively applied to a variety of mental health problems, including addictive behaviors. According to the ACT model, at least four processes contribute to mental health problems, including (1) *cognitive fusion*, (2) *experiential avoidance*, (3) *poorly defined values*, and (4) *lack of commitment to behaviors that support well-defined values.* As the title indicates, the primary aims of ACT are to help patients flexibly accept what they cannot change and commit to changing what they can, in accordance with their deeply held values. When applied to people with addictions, an example of cognitive fusion is the idea that, "I am trapped in my addiction and cannot escape from it." Experiential avoidance involves a pattern of evading rather than facing challenges, for example by continued engagement in addictive behaviors. As discussed earlier, many people with serious addictions have lost sight of and, therefore, have compromised their values.

It is appropriate to focus on acceptance and commitment when patients have difficulty changing problematic thoughts, beliefs, feelings, situations, relationships, circumstances, and so forth (in other words, when they are overly *attached* to—or fused with—these processes). This attachment may be to the addictive behavior itself, but it can also be attachment to beliefs that activate the triggers themselves. For example, many cigarette smokers are attached to the idea, "I must smoke" when they have an urge. In addition, they may be attached to an idea like, "I must be perfect at all times," which will inevitably cause them substantial tension, which may lead to thoughts like, "I need a cigarette to relax," which may trigger smoking.

For example, Rich comes to therapy saying he wishes to quit smoking. He explains that he tends to smoke when he is angry, which is often. After a lengthy discussion it is apparent that Rich's anger is a result of his tendency to have numerous rules for others, and his judgment that they should change their behaviors to suit him. He describes anger toward his coworkers, slow drivers, his neighbors, and others. The therapist realizes quickly that Rich has this tendency to judge others. The following dialogue between them illustrates how Rich's therapist addresses this tendency:

THERAPIST: Hello Rich, what would you like to work on in our session today?

RICH: I don't know. I'm really pissed. I would have been on time, but this damn coworker of mine, Russ, called in sick again and I had to pick up the slack.

THERAPIST: Rich, it sounds like you're angry at Russ.

RICH: Yeah, Russ is the biggest slacker in the world. And he only cares about himself.

THERAPIST: I'm wondering Rich, if there is any benefit to your feeling so angry.

RICH: How would you feel if, well like . . . your secretary wasn't doing her job?

THERAPIST: You mean if she was not coming to work or breaking rules? I guess I would need to make a choice about whether to keep her on the job.

RICH: Yeah, but wouldn't it make you angry?

THERAPIST: It would certainly make me angry if I couldn't accept that all people are fallible, imperfect, and they are likely to do things differently from me.

RICH: Sounds like you live in a perfect world.

THERAPIST: No Rich, I just try to think in ways that are least likely to make me upset.

In addition to accepting what cannot be changed, a major task necessary for recovery is the process of making commitments to achieve what is valued. In the example above, it was eventually determined that Rich had no close relationships and he was very lonely. His therapist helped him understand this about himself and then commit to learning to care for and get close to people, rather than judging them.

RELAXATION TRAINING

Addictive behavior is often associated with the experience of hyperarousal. This is seen in individuals with posttraumatic stress disorder who perpetually oversedate themselves with benzodiazepines, people with chronic anger who seek relief in alcohol or cigarettes, individuals who feel panic and smoke marijuana to reduce anxiety, and many others. As such, addictive behaviors have become a form of self-medication in response to hyperarousal.

Relaxation training is a useful technique that provides patients with a safe method of reducing the arousal and tension associated with urges and craving. Engaging in relaxation provides patients with a time lag after the initial craving experience, during which the craving might subside. Hence, this method can be one of those that patients use as part of their D&D strategy.

Relaxation training can take many different forms. The two most common are controlled breathing and progressive muscle relaxation. Training in these two processes is introduced by explaining the rationale and then teaching the practices of controlled breathing and progressive muscle relaxation. Prior to initiating relaxation training, therapists teach patients that people are most likely to make mistakes and cause themselves serious problems when they make important decisions and try to accomplish important tasks while hyperaroused. They explain that there are at least two effective strategies for countering tension: controlled breathing and progressive muscle relaxation. Patients are taught that breathing tends to become shallow and fast and muscles tend to tense up when people are upset or nervous. For example, upon being exposed to an opportunity to lapse or relapse, they are likely to start feeling tense. They may describe or experience this tension as "revved up" or "energized," and they will most likely associate it with urges to use, craving, lapses, and/or relapses. Therapists explain that these feelings are incompatible with relaxation, and so techniques that produce relaxation will relieve hyperarousal and may help to avoid relapse.

Controlled breathing is taught simply as paying attention to each breath and making the process of breathing deep, slow, and rhythmic. Progressive muscle relaxation is taught (as the name suggests) as focusing on specific body parts, one at a time, noticing whether they are tense or relaxed, and progressively tensing and relaxing each body part. Some therapists prefer to start by recommending that patients relax facial muscles, others start with the hands, and others still recommend starting with the muscles in the feet. The process begins with individual areas of the body in order to help patients identify tension systematically.

Relaxation training may be appropriate for all patients who struggle with hyperarousal symptoms, regardless of their interest in or motivation to change addictive behaviors. The process enables patients with a variety of mental health problems to reduce their arousal in a wide range of challenging situations. In other words, when patients are not willing, able, or interested in changing addictive behaviors, relaxation training can be helpful in emotion regulation and behavioral self-regulation. During the process of conceptualizing patients, it is important to consider that hyperarousal might be a problem for individuals across the spectrum of mental health problems. Patients with histories of trauma, anxiety diagnoses, anger problems, impulse control problems, relationship problems, and more may benefit from relaxation training.

It is important to note that relaxation training has the potential to make some patients more anxious or upset. The process requires that patients disengage from their desire for control, which requires a certain amount of trust. Some patients with histories of trauma, while learning to relax, are reminded of triggers that contributed to their trauma, which may result in a wide range of psychological and even physiological symptoms (e.g., depression, crying, anxiety, shaking, hyperventilation, and so forth). While these are not common occurrences, it is important for therapists to be aware of these risks and discuss them prior to introducing relaxation exercises. Simply stated, relaxation training may be contraindicated for some patients.

MINDFULNESS AND MEDITATION TRAINING

For the past 25 years, cognitive-behavioral therapists have increasingly been applying the skills of mindfulness and meditation to help people gain mastery over their cognitive processes. In fact, mindfulness-based approaches have been developed for depression (Segal, Williams, & Teasdale, 2013) and relapse prevention (Bowen et al., 2021; Witkiewitz et al., 2005). Mindfulness-based approaches involve a blending of CBT and meditative principles and practices that include such activities as controlled breathing, body scanning, stretching, yoga, and mindfulness. Meditation takes various forms and follows from various traditions, but the ultimate goal of meditation is to cultivate mindfulness. Meditation can be practiced in various ways (e.g., sitting, standing, walking) and in various settings (e.g., indoors, outdoors). A primary aim of mindfulness and meditation training is to encourage individuals to be aware of their *present* and *moment-to-moment* experiences in ways that are conscious and accepting. Earlier in this chapter we discussed the role of acceptance in CBT for addictions. Mindfulness and meditation are techniques aimed at helping people to observe sensations (e.g., tension, anxiety, sadness, urges, craving) and accept them with the understanding that all such states are impermanent (i.e., temporary).

It has been well established that mindfulness and meditation are important life skills. Cognitive-behavioral therapists who are interested in teaching these skills should seek specialized training in order to do so. However, therapists who wish to introduce patients to these approaches may recommend that patients conduct research to learn about potential resources (e.g., live or Internet-based meditation or yoga classes). In addition, therapists who teach patients progressive muscle relaxation and controlled breathing techniques can explain that these activities help prepare people for mindfulness and meditation.

CONTINGENCY MANAGEMENT

Earlier in this chapter we discussed the advantages–disadvantages analysis. In doing so we reflected on the fact that people engage in addictive behaviors to achieve certain desired outcomes. Some engage in addictive behaviors to pursue desired rewards, while others seek to avoid punishment. It has been well-established that *contingency management* (CM), which involves the process of rewarding positive changes, is effective in the treatment of substance use disorders (Higgins, Silverman, & Heil, 2007; Prendergast, Podus, Finney, Greenwell, & Roll, 2006).

While most CM programs are offered by addiction service providers (e.g., on an agency level), individuals can create their own CM strategies by rewarding themselves with resources otherwise spent on addictive substances and activities (contingent on their success at change). Examples of such rewards can include money saved as a result of smoking cessation, as well as the purchase of new clothing as a reward for weight loss following cessation of binge eating. It is well understood that making such changes should be intrinsically rewarding, but it is also understood that such intrinsic rewards may be less immediate or noticeable.

Formulating an accurate case conceptualization for effective CM is essential. The case conceptualization should include the determination of appropriate incentives for achieving chosen goals, but also the incentive magnitude (i.e., how much), frequency (i.e., how often), and timing (i.e., when and for how long the incentive should last). For example, should the reward for weight loss be new clothing? At what weight goal? How much clothing? And how often should new clothing be purchased? These choices are not easy to make. Again, they require a careful and accurate case conceptualization to be effective. But again, when CM is done well, it is likely to be helpful and effective.

ROLE PLAYING

Role playing is a potentially powerful technique that is certainly underutilized in therapy. Role playing is best described as an interaction between individuals wherein one or both act as a character other than themselves, in order to facilitate a learning process. For example, a therapist might act as an acquaintance who offers the patient a drink at a party so the patient might practice saying, "No thank you, I prefer not to drink tonight." Or a patient might act like an angry spouse, so the therapist can demonstrate effective conflict de-escalation strategies. Role playing can be used to teach a variety of skills, including active listening, assertiveness, empathy, emotion regulation, and others. When executed well, role playing enables patients to practice interpersonal skills without adverse consequences that might occur in actual situations.

For example, Nora expected that her attempts at stopping methamphetamine use would be challenged by some acquaintances with whom she previously used. When her therapist asked what sort of upcoming situations she imagined, Nora said she would be "manipulated and guilt-tripped" by a particular person who would look at Nora's abstinence as saying, "I'm superior to you now." The therapist, having a comfortable and well-established positive relationship with Nora, suggested that they role-play, as reflected in the following dialogue:

THERAPIST: So, you expect this person is going to try to convince you to use again by saying things to push your buttons. Maybe by saying things like, "You're going to meet us later for some fun, right? You're not going to let us down, right?" Nora, how would you respond to that?

NORA: I might say, "No, you can all go ahead and have a good time without me. I'll be fine."

THERAPIST: [*Continuing the role play.*] "You'll be *fine,* huh. You'll be *fine.* You'll be fine if you don't forget who your friends are! You're not thinking of bailing on us, are you?"

NORA: "Don't be reading into what I'm saying now. I'm on parole, I'm in treatment, and I need to watch myself. That's all. No disrespect to you."

THERAPIST: "Oh, I get it. Now you're too good for your old friends. I get it.

Fine, if that's the way you want to be. All high and mighty. Yeh, I understand real good."

NORA: "I'm not sure you understand. I feel uncomfortable when you give me a hard time for trying to take care of myself."

THERAPIST: "Listen, Nora, we can still hang out. We don't use all the time."

NORA: "Truthfully, I can't be around drugs *any* of the time. I hope you can understand that."

THERAPIST: [*Role play ends.*] Nora, how do you feel right now?

NORA: Annoyed!

THERAPIST: Uh-oh. Annoyed? Are you upset that we did that role play?

NORA: No, I mean I'm annoyed at that situation. That's what's probably going to happen, and I don't need that kind of aggravation.

THERAPIST: How do you think you handled the situation? I thought you were strong, assertive, and direct.

NORA: [*Smiles.*] Well, I'm glad you think so, but it's hard to keep that up. They'll just keep coming after me.

THERAPIST: We'll just keep on working on what you'll say to them, and to yourself, so that you can stay on track. In the meantime, I hope that we can focus your attention on the people in your life who share your goals and values, so you don't feel isolated.

In another role play, the therapist took the role of "devil's advocate" by acting like a caricature of the patient's previously held automatic thoughts and beliefs, whereas she was given the challenge of rebutting the therapist's problematic comments with her new adaptive responses. The role play was set up so both parties used the first-person "I" in order to indicate that this dialogue was between Nora and herself (i.e., her previously held dysfunctional thoughts and beliefs, and her newly generated adaptive responses):

THERAPIST: [*As devil's advocate.*] "I'm not even going try to stay clean, because it's a losing battle, so what's the point of trying?"

NORA: "I won't let myself think like that. That's being defeatist, and I'm done with that whole defeatist thing."

THERAPIST: [*Continuing as devil's advocate.*] "I have no control over my feelings, so who am I kidding? Things don't work out for me, and the only thing that's fun in my life is partying with friends. Staying clean means I'm going to be alone and relapse eventually."

NORA: "That's not true. I am learning how to do things that will help me feel better that don't involve getting high, and I'm already feeling better about myself because I've been clean for a while. And that's helping me get over my depression better than anything I've tried before."

Therapist: "I just know that the cravings will eventually get me, I'll have a big crash, and then all my hopes will go up in smoke."

Nora: "Trying to improve my life is the better way to go. I'm willing to take the risk that I will have some slips along the way. I accept that I'm not perfect. I don't accept that I'm trapped in a life of addiction. Even if I slip, I'll keep working the program."

Following this role play, the therapist helped Nora process the experience and highlight what she learned from it. Like many patients skilled enough to take part in this type of role play, Nora felt strengthened by enacting adaptive responses while under fire from negative cognitions that would typically demoralize her and reduce her resolve to remain abstinent. She felt prepared for the possibility that she might have these devil's advocate thoughts, and she wrote down a number of the constructive things she said in the role play, to make sure that she practiced them and remembered them for further use.

Like ATRs and activity monitoring and scheduling, role playing is appropriate for all therapy patients, regardless of readiness to change addictive behaviors. Role playing enables patients to imagine and practice important interactions with others. When patients are actively involved in changing addictive behaviors, role playing helps them to sharpen empathy skills and effectively respond to others in ways that minimize their being triggered by negative interactions. When they are not willing, able, or interested in changing addictive behaviors, role playing may be generally helpful in developing interpersonal skills and talking back to depressing or anxiety-provoking thoughts and beliefs.

Understanding the Impact of Standardized Techniques and Interplay between Them

It is vital for therapists to recognize that patients' positive changes may be accompanied by substantial discomfort that does not entirely abate just because patients change their thoughts and behaviors. Hopefully, positive changes increase patients' self-empathy, compassion, insight, self-respect, and hope that an honest, committed, concerted effort will eventually lead to a better life.

It is tempting to organize standardized techniques into distinct cognitive and behavioral categories. However, in reality, most techniques contain both cognitive and behavioral components. For example, identifying and challenging beliefs is most effective when patients make behavioral changes that reinforce new, more adaptive beliefs. And behavior change techniques are most effective as they change patients' views of their personal lives.

Although the techniques in this chapter are described as separate entities, in reality there is substantial overlap between them. For example, some components of relaxation training are essential to mindfulness and meditation training. Activity monitoring and scheduling are central to behavioral activation. Stimulus management is vital to delay and distract techniques. Advantages–disadvantages analyses often reveal general problematic thoughts and beliefs that are effectively addressed with automatic thought records. We have presented a nonexhaustive array of CBT techniques. For a more complete collection of CBT techniques we recommend *Cognitive Therapy Techniques: A Practitioner's Guide* (Leahy, 2017).

FACILITATING LIFE-ENHANCING SKILLS

Professionals who serve people with addictions understand that recovery is about more than abstaining from addictive behaviors. It is also about effecting positive lifestyle changes that promote general well-being, which in turn reinforces confidence that life can continue without addictions. Thus, CBT for addictions inherently includes techniques for cultivating skills that will enhance patients' lives (e.g., communication, problem solving, time management, living a balanced life).

Communication Skills

Communicating effectively is its own reward. Conversely, communication problems can be quite punishing. Both expressive (speaking) and receptive (listening) communication skills can be addressed directly in CBT sessions. Role playing is an excellent way to practice these skills, and homework can be assigned to reinforce them. Patterns of communication between therapist and patient in session can be used as a microcosm for understanding how patients function outside of therapy. Therapists tend to be reluctant to comment on patients' in-session communication patterns, as many believe that it is not "polite," or it is too confrontive to do so. However, when framed effectively, such in-session feedback can be extremely valuable to patients who wish to develop and maintain close relationships.

Problem-Solving Skills

Problem-solving skills may be lacking in patients who have learned over time to follow their impulses, rather than reflect and make careful decisions about their actions. To make matters worse, many people with addictions increasingly avoid problem solving, as their problems grow and become more complicated. Furthermore, addictive behaviors themselves tend to cause their own unique problems, resulting in an accumulation of problems that may become unresolvable. Patients with histories of severe addictive behaviors (perhaps beginning in childhood or adolescence), tend to have little experience in recognizing and solving vital problems constructively. At the risk of oversimplifying a complex process, the following six steps comprise the basic sequence of problem-solving procedures (Nezu, Nezu, & Perri, 1989):

1. Defining the problem in clear, specific terms
2. Brainstorming a number of possible solutions
3. Examining the pros and cons of each brainstormed solution (for the patient, and for the patient's loved ones, now, and in the future)
4. Choosing a solution that is well supported by the "pros," even if it is difficult
5. Implementing the solution after appropriate planning, preparation, and practice (perhaps in session)
6. Evaluating the results and assessing for further solutions that are required

The acquisition of problem-solving skills requires a long, tedious process that demands patience and endurance. Therapists are advised to remain supportive and encouraging as patients persevere in learning these skills.

Living a Balanced Life

Most people understand that living a balanced life is important, though most would likely say that they are not doing so. It is common to hear people say things like, "There are never enough hours in the day" and "If only I had time for _____." The SMART Recovery program (www.smartrecovery.org), based on CBT principles and practices, has four focal points. These include:

1. Developing and maintaining motivation
2. Coping with urges and craving
3. Managing thoughts, feelings, and behaviors
4. Living a balanced life

It is not a coincidence that *living a balanced life* is last on this list. As mentioned earlier in this chapter, people with addictions spend disproportionate amounts of time obtaining, using, and recovering from their addictive behaviors. Hence, loss of balance in their lives seems to be inevitable. The first three points listed above are essential for the sake of recovering from addictive behaviors. The process begins with motivation to change. Change itself requires coping with urges and craving. And the skills necessary for maintenance of an addiction-free life include managing thoughts, feelings, and behaviors. As these basic skills are acquired, a person in recovery can begin to seek meaning and fulfilment by living a balanced life.

The degree to which a person is living a balanced life can be determined by the extent to which they are living according to their most deeply held values. Reflecting back on the hierarchy of values exercise, one of the goals is to list at least five values central in a person's life. After generating this list, patients are asked to compare whether their values and behaviors align. In a well-balanced life, values and behaviors are well aligned. For example, people who say they value marriage, parenting, physical health, financial security, and community relationships are living balanced lives if their actual behaviors are proportionate to these values. Truly effective time management exists when people fill their time with an array of activities that are meaningful to them. These are individuals who are true to their values but also know they must accept that they will never be able to fully accomplish all value-related goals.

HOMEWORK AS A MEANS
OF PRACTICING AND GENERALIZING SKILLS

Cognitive-behavioral therapists help patients to help themselves. The techniques presented in this chapter are meant to be practiced both in session and as homework aimed at providing skills for changing addictive behaviors and creating richer, fuller lives. In session, therapists teach patients to accurately and effectively define their problems, facilitate skill building to resolve these problems, and encourage patients to live healthy, adaptive lives. By the end of each session, therapists give homework to help patients practice and generalize skills learned in that session. When patients practice newly acquired therapy skills as homework, they maintain therapeutic gains long after the completion of formal sessions (Burns & Spangler, 2000; Kazantzis, Whittington, & Dattilio, 2010; Rees, McEvoy, & Nathan, 2005). Techniques practiced in session should lead to homework assignments between sessions (e.g., brainstorming solutions to problems; rationally responding to maladaptive thoughts and beliefs). Additional assignments may require that patients take what they learn in the "lab" (the therapist's office) and apply it in the "field" (the patient's everyday life), such as the delay and distract technique, or stimulus control to reduce exposure to high-risk situations.

Homework assignments should ideally stem from work done in sessions, so patients understand their relevance. It is essential for therapists to provide a rationale for assignments, along with any necessary instructions. All homework assignments should be chosen collaboratively, by therapists and patients together. Whenever possible, therapists and patients should *start homework assignments in the therapist's office* as a way to initiate momentum for completing tasks. For example, if automatic thought records are assigned as homework, therapists and patients should always begin working on them in session together.

SUMMARY

The process of choosing a CBT technique should be deliberate and intentional. It should be based on an accurate conceptualization of each individual patient, with careful consideration given to their existing problems, strengths, limitations, resources, beliefs, values, fears, hopes, and goals. Put simply, the choice of a specific technique should be patient-dependent, rather than therapist-dependent. Regardless of the chosen technique, the process should always be consistent with the principles of guided discovery and motivational interviewing (e.g., active/reflective listening, accurate empathy, supportive responding, and so forth). And finally, all techniques learned in session should be followed by homework between sessions, to ensure that they become skills that are generalizable to the real world.

Advantages–Disadvantages Analysis

Instructions: In the four-panel grid below, list the ***advantages*** and ***disadvantages*** of ***using*** (continuing) versus ***not using*** (discontinuing) your addictive behavior. For example, you might list an **advantage** of using marijuana as "relaxing" and a **disadvantage** as "becoming dependent." List as many responses as possible in each panel.

Behavior of concern (e.g., alcohol, marijuana, opioid, tobacco use): _____

	Advantages	**Disadvantages**
Using		
Not using		

FORM 7.2. Sample Daily Activity Schedule

Instructions: Using the grid below, list your activities during the time block when they occurred along with a rating (0–10) to indicate how much mastery (*M*) and pleasure (*P*) you experienced while engaged in the activity. Mastery relates to *skill development* and pleasure relates to *enjoyment* (see examples provided). You may list specific times when an activity begins or ends in a new time block or in the middle of a time block.

	Examples	Monday	Tuesday	Wednesday	Thursday	Friday	Saturday	Sunday
Early morning 5:00 A.M.–9:00 A.M.	Woke up 6 A.M., showered, ate breakfast, walked dog (M=0; P=5) Watched TV news, dressed, drove to work (M=2; P=2)							
Midmorning–early afternoon 9:00 A.M. – 1:00 P.M.	At work, completed overdue project until 3:00 P.M. (M=6; P=2)							

(continued)

From *Cognitive-Behavioral Therapy of Addictive Disorders* by Bruce S. Liese and Aaron T. Beck. Copyright © 2022 The Guilford Press. Permission to photocopy this form is granted to purchasers of this book for personal use or use with clients (see copyright page for details). Purchasers can download and print enlarged versions of this form (see the box at the end of the table of contents).

Sample Daily Activity Schedule *(page 2 of 3)*

Examples	Monday	Tuesday	Wednesday	Thursday	Friday	Saturday	Sunday
Late afternoon 1:00–5:00 P.M. 3:00 P.M.—Got coffee, sat at my work desk, surfed the Web, checked social media (M=0; P=4) Texted friends (M=2; P=8)							
Evening 5:00 P.M.–9:00 P.M. Drove to 6 P.M. therapist appointment, stuck in traffic (M=0; P=0) Came home, watched TV for two hours (M=0; P=6)							

(continued)

Sample Daily Activity Schedule (page 3 of 3)

Examples	Monday	Tuesday	Wednesday	Thursday	Friday	Saturday	Sunday
Late night 9:00 P.M.–1:00 A.M. _Got ready for bed, watched some more TV, went to bed at 11:00 P.M. (M=0; P=4)_							
Predawn 1:00 A.M.–5:00 A.M. _Slept until 6 A.M. (M=0; P=8)_							

FORM 7.3. Automatic Thought Record

Instructions: In the table below, enter the date, time, location, situation, thoughts or beliefs, emotions, alternative beliefs, and outcomes (as in the examples provided). Be sure to rate your confidence in your thought and intensity of your emotion on a 0–100 scale. This information should be recorded each time you feel a craving or experience an urge to engage in your addictive behavior, using an entire row for each entry.

Date, time, location	Situation	Automatic thoughts or related beliefs (0–100% confidence)	Emotions (0–100 intensity)	Alternative beliefs or responses (0–100% confidence)	Outcomes
Example: Saturday 7 P.M., home alone	Example: Decided **not** to attend a social event where alcohol is served because I'm trying to quit drinking	Example: "I hate being home on Saturday night." (75%) "It's not fair that everyone else gets to drink." (65%)	Example: Tense (90) Irritated (95) Craving a beer (65) Worried about risk of drinking (90)	Example: "Alcohol is ruining my life." (90%) "I'll feel so much better tomorrow if I don't drink." (85%)	Example: Decide to stay home and watch a movie Plan for next Saturday night with sober friends

(continued)

Automatic Thought Record *(page 2 of 2)*

Date, time, location	Situation	Automatic thoughts or related beliefs (0–100% confidence)	Emotions (0–100 intensity)	Alternative beliefs or responses (0–100% confidence)	Outcomes

CHAPTER 8

SETTING GOALS

In the words of celebrated baseball player Yogi Berra, "If you don't know where you're going . . . you might not get there." This statement is especially true when working with patients struggling with addictions. Goals help therapists and patients establish where they are going, or at least where they wish to go with therapy. As noted in Chapter 3, establishing goals is among the essential components of the case conceptualization. And since goal setting is associated with readiness to change, patients' goals may change from moment to moment. It is for this reason that therapists need to be keenly aware of patients' goals from moment to moment and session to session. For example, some patients enter therapy in crisis, proclaiming a full commitment to abstinence from alcohol, and then one week later announce that moderate drinking is their preferred goal. It is conceivable that this same patient might change goals (e.g., from moderate drinking to abstinence and back again) several times *during a single session.*

When collaboratively set, goals reflect a mutual understanding between patients and therapists. Generally, patients enter therapy wanting to feel better. Most want to alleviate feelings of worry, frustration, despair, loneliness, restlessness, or other negative emotional states. Many are willing to make substantial behavioral changes, but impose limits on what they are ready to change. After patients and therapists set goals together, they are in a position to consider cognitive and behavioral skills necessary for achieving these goals.

In the absence of clearly defined goals there is a risk of therapist and patient working at odds with each other. For example, consider a patient with severe cocaine use disorder who states, "I want to feel better." In the absence of an active, open, collaborative process, this patient might plan to feel better by using *less* cocaine, while at the same time the therapist assumes the patient's goal is *no* cocaine. Only by carefully questioning and actively listening to each other, can therapist and

145

patient establish mutual goals. Eventually the therapist might help the patient see that cocaine is interfering with feeling better, but first the therapist needs to understand and accept that the patient is not yet ready to stop using cocaine. In cases like this, harm-reduction goals may be more practical than abstinence goals.

HARM REDUCTION AS A THERAPY GOAL

Sandra was a patient who benefited from harm-reduction goals. She was severely depressed when she entered therapy. She attributed her depression to the fact that she "lost everything" because of her gambling disorder, including her home, savings, family, and friends. Sandra had succeeded at overcoming various chemical addictions in the past, but she was convinced she could never quit gambling. She described gambling binges where she would spend her entire paycheck playing slot machines and then borrow money from family members and friends to pay monthly bills. When her therapist asked Sandra whether she would even consider abstaining from gambling, the most she offered was, "I'll try to cut back."

Sandra's therapist was patient, and spent several sessions learning about Sandra's triggers, thoughts, feelings, and behaviors relating to gambling. Realizing that Sandra is unprepared to completely abstain, she introduces Sandra to harm-reduction goals. Their discussion is productive:

THERAPIST: Sandra, based on what I know about your current thoughts and beliefs about gambling, quitting is clearly not your goal right now . . .

SANDRA: [*Interrupts.*] You got that right.

THERAPIST: . . . despite the fact that your situation is dire, and you continue to lose money, family, and friends.

SANDRA: I don't always lose money. That's just the thing. There are times when I win hundreds of dollars in a day. If I could just keep that rally going.

THERAPIST: Yeah, that is the very belief that gets you back to the casino: that you will eventually have a run of good luck or hit the jackpot and be able to resolve all your problems.

SANDRA: Exactly.

THERAPIST: You've told me that you gamble whenever you have any extra money available, right?

SANDRA: Right. Sometimes I panic when I receive a shutoff warning from a utilities company, or a collection letter. That's when I might pay a bill. But more often than not, I think I have extra money when I still owe a lot of money.

THERAPIST: What are your paydays, when you get a paycheck?

SANDRA: On the first and fifteenth of every month.

THERAPIST: And when are you most likely to gamble?

SANDRA: On the first and fifteenth of every month.

THERAPIST: So, whenever you get a paycheck.

SANDRA: Yeah, that's right.

THERAPIST: Would you be willing to pay your essential bills each month prior to gambling?

SANDRA: That's what I try to do, but I just can't get myself there.

THERAPIST: Have you ever heard of automatic withdrawal?

SANDRA: Is that where your bank pays your bills?

THERAPIST: [*Chuckles.*] They pay your bills with *your* money.

SANDRA: So, you think I should do automatic withdrawals?

THERAPIST: That seems like a reasonable goal to me.

SANDRA: Yeah, I guess it makes sense: pay some bills and then do some gambling.

In this exchange, Sandra's therapist understood that the intermittent reinforcement of occasionally winning keeps Sandra returning to gamble, despite the losses she has suffered. Sandra clearly believes she will eventually win big and recoup her losses. Hence, Sandra's therapist suggested a harm-reduction goal that does not require abstinence from gambling: paying some bills before gambling. This strategy makes sense whenever therapists encounter patients who do not accept abstinence as a solution to their addictive behaviors. Simply stated, when patients are not interested in "Plan A" (abstinence), it's time to enthusiastically support "Plan B" (harm reduction). We discuss harm-reduction approaches in greater detail in Chapter 13.

SOME THERAPISTS NEED TO CHANGE THEIR GOAL-RELATED ATTITUDES

Most people with addictions experience unsuccessful change efforts, lapses, and relapses. Some therapists become frustrated, disappointed, or even irritated when patients do not succeed at achieving their addiction-related goals. These negative feelings toward patients are typically counterproductive, and of course they result from negative thoughts. The following is a list of such thoughts that might occur when therapists' goals for patients are unmet:

"It's terrible when patients set goals and fail to achieve them."
"They should know better."
"They should do what they say they're going to do."
"If it were me, I would have kept my commitment to change."
"They're wasting precious therapy time by failing to achieve their own goals."
"It's awful when patients don't do what's right for themselves."
"I can't stand when my patients relapse."
"Nothing good results from a relapse."
"I don't want to encourage my patients by saying it's okay to relapse."
"My patients' continued drug use reflects a lack of commitment to therapy."

Thoughts like these inevitably lead to negative therapist emotions (e.g., irritation, frustration, annoyance, disgust). And *patients can tell when therapists have negative feelings toward them.* Therefore, therapists are encouraged to monitor themselves for negative thoughts and feelings when patients set goals and fail to achieve them. When identified, such negative thoughts and feelings should be modified, to enable therapists to collaboratively refocus on learning, problem solving, and goal setting. The following is a list of alternative thoughts that counter the thoughts listed above. Thoughts such as these are likely to prepare therapists for collaborative goal setting:

"It's perfectly normal for people to set goals and fail to achieve them."
"Sometimes people disregard what's best for them."
"At times, all people find they don't do what they say they're going to do."
"If I were in their position, I might make the same choices and mistakes."
"Every minute spent in therapy has the potential to be valuable."
"Human beings don't always do what's in their best interest."
"I want to help my patients when I learn they have relapsed."
"Relapses provide opportunities for learning."
"Encouraging patients to learn from relapses is a good practice."
"My patients' continued drug use reflects the importance of their being in therapy."

Thoughts like these are likely to lead to more positive therapist feelings and more of a collaborative spirit. In addition, these thoughts are likely to reduce, or even eliminate, the risk of patients feeling stigmatized by therapists.

FORMULATING REALISTIC GOALS AND AVOIDING THERAPY DRIFT

Just as therapists may have unrealistic expectations of their patients, their patients' expectations regarding therapy may be unrealistic. Gina came to her first visit describing her goal as, "Getting custody of my children back after they were taken away by the court." Several months before, Gina left her three children home alone while she went to her dealer's apartment to buy methamphetamine. While there, Gina's 4-year-old daughter walked to a neighbor's apartment and asked if she could live with the neighbor. State authorities were called, and Gina's children were taken away. She was subsequently court-ordered to get treatment and completely abstain from drugs and alcohol before the court would even consider returning custody to her.

When Gina arrived at the therapist's office, she expected the therapist to intervene to get her children back. This of course was an unrealistic goal. The therapist was warm and caring but explained to Gina that getting custody of her children would necessarily be a future therapy goal. Gina's therapist suggested that more realistic short-term goals might be abstinence and improving her parenting skills. Upon hearing this Gina became visibly upset, but eventually admitted, "I knew you would tell me that. I hate that you can't get my children back for me."

Formulating goals helps to make explicit what patients can expect from therapy. By initially discussing desired outcomes of therapy and defining them in concrete terms, patients know where therapy is headed, and they begin to understand how their goals might be achieved. In other words, therapy is more focused when patients and their therapists know where they are going and how they are going to get there.

Focusing on *realistic* outcome goals also helps patients feel hopeful about potential changes. Well-defined goals can direct patients' attention to possibilities beyond abstinence. During Jack's first therapy session he admitted to current daily alcohol consumption, saying he could not imagine being abstinent forever, even though he recently completed an alcohol detox program and achieved abstinence for several weeks. It was difficult for him to stay focused on the possibility of long-term abstinence and imagine himself abstinent again. Eventually, therapy was successful because Jack's therapist facilitated gradual goals that were acceptable to Jack. For example, Jack readily agreed not to drink before driving. He also agreed to avoid heavy alcohol consumption, defined as more than four standard drinks per day, or more than 14 standard drinks per week. In fact, it was only after failing to achieve these goals that Jack agreed he needed to revise his goal to complete abstinence—and he quit drinking. After being "clean and sober" [his words] for several months, Jack realized his difficulty keeping a job had been a result of his heavy drinking. With the help of his therapist, Jack set a goal of finding and keeping a job, and within 6 months he achieved this goal, partly by improving interpersonal and self-regulation skills he had neglected while drinking.

Setting goals also helps prevent therapy drift. Many people with addictions enter therapy after accumulating serious troubles such as job, family, legal, and health problems. These problems contribute to patients' emotional distress, which often leads to the pursuit of therapy. With so many concerns, it is easy to shift haphazardly from one topic to another *within and between sessions.* Setting specific long-term and short-term goals for therapy and determining the order in which they need to be accomplished helps prevent such drift. Therapists and patients can focus during sessions on one or two of the most immediate and pressing goals, yet still fully realize that there are additional goals that will be addressed as therapy progresses.

Goals can function as points on a compass and thus make it more evident when therapy is on or off course. Bill was in therapy for opioid use disorder. He had begun taking oxycodone for back pain following an injury at work. As Bill's physician reduced his narcotic pain medication, Bill became increasingly anxious about living without opioids. The initial goal of therapy was to help Bill develop strategies for living without opioids; however, it became evident after several sessions (when Bill had become somewhat less anxious about his medication) that he was also experiencing severe marital discord. He disclosed that his wife had also been taking his medication, and this was causing a great deal of strife between them. While fully aware of the original goal of therapy, which was to help Bill address his addiction, Bill and his therapist were able to add the goal of improving his marriage. It would have been easy to drift aimlessly into working on Bill's marital problems at the expense of working on his addiction. Instead, Bill and his therapist put both topics on the agenda and acknowledged the strong link between them. They allotted time for both and explored the much more complex problems between Bill's addiction and his wife's problems. (To complicate matters, Bill's wife initially insisted that he not talk about her in therapy.)

Setting mutually established goals reinforces the therapeutic alliance and the spirit of collaboration between patient and therapist. It also gives the patient a sense of responsibility for therapy outcome. This is especially important for patients who see their lives in disarray and feel out of control and at the mercy of their dependency. Collaborative goal setting aids in fostering the patient's sense of self-efficacy and confidence to overcome addictions and other problems. For example, a patient stated the following after achieving several small therapy goals: "For the first time since trying to stop on my own I have a sense of control over my life. I'm clear about what I want from therapy. I want to learn how to cope with cravings, but I also want to learn better ways of living. I feel like my therapist and I are a team, and therapy is not just being done *to me*."

Reviewing goals is an essential part of each CBT session. As patients list agenda items, therapists can relate each item to established goals, or they can determine that a new agenda item calls for a new goal. For example, goals associated with preventing lapses or relapses will inevitably be included alongside other goals regarding abstinence from addictive behaviors. Previously undisclosed anger, on the other hand, might necessitate a new goal regarding anger management. So, setting and reviewing goals can occur during the agenda-setting stage of a session, but they may also occur while bridging from prior sessions, or even during the process of prioritizing or discussing agenda items.

Therapists need to be flexible in setting and reviewing goals. Patients often become discouraged as a result of slow progress, setbacks, lapses, and relapses. This may, in turn, result in all-or-none thinking about therapy (e.g., "Therapy is worthless"). Reviewing and reestablishing therapy goals potentially decreases patient hopelessness about change. For example, Richard and his therapist agreed to two major goals at the beginning of therapy: (1) abstain from cocaine and (2) get and keep a steady job. Over a period of 6 months, Richard succeeded at abstaining from cocaine. However, he was unable to find employment. He became frustrated and began making negative comments about therapy. For example, he told his therapist, "I'm stuck. This just isn't working for me anymore." Richard's therapist pointed out that Richard's attitude about life and his mood had improved substantially since starting therapy, and he had a sense of pride about abstaining from cocaine, despite his difficulty finding a job. Richard's therapist suggested that they revise their original goal of full employment and set shorter-term goals, like improving Richard's job-seeking strategies and interviewing skills. They also agreed that Richard needed to create a resume. After making gains in these areas, Richard revived his positive thoughts about therapy. He felt more hopeful and motivated to continue working with his therapist. And a month after sounding so discouraged, he found a fulfilling job that he continues to hold.

Richard's case provides an opportunity to emphasize an important point: namely, that goals for therapy do not exclusively entail abstinence from addictive behaviors. Criteria for success in therapy must be assessed across a number of important life domains, including personal relationships, physical health, emotion regulation, and vocational development, to name just a few. There are numerous problems that may be discussed in therapy. With goals for each problem, therapists and patients can make optimal use of therapy time and address problems in an organized and systematic manner.

STRATEGIES FOR SETTING GOALS

When patients enter therapy, they are often ambivalent about abstinence, so therapists should certainly not insist on abstinence as a requirement for being in CBT. Instead, therapists should explore the advantages and disadvantages of patients' addictive behaviors. This might be accomplished by simply asking, "What were the benefits of engaging in your [addictive behavior] and what were the drawbacks?" When patients describe advantages that seem vital to them (e.g., amelioration of physical pain), therapy goals might include the acquisition of skills that accomplish the same advantages (e.g., psychological pain management). Indeed, there are some behaviors that preclude abstinence. For example, therapists who treat overeating and binge eating understand all too well that patients cannot abstain from eating. When abstinence is not an option, it is especially important to determine advantages of the behavior (e.g., anxiety reduction) and establish goals (e.g., improved anxiety management) that enable patients to accomplish similar, albeit healthier, advantages without engaging in their addictive behaviors.

In setting goals, therapists might highlight the reciprocal relationship between abstinence and improved quality of life. For example, therapists might acknowledge that abstinence can contribute to improved relationships—and improved relationships can support abstinence. However, therapists might also emphasize that abstinence alone will not solve other problems; it merely makes success more likely. Martha entered CBT for the express purpose of ending her methamphetamine use. She said abstaining would enable her to save money, pay her bills, and motivate her to go to work each day. Upon hearing this, Martha's therapist responded, "So being drug-free is just one of your goals. Your other goals include saving money, paying your bills, and keeping your job. You seem to understand that abstinence alone will not guarantee success at these other goals. It will certainly help you to be in a better position to learn how to get what you want in these other areas of your life. Can we work on other skills as well? I want to help you succeed at all of your goals."

Goals are best stated in concrete, specific, measurable terms. At the beginning of therapy, many patients present abstract, nonspecific goals, such as, "I want to get my life in order," "I want to be my old self again," or "I want this anxiety to go away." Therapists help patients define therapy goals in more measurable behavioral terms, such as avoiding specific people, places, and things associated with drugs; choosing specific healthy, rewarding activities that do not involve addictive behaviors; or reestablishing important relationships. As an example, Joe enters CBT with severe opioid use disorder. He says he wants his world to "stop falling apart." In order to encourage more concrete goals, Joe's therapist asks what he would like to change in his life. Joe responds, "I'm separated from my wife right now and she doesn't allow me to see the kids. I would like to see my children more often. I guess I need to stop using drugs. I want to get involved with the church again. I used to be really into it. I would like to have a regular job. I'm tired of doing odd jobs. I want more excitement in my life. I'm bored most of the time except when using drugs." The therapist facilitates this process by periodically asking, "What else would you like to change in your life?" As a result, Joe's goals are transformed from vague statements to much more concrete, measurable events. The therapist summarized Joe's goals as follows:

- Completely stop using opioids
- See children at least once a week
- Find and hold down a full-time job
- Find a church and attend it weekly
- Find at least one substance-free activity that feels exciting

Upon collaboratively agreeing to concrete goals, therapists can help patients consider strategies for achieving them, as well as criteria on which to assess therapy outcome. In addition to abstinence from opioids, an example of goal attainment was Joe's finding a permanent job with a construction company. Another goal was reached when, after getting a job, his wife allowed him to see their children each weekend. These accomplishments solidified Joe's commitment to abstaining from opioids. Finally, Joe and his therapist worked on developing sources of nondrug positive reinforcement, such as hobbies and physical recreation.

Having these specific goals in the foreground helped keep Joe and his therapist from drifting in each therapy session. Also, having these goals written down at the beginning of therapy proved to be a powerful motivator for Joe, as he was able to compare his situation at the beginning of therapy with his functioning at later stages in therapy, and thereby to recognize his progress in therapy.

Two common goals of CBT for addictions are: (1) to reduce or abstain from addictive behaviors, and (2) to cultivate effective strategies for coping with life's challenges. As we've mentioned, when people with addictions enter therapy, they are typically ambivalent about stopping their addictive behaviors. Increasing their motivation to change tends to be an important focal point early in therapy. As noted earlier, an approach to assessing and potentially enhancing motivation is to focus on the advantages and disadvantages of engagement versus nonengagement in addictive behaviors. The following is a discussion between Roger and his therapist regarding the advantages and disadvantages of using cocaine:

THERAPIST: Roger, would you be willing to discuss the advantages and disadvantages of using cocaine?

ROGER: Sure.

THERAPIST: What are some advantages or benefits you get from using cocaine? What makes it appealing to you?

ROGER: It ain't good, but it makes me feel good.

THERAPIST: Okay. It makes you feel good.

ROGER: Yeah, that's an advantage of using. It makes me feel good for a while.

THERAPIST: What's another advantage?

ROGER: I don't know, my friends get high and that's what we do together.

THERAPIST: So, are you saying that it helps you fit in with friends?

ROGER: Yeah, it helps me fit in. It's what we do. If I had a choice, I'd probably have different friends.

THERAPIST: It sounds like you're almost saying that they're not real friends. Maybe this is actually a *disadvantage* to using: You end up with friends you don't really want.

ROGER: Yeah, it seems like they're my friends, but they're not. Spending time with them and using just go together.

THERAPIST: Okay. Now let's focus on certain advantages of *not* using. What would be a benefit to not using cocaine?

ROGER: You mean if I quit? I'd save money.

THERAPIST: You'd save money.

ROGER: I might think more clearly. It messes with my brain. I'd probably do better at work.

THERAPIST: Some people say that they can function better at work when they're on cocaine. What do you think about that?

ROGER: Oh, I don't function better. It makes me want to take days off. I don't feel like working.

THERAPIST: So, another advantage of not using is that you might feel like going to work?

ROGER: Yeah, I might want to go to work. Then I'd be able to pay my bills. Yeah, because when I was doing coke I was taking days off. You just don't have the motivation to do nothing but coke.

THERAPIST: Some advantages of not using are that you can save money, think more clearly, feel like going to work, and pay your bills.

ROGER: Yeah, so I might feel better about me.

THERAPIST: Are you saying that sometimes when you don't use coke you feel better about yourself? In other words, you feel proud of yourself when not using?

ROGER: Yeah, that's the feeling I'm talking about. And when I use, later I feel depressed and guilty that I gave in.

THERAPIST: Okay, let's put aside your addiction for a moment and think about some possible goals. If you agree, I'll write them down.

ROGER: That's fine.

THERAPIST: First, you would like to think clearly. Second, you would like to have more positive thoughts about yourself. Third, you would like to be responsible at your job—and keep your job. Fourth, you would like to save money. I've written these goals down along with your goal of being abstinent from cocaine. Did I get these right?

ROGER: Yeah, that's a tall order.

THERAPIST: I'm glad you mentioned that. It is a tall order, but one that seems doable. None of these things will happen overnight, so we'll just work toward them at each session, and decide together if your thoughts and behaviors are consistent with these particular goals.

ROGER: That makes sense. It's less overwhelming to think about it that way.

In this example, reviewing advantages and disadvantages enabled the therapist to uncover potential goals for therapy, including: having more money, being able to think more clearly, being able to pay bills, and so on. However, there is another set of goals that was highlighted as a result of discussing advantages of using; that is, the patient viewed the cocaine as making him feel good and having more friends. A set of goals can be derived from these statements, with the therapist saying, "If we could work on helping you to feel good, to be able to fit in and have friends, but *without* using cocaine, would these be important goals for us to try to achieve in therapy?" By using this strategy, the therapist focuses on the positive aspects of abstaining from cocaine and presents the goals in a positive manner, while still empathizing with the patient's desire for the drug. This is important since many patients view abstinence as a form of deprivation (i.e., something that everyone can have but them). The therapist collaboratively helps the patient to reframe the goal in a more positive way. Therefore, the patient can work on attaining the perceived positive aspects of using cocaine but without incurring the disadvantages involved in actually using the drug.

Addressing Patients' Ambivalence Regarding Goals

As noted, most patients are ambivalent about being in therapy and giving up established addictive behaviors. Ambivalence can be addressed as part of the early process of establishing therapeutic goals, as in the following discussion between Pam and her therapist:

THERAPIST: Pam, welcome back to your second session. In your first session you said you want to quit smoking marijuana. You said quitting was your primary goal. Would you like to continue discussing that with me?

PAM: That's why I'm here. If I screen positive for weed, I lose my job. It's the best job I've ever had and I can't afford to lose it. I'm already having financial problems, and I don't want to be a bad role model for my kid.

THERAPIST: Even though you say you want to quit smoking marijuana, I sense some hesitation.

PAM: When I'm honest with myself I really don't want to quit. Sometimes it seems like quitting is the most important thing in my life. But then I think it would be nice to pick up every now and then. You know what I mean? Control it, like when I first started smoking. I'm thinking, if I only smoke on Friday nights it should be out of my bloodstream by Monday, when I'm back at work.

THERAPIST: So, you're ambivalent: On one hand you want to quit, and on the other hand you don't. In other words, you have two competing sets of goals that shift back and forth.

PAM: Yeah, that's me: ambivalent.

THERAPIST: What would it be like to stop completely?

PAM: I'm not sure. My friends all smoke, and that's the first thing we do when we get off work on Fridays.

THERAPIST: It would be hard to quit when you're surrounded by friends who smoke. Are there any benefits to stopping besides job security, finances, and being a good role model?

PAM: I might be in a better place in my life.

THERAPIST: What do you mean by "better place"?

PAM: This has been a tough year. I actually tried to quit a few times, but each time I failed. I know if I stopped, I'd have more money. I'd worry less about my kid finding my weed. I certainly wouldn't have to worry about random pee tests at work.

THERAPIST: Those would certainly be benefits. Maybe this would be a good time to carefully consider your goals for seeing me in therapy. Does that sound okay?

PAM: Yeah, that's okay.

THERAPIST: You thought by quitting you'd be a better mom, right?

PAM: Yeah, when I'm high I think my kid doesn't know, but he's getting to the age that he does.

THERAPIST: I seem to recall that, in our first session, you also thought you'd be in better physical shape if you stopped smoking marijuana.

PAM: I definitely wouldn't get the munchies and eat so much junk food. And I'd probably get my ass off the couch.

THERAPIST: Would you be interested in setting some goals related to parenting and getting in better physical shape?

PAM: You know, those are great goals, but I think the best solution is to stop smoking weed. Your questions are helping me to see that. Let's get back to the idea that I need to quit using.

This exchange is similar to countless exchanges between ambivalent patients and their therapists. Pam was clearly not ready to set the goal of abstinence, but she was not ready to abandon that goal either. This exchange illustrates how patients may vacillate between goals from moment to moment. The lesson to be learned here is that therapists should be ready at any time for new goals or changes to past goals and accept that patients will set firm goals only when they are ready to do so.

Reframing Patients' Beliefs about Their Ability to Achieve Certain Goals

Patients become overwhelmed during goal setting when they magnify their weaknesses and minimize their personal strengths. Such thinking may lead to the belief that change is impossible and goals might as well be given up. In response, therapists can help patients reframe problems in a more hopeful way. Reframing involves (1) getting the patient to collect objective data about situations, (2) generating alternative ways of looking at situations, and (3) brainstorming new goals. The process of reframing goals in order to overcome patients' hopelessness is illustrated in the following exchange between Chris and his therapist:

THERAPIST: Let's discuss this problem of your girlfriend calling you when she's drunk, since you've put it at the top of today's agenda.

CHRIS: There's no use in talking about it. There's nothing I can do. She's my son's mother and she's always been like this.

THERAPIST: You believe there's nothing you can do about it. You think it's pretty hopeless.

CHRIS: It is.

THERAPIST: Can you tell me more about what happens?

CHRIS: She goes out and gets drunk. Then when she is smashed, she calls me crying and complaining. She wants me to come over and that's what I usually do. And the next part is predictable.

THERAPIST: What happens?

CHRIS: I obviously go and try to calm her down.

THERAPIST: And that's when you're at risk for relapsing.

CHRIS: Yeah.

THERAPIST: How do you end up feeling when that happens?

CHRIS: Like hell. First I get angry at her. Then I feel sorry for her. Then I think, "Here we go again. I'm tired of this." And before you know it, I'm drinking with her.

THERAPIST: You said earlier there is nothing else you can do about her calls. What would you *like* to see happen?

CHRIS: For her to stop calling me when she's drunk.

THERAPIST: Let's think about this for a few minutes. Her calling you is for the most part out of your control. I was wondering, are there things that are still within your control?

PATIENT: I don't have to talk with her. I don't have to go over.

THERAPIST: True. But, what would it mean if you didn't talk with her and you didn't go over?

PATIENT: She's the mother of my son. It would mean that I'm not helping her.

THERAPIST: So you believe, at this point, that by talking to her and going over you are helping her? Is that really true?

PATIENT: Not really. I keep doing the same thing over and over again. She still doesn't stop and she won't get any help.

THERAPIST: So, maybe an alternative way of looking at this is that it's best if you decide to steer clear of her when she's drinking. You believe you are helping her by talking to her and going over to her place. But, when you look back, you are really not helping her situation and you set yourself up for a relapse.

PATIENT: That's right.

THERAPIST: Would not talking to her and not going to her house be part of a solution to this?

PATIENT: Easier said than done.

THERAPIST: When she calls this belief within you gets activated, fired up, and you behave as if it were true. The belief is that you must go over and help or, somehow, you've failed.

PATIENT: That's right. It's only afterward that I see I'm not really helping and it's the same thing over and over again.

THERAPIST: I think this gives us something to work on to help you solve this problem. First thing we'll do is to help you deal with her calling and the second is to explore *other* things you might do to help her. Perhaps we can come up with some new goals that address this problem.

In this scenario, the patient's problems had less to do with his addictive behaviors and more to do with problem solving and conflict resolution. Even if this patient is currently engaging in addictive behaviors, it might be more important to focus on his relationship. In doing so, he learns to face problems rather than running from them, he addresses a major source of frustration, and the therapist demonstrates a willingness to focus on what's most important to the patient.

SUMMARY

This chapter has focused on the value of setting and reviewing goals for patients receiving CBT for addictions. Patient goals are most likely to be achieved when they are:

- Deliberately and intentionally determined and reviewed on a regular basis
- Collaboratively set, with both patients and therapists sharing in their formulation
- Meaningful to the patient
- Realistic (i.e., based on patients' skills and resources)
- Used as guides in each session so that discussions do not drift from topic to topic
- Operationalized in positive behavioral terms
- Flexible, since most patients with addictions tend to be ambivalent about change

When these guidelines are followed, CBT is most likely to be gratifying for both patients and therapists. Since experienced cognitive-behavioral therapists accept the inevitability of lapses and relapses in treating people with addictions, they patiently establish and reestablish goals with patients who struggle to achieve goals. And they assure patients that much can be learned from failure to achieve goals.

CHAPTER 9

PSYCHOEDUCATION

Psychoeducation involves the transmission of knowledge or skills, either directly or by modeling. Patients with addictions have overlearned cognitive and behavioral patterns that perpetuate their addictive behaviors. Hence, a primary goal of CBT is to help patients learn alternative cognitive and behavioral patterns that enable them to overcome addictive behaviors.

The number of potential psychoeducational topics to be addressed by therapists is vast. In the following sections we discuss some of the more salient topics (i.e., the *what*) and then we discuss the process (i.e., the *how*) of psychoeducation.

POTENTIAL PSYCHOEDUCATION TOPICS

We find it helpful to divide potential psychoeducation topics into four categories: (1) the science of addiction, (2) the science of recovery, (3) the CBT model of addiction, and (4) the CBT process.

The Science of Addiction

Over the course of CBT, it is common for patients to ask questions like:

"What exactly is an addiction?"
"How do I know if I'm addicted?"
"Why can't I drink like everyone else?"
"Is marijuana addictive?"
"Can I really get addicted to love? Or sex? Or chocolate?"

Some patients will ask specific questions like these and some will express general interest in the nature of addictions. Regardless, therapists have opportunities to address such issues whenever patients disclose misconceptions regarding addictions. For example, a patient might say, "Marijuana is natural, so I figure it can't be that bad for me," or "I can't have an alcohol problem as long as I only drink beer or wine." Statements such as these offer opportunities for sharing knowledge and facts based on the science of addiction.

The fifth edition of the *Diagnostic and Statistical Manual of Mental Disorders* (DSM-5; American Psychiatric Association, 2013) provides useful information for psychoeducation. For example, many patients find the DSM-5 diagnostic criteria to be helpful. Besides providing standards for classifying various addictions, the DSM-5 provides for an estimate of severity (i.e., 2–3 symptoms for mild SUDs; 4–5 symptoms for moderate SUDs; 6+ symptoms for severe SUDs). The following exchange reflects how a therapist provides psychoeducation to a patient (Jim), who is asking whether he is an "alcoholic." This is Jim's second CBT visit, and his therapist has just learned that Jim drinks "three or four beers every evening."

JIM: You seemed surprised when I said I drink beer every day.

THERAPIST: That's when I realized I needed to learn more about your drinking pattern.

JIM: Does drinking every day make me an alcoholic?

THERAPIST: Not necessarily. And actually, the term *alcoholic* is no longer used by health care professionals to describe alcohol problems.

JIM: What do you mean?

THERAPIST: A person with a drinking problem is now understood to have an *alcohol use disorder* that may be mild, moderate, or severe.

JIM: What's the difference between mild, moderate, and severe?

THERAPIST: Severity is determined by the number of symptoms a person has. For example, a person with two or three symptoms might have a mild alcohol use disorder. A person with a moderate alcohol use disorder might have four or five symptoms. A person with a severe alcohol use disorder might have six or more symptoms.

JIM: So how does that relate to me?

THERAPIST: To answer that question I need more information. You've told me that you drink three or four beers a day. I don't yet know how your drinking has affected you. For example, have you ever tried to cut down or quit drinking, but were unsuccessful?

JIM: Doesn't everyone cut down their drinking sometimes?

THERAPIST: A lot of people do try to cut back on their drinking at times. How about you?

JIM: Well actually I've tried to cut down but always go back to normal.

THERAPIST: What do you consider "normal"?

JIM: Like I said, three or four beers a day.

THERAPIST: Are there periods of time when you drink more than that?

JIM: Yeah, that's when I've tried to cut back.

THERAPIST: And did you try to cut back because drinking caused problems?

JIM: No more than you would expect. Everyone gets hangovers, right?

THERAPIST: Have you had some serious hangovers?

JIM: Yeah, but for the most part I've always been able to function the next day.

THERAPIST: "For the most part"?

JIM: Truth be told, I've missed more than a few days of work because I couldn't get out of bed.

THERAPIST: With a hangover?

JIM: Yeah.

THERAPIST: And what about your relationships? Has anyone else ever complained about your drinking?

JIM: My wife has gotten pissed off at me when I can't remember what I've done the night before.

THERAPIST: You've had blackouts?

JIM: No, I've never passed out.

THERAPIST: Actually, a blackout is when you can't remember things you've done while drinking.

JIM: Oh, I didn't know that was *a thing*. I guess I've had some blackouts.

THERAPIST: What was the longest period of time you've gone without drinking—recently?

JIM: I stopped when I wanted to lose weight, maybe for a couple of weeks. It actually helped me lose weight. And when I started drinking again, it hardly took anything to get a buzz. You might say I was a cheap date [*laughs*].

THERAPIST: Did you feel physically uncomfortable when you quit?

JIM: No, actually I felt more rested during the day. But I missed drinking and was happy to go back to it.

THERAPIST: What do you mean when you say that you "missed drinking"?

JIM: I just felt like I wanted a drink.

THERAPIST: Kind of like a craving?

JIM: Yeah.

THERAPIST: Jim, you asked whether you are an alcoholic. Again, the term I'd prefer to use is *alcohol use disorder*. It sounds like you have a moderate alcohol use disorder, based on at least five symptoms related to your drinking.

JIM: What are the five symptoms?

THERAPIST: You drink every day, which is more often than most people consume alcohol. At times you drink more than you think you should. It's hard for you to cut back on your drinking, and when you do, you crave alcohol. Your wife has been concerned about your drinking. You've had some blackouts and you've missed work because of hangovers.

JIM: You're telling me I have an alcohol disorder?

THERAPIST: You asked if I thought you are an alcoholic and I explained that you might have a moderate alcohol use disorder. Let's talk about what that means.

In this exchange Jim's therapist provided psychoeducation in several ways. First, he explained that the term *alcoholism* had been replaced by the term *alcohol use disorder* (AUD). Second, he explained that there is a standard procedure for diagnosing AUD and estimating its severity (via DSM-5). Third, he defined the term *blackout*. Fourth, he listed specific symptoms of AUD and confirmed that Jim had these symptoms. And finally, he shared his impression that Jim had moderate AUD. This was all aimed at transmitting knowledge, so Jim better understood how his drinking pattern was problematic.

Fortunately, many years and millions of dollars have been spent on the scientific study of addictions. Much of the literature, including many hundreds of available published articles, chapters, and public websites, is available to the public. The following websites are all considered reliable resources for both therapists and patients who seek answers to questions about the nature of addictions:

- National Institute on Drug Abuse (NIDA): *www.drugabuse.gov*
- National Institute on Alcohol Abuse and Alcoholism (NIAAA): *www.niaaa.nih.gov*
- Substance Abuse and Mental Health Services Administration (SAMHSA): *www.samhsa.gov*
- Office of the Surgeon General: *www.hhs.gov/surgeongeneral/reports-and-publications/addiction-and-substance-misuse/index.html*
- Addiction Technology Transfer Center (ATTC) Network: *www.attcnetwork.org*

These websites address many of the questions relating to the science of addiction. For example, each website defines *addiction* and delineates problematic use of psychoactive substances. The NIDA website directly addresses questions regarding marijuana, illicit drugs, tobacco use, vaping, and more, while the NIAAA website provides extensive information about the effects of alcohol consumption, and guidelines for safe drinking limits.

In addition to the many *facts* about addiction, there are many diverse *theories* regarding the development and maintenance of addictive behaviors, based on scientific studies of addiction. For example, one popular theory is the brain disease model (e.g., Volkow & Koob, 2015). Another theory has been referred to as cognitive social learning theory (e.g., Niaura, 2000). And yet another theory is the syndrome model of addiction (Shaffer, 2012), described in Chapters 1 and 2. It is common for patients to ask therapists whether they view addiction as a medical illness, or a disease. In response to this question, therapists should acknowledge that addictive behaviors have both neurochemical and psychosocial roots. Attention should be paid to the potential role of genetics in addictions. Specifically, therapists should ask whether patients have a family history of addiction, and then follow up by explaining that a family history of *any* addiction places individuals at greater risk for *all* addictions. A therapist could also emphasize that addictive behaviors are learned, and that CBT focuses on changing the thoughts, beliefs, and behavioral patterns that underlie addictions. Our approach to teaching the CBT model is discussed in detail later in this chapter.

The Science of Recovery

Just as there are numerous theories of addiction, there are numerous potential approaches to recovery. Over the course of CBT, it is common for patients to ask questions like:

"What is the best path to recovery?"
"Is there medicine I can take for my addiction?"
"Should I go to AA?"
"Can I still be a recreational user?"
"Do I need inpatient treatment?"

Answers to these questions are largely dependent on individual differences, including specific addictive behaviors, severity, co-occurring disorders, financial resources, support systems, social circumstances, personal values, and readiness to change. Some individuals are most likely to benefit from abstinence-based approaches to treatment. Others are most likely to benefit from replacing more dangerous drugs (e.g., heroin sold on the street) with less dangerous drugs (e.g., methadone or buprenorphine prescribed by a physician). And still others are most likely to benefit from reducing the quantity and frequency of their addictive behaviors. The following exchange between Jim and his therapist continues from their earlier conversation.

JIM: So now that I have an alcohol use disorder, what am I supposed to do about it?

THERAPIST: That depends on a lot of variables. For starters, are you interested in completely abstaining from alcohol?

JIM: Not if I don't have to. So far, you haven't convinced me that I have to.

THERAPIST: I don't intend to convince you to make any particular choices. I'm more interested in discussing options. I can explain that there are safe limits to alcohol consumption for people who want to make sure they are drinking safely.

JIM: What are these safe limits?

THERAPIST: For starters, it is important to know how to measure a standard drink. Since you drink beer, a standard drink of regular beer is 12 ounces. If you were a wine drinker, a standard drink of wine would be 5 ounces. And if you were drinking hard liquor, like vodka or whiskey, a standard drink of alcohol would be 1.5 ounces, plus any mixer. And generally speaking, men shouldn't drink more than seven drinks per week, and never more than five drinks in a 2-hour period of time.

JIM: How am I supposed to remember all that?

THERAPIST: Actually, I'll write down the URL of a helpful website known as the Alcohol Treatment Navigator. [*Writes* www.alcoholtreatment.niaaa. nih.gov *on a piece of paper and hands it to Jim.*]

JIM: Did you say that five drinks in two hours is okay?

THERAPIST: No, actually more than five drinks is considered binge drinking, and four drinks is considered heavy drinking. Again, safe drinking would be less than seven standard drinks per week for men, and fewer than four standard drinks on any occasion.

JIM: That doesn't sound too hard.

THERAPIST: It will be a big change from four to five beers every night.

JIM: Yeah, I guess so.

THERAPIST: The Treatment Navigator website should give you some additional ideas if you decide that safe drinking limits are too difficult to maintain.

JIM: Do they offer easier approaches?

THERAPIST: No. In fact, moving from heavy drinking to safe drinking, as you wish to do, can be more difficult than completely abstaining. So, it's good to have options.

Jim: I guess so.

Therapist: It may be helpful to consider a few possible homework assignments: (1) observe the safe drinking limits we just discussed, (2) spend at least 30 minutes reading the Treatment Navigator website, and (3) come in with at least two questions based on your reading. What do you think about this homework?

Jim: I can try those things. I'm still trying to make sense of this whole alcohol use disorder thing.

Therapist: A goal of the homework is to help you do just that.

Jim: I guess I'll give it a shot.

Another common question raised in therapy is whether a patient should consider a mutual-help group as part of the recovery process. Mutual-help groups include Alcoholics Anonymous (AA; *www.aa.org*), Narcotics Anonymous (NA; *www.na.org*), and other 12-step options, as well as Self-Management and Recovery Training (SMART Recovery; *www.smartrecovery.org*). Just as some patients benefit from abstinence-based approaches and others benefit from harm-reduction approaches, some patients benefit from AA, while others benefit from SMART Recovery. Both have their advantages and disadvantages, and some savvy consumers attend and receive benefits from both approaches. Mutual-help programs are available worldwide, and as a result, patients tend to have questions and (of course) misconceptions about them. The following exchange between Jim and his therapist occurs at a later visit.

Jim: Do you think I need to go to AA? I'm not even sure what AA is all about. I just know it's for alcoholics.

Therapist: Lots of people benefit from attending AA and other mutual-help groups.

Jim: What's a mutual-help group?

Therapist: It's where people get together to help each other with a problem, like an addictive behavior. Besides AA, another mutual-help group is SMART Recovery. Both can be helpful, but some people prefer one over the other.

Jim: I think you're telling me to check them out.

Therapist: I would recommend that you check both out. You can start by reading about them online, and then you can attend a few meetings of each.

JIM: Can you tell me anything about them?

THERAPIST: Sure. AA focuses on 12 steps, including admitting to powerlessness over alcohol; believing in a power greater than oneself; turning one's life over to God; making a searching and fearless moral inventory; and making amends to others. SMART Recovery focuses on building and maintaining motivation to change; coping with urges to use; managing thoughts, feelings, and behaviors; and living a balanced life. AA has been known to focus more on spiritual issues, while SMART Recovery places more emphasis on the science of addiction and recovery. SMART Recovery is based on the principles of CBT and skill acquisition, while AA is more focused on spiritual and interpersonal matters.

JIM: I don't know whether I need either of them.

THERAPIST: I recommend that you at least learn more about both. Would you be willing to check them out online as homework, and maybe even consider attending a meeting of each prior to our next visit?

It is important for therapists to familiarize themselves with available addiction recovery options. It should be obvious that no single approach is necessarily better than others. Furthermore, it is difficult to predict which services will best fit particular patients. Hence, it is important to provide patients with a variety of options, so they can choose those that best meet their needs. In fact, many patients try several options before finding a resource that meets their needs. And many people with addictions engage multiple services concurrently (e.g., outpatient treatment and AA meetings, or even AA meetings and SMART Recovery meetings).

As mentioned earlier, there is a vast number of topics that can be addressed as part of CBT psychoeducation. Thus far we have discussed only a few specific topics. Information about most topic areas and answers to most questions can be found in print literature and on the Internet (for example, on the websites listed above). We encourage therapists to learn about the most reliable resources and share these with patients. In some cases, entire sessions can be spent discussing specific topic areas. In the two sections that follow, we shift our attention to teaching patients about the CBT model and what they can expect from the CBT process.

The CBT Model of Addictions

The CBT model of addictions was introduced in Chapter 2. When talking to patients, we often refer to the CBT model as "The ABC model," explaining that *A* stands for *A*ntecedents or *A*ctivating events, *B* stands for *B*eliefs or thoughts, and *C* stands for the behavioral and emotional *C*onsequences of thoughts (see Figure 9.1; originally presented as Figure 2.2). Most of our patients find this model to

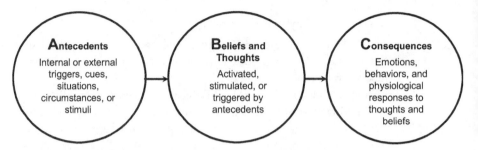

FIGURE 9.1.   The ABC model.

be helpful, so we recommend that therapists orient patients to this model early in therapy, and regularly apply this model when talking about patient choices. The ABC model is perhaps the most important of all psychoeducation topics, as we use it to explain how addictive behaviors are maintained and potentially changed. Patients find it helpful to see the links between their beliefs and thoughts and the behavioral and emotional consequences of these beliefs and thoughts. We explain that people with addictions possess numerous beliefs and thoughts about addictive behaviors (e.g., "I'd really like to drink/smoke/gamble right now") that are foreign to people who do not have addictions. We emphasize that internal and external triggers are likely to activate these thoughts and it is important to identify triggers and avoid or effectively cope with them.

To illustrate relationships between triggers, beliefs (or thoughts), and consequences, we encourage therapists to use *concept maps* (Liese & Esterline, 2015) whenever possible. A concept map is simply a flowchart that illustrates these relationships (e.g., Figure 9.1). Most cognitive-behavioral therapists have this model indelibly fixed in their minds, so preprinted concept maps are not necessary. However, especially for those who are new to CBT, preprinted ABC models can be helpful. In the following exchange, Jim's therapist explains the ABC model of addictive behavior:

THERAPIST: Jim, you've asked some good questions about alcohol use. Would you be interested in discussing why you drink?

JIM: I already know why I drink: I like to drink.

THERAPIST: That's clearly the case, but are you interested in looking more carefully at the dynamics that underlie your drinking?

JIM: That's fine, if you think it will help.

THERAPIST: Good. Let's start with this blank piece of paper. As you can see, I am drawing three circles with two arrows between them, and placing an *A, B,* and *C* in the circles (as in Figure 9.2). Let's start with the last circle, labeled *C.* The letter *C* stands for the word *consequences,* which can be either an emotional, behavioral, or physiologic consequence. As we think about your situation, let's imagine that your behavioral consequences include going to the bar and drinking. Now let's look at circles *A* and *B.* Can you recall what you think right before you take a drink?

JIM: Yeah, sure. My thought is, "I want a drink." Is that really important?

THERAPIST: Well actually, it might be important if you want to gain control over your drinking.

JIM: I don't get it.

THERAPIST: It's the *thought,* "I want a drink," that leads to your drinking. If you thought something radically different, you probably wouldn't want a drink.

JIM: What do you mean by "radically different"?

THERAPIST: I mean other thoughts might lead to behaviors other than drinking.

JIM: You'll have to explain that.

THERAPIST: Okay, but first I'll need to ask more questions. When do you take your first drink of the day?

JIM: It depends on the day of the week.

THERAPIST: How about weekdays?

JIM: [*After a long pause.*] I've never told my wife this, but when I'm having a stressful day, I'll leave work early, stop at a local bar, and have a few drinks before I go home.

THERAPIST: Thank you for being honest with me. Do you mind if I ask more about that?

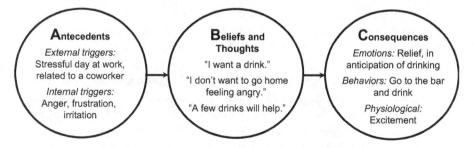

FIGURE 9.2.   The ABC model applied to Jim.

JIM: I guess not.

THERAPIST: Good. You mentioned a stressful day at work. What makes a day at work stressful?

JIM: I have a coworker who doesn't do his share of the work, so the rest of us pick up his responsibilities. It really pisses us all off.

THERAPIST: So, a trigger for you is added pressure at work, but also your anger.

JIM: Did I say I was angry?

THERAPIST: You said, "It really pisses us all off."

JIM: I guess I'm angry before I go to the bar, but I'm not angry after a few drinks.

THERAPIST: So maybe your thought is, "I don't want to go home feeling angry."

JIM: That's for sure.

THERAPIST: And before that you said, "I'm not angry after a few drinks," so you must think that "A few drinks will help."

JIM: I don't just think it—I know it.

THERAPIST: I'll draw all this out. [*Draws the concept map in Figure 9.2 and explains how he decides what to write in each circle.*]

JIM: When you draw it out like that it makes more sense.

THERAPIST: Good. The next step might be to consider alternative ways of dealing with your stress, anger, frustration, and irritation.

JIM: Like how?

THERAPIST: Let's talk about that. Besides drinking, what else has helped to reduce your stress?

This is just one example of psychoeducation regarding the CBT model. There are many other related concepts that can be taught in the spirit of CBT psychoeducation. For example, patients can be taught that certain automatic thoughts (e.g., "I hate when people are stupid") lead to certain emotions (e.g., irritation, anger), which may then function as triggers for addictive behaviors. Patients also might be taught that cognitive distortions (e.g., all-or-none thinking, overgeneralizing, should and musts, labeling, and so forth) may lead to anxiety, depression, anger, tension, restlessness, boredom, or other emotions that can trigger addiction-related automatic thoughts. Patients may also benefit from learning about their *conditional beliefs* and *assumptions* that drive addictive behaviors; for example, "*If* I drink, *then* I won't be anxious" and "Drinking is the only way I can handle my feelings" respectively.

Applying the CBT Model to Patients' Craving Experiences

Therapists can also teach patients about the relationships between triggers, thoughts, and craving by diagramming a *craving scenario*. In a craving scenario, the ABC model is applied to patients' cognitive, behavioral, and emotional experience of craving. While working with his therapist, Jim eventually decides to quit drinking alcohol. However, during his ninth session Jim tells his therapist, "I had a close call last week." In response, the therapist discusses Jim's close call and maps out his craving scenario (see Figure 9.3), which highlights the sequence of events and thoughts that put Jim at high risk for relapse:

THERAPIST: Hi Jim, let's set an agenda. What do you want to work on?

JIM: I had a close call last week.

THERAPIST: What do you mean by a "close call"?

JIM: I almost went back to the bar.

THERAPIST: Tell me more.

JIM: It was Friday afternoon. I'd just gotten home from work and was looking forward to relaxing. It had been a hard week and I was relieved to have nothing on the schedule. I finally had some free time to relax.

THERAPIST: And then what happened?

JIM: My wife met me in the driveway and, instead of a hug and kiss, she hands over a list of chores. I was pissed.

THERAPIST: And what happened next?

JIM: I walked into the house. It was a freaking mess. The kids were screaming their heads off. I couldn't stand it!

THERAPIST: And then what happened?

JIM: I immediately thought, "I've got to get away from here." And after that I started to feel intense craving.

THERAPIST: Can you recall whether there were any other thoughts before the craving started?

JIM: The craving actually started when I imagined a strong drink. All I could think of was drinking. I thought, "I need a drink!"

THERAPIST: And that's when you started craving.

JIM: Yeah, intensely.

THERAPIST: [*Pointing at his concept map in Figure 9.3.*] Does this drawing accurately reflect what happened that day, leading up to your intense craving?

JIM: Yeah, exactly.

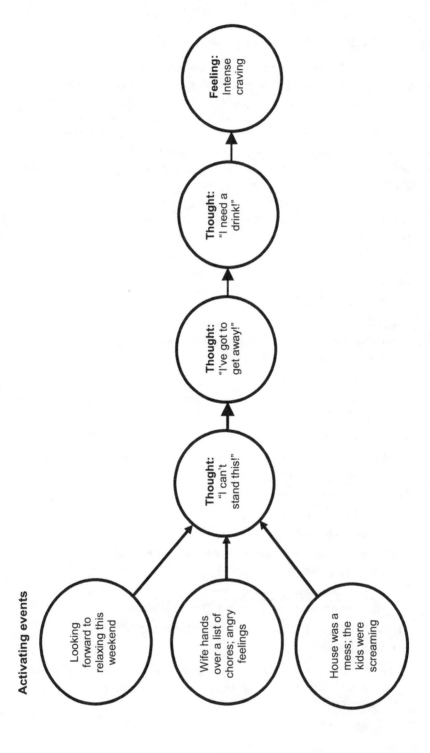

Activating events

Looking forward to relaxing this weekend

Wife hands over a list of chores; angry feelings

House was a mess; the kids were screaming

Thought: "I can't stand this!"

Thought: "I've got to get away!"

Thought: "I need a drink!"

Feeling: Intense craving

FIGURE 9.3. Jim's craving scenario.

Next, Jim's therapist used this concept map to review the relationships between Jim's triggers, thoughts, and feelings (i.e., the ABC model). And since Jim had chosen not to go to the bar and drink, they discussed the thoughts that kept him from doing so. Jim's therapist emphasized that much can be learned from *near misses* like the one Jim had experienced. This was particularly true in this case, as Jim's therapist used this situation to provide timely, appropriate psychoeducation.

Using the CBT Model to Describe the Development of Addictive Behaviors

As part of the psychoeducation process, we often help patients understand the origins of their addictive behaviors. We explain that early life experiences (i.e., distal antecedents) tend to influence later life thoughts, feelings, and behaviors— including addictive behaviors. As mentioned earlier, we regularly ask patients about any family history of addictions. We also explain that many people who struggle with addictions are genetically predisposed to becoming addicted to alcohol, tobacco, opioids, amphetamines, gambling, online gaming, and so forth. We clarify that the process of becoming addicted is complex and it involves multiple factors, including genetic, psychosocial, and environmental factors. We often find ourselves drawing a concept map to depict this developmental process for individual patients (see Figure 9.4).

The generic version of this model was presented in Chapter 2 (see Figure 2.5), while the concept map in Figure 9.4 is based on a discussion between Jim and his therapist. In this exchange Jim wants to better understand the origins of his alcohol use disorder.

JIM: I'm doing everything to keep from drinking, but I still ask myself "Why me? Why am I having all of these problems? Why can't I drink like everyone else?"

THERAPIST: I can share my ideas about how you developed your alcohol problems if you like.

JIM: I'm listening.

[*As the therapist shares his thoughts, he also draws the concept map in Figure 9.4.*]

THERAPIST: In past sessions you've shared that you come from a family of heavy drinkers and people with alcohol problems. Alcohol was all around you. There was always alcohol in your home and people in your community willing to share their alcohol. Is that right so far?

JIM: Yeah.

THERAPIST: You've told me that your father was angry and intimidating during frequent conflicts at home. You've shared that you don't want to become the angry man your father was.

JIM: Yeah, that's for sure.

THERAPIST: Though you thought you'd never be like your father you may have inherited his genetic predisposition for alcohol problems. When you were young and drinking only on weekends you found the effects of alcohol to be reliably rewarding, but that was prior to escalating into

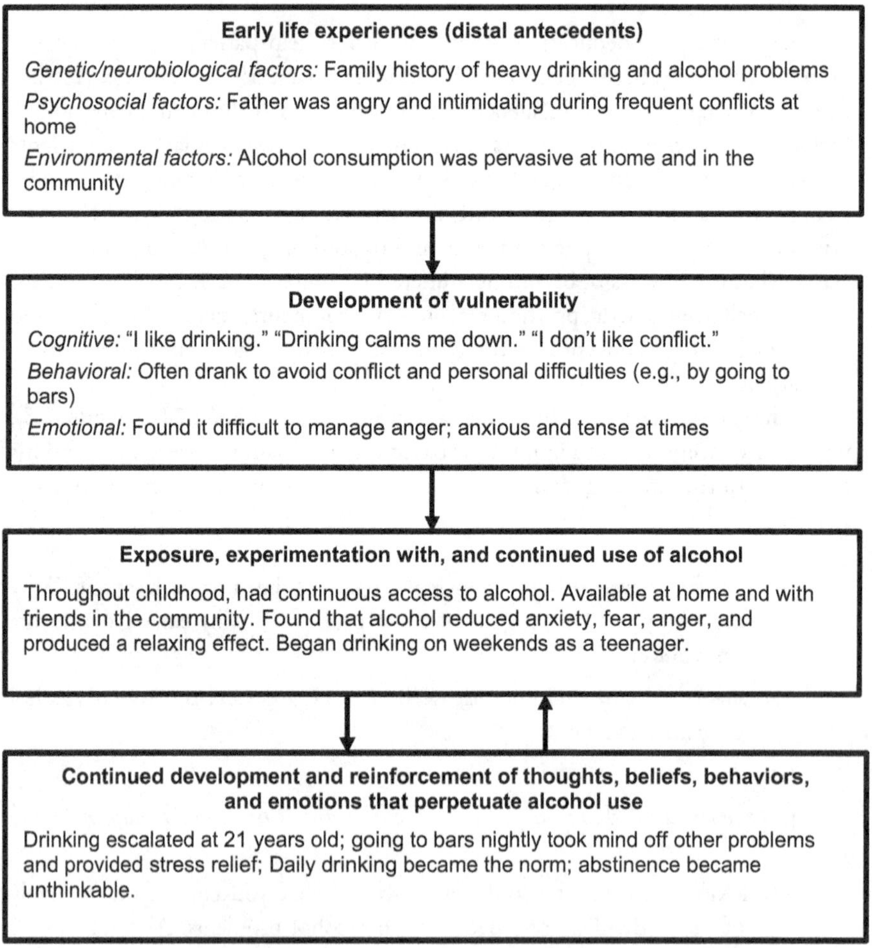

Early life experiences (distal antecedents)

Genetic/neurobiological factors: Family history of heavy drinking and alcohol problems

Psychosocial factors: Father was angry and intimidating during frequent conflicts at home

Environmental factors: Alcohol consumption was pervasive at home and in the community

↓

Development of vulnerability

Cognitive: "I like drinking." "Drinking calms me down." "I don't like conflict."

Behavioral: Often drank to avoid conflict and personal difficulties (e.g., by going to bars)

Emotional: Found it difficult to manage anger; anxious and tense at times

↓

Exposure, experimentation with, and continued use of alcohol

Throughout childhood, had continuous access to alcohol. Available at home and with friends in the community. Found that alcohol reduced anxiety, fear, anger, and produced a relaxing effect. Began drinking on weekends as a teenager.

↓   ↑

Continued development and reinforcement of thoughts, beliefs, behaviors, and emotions that perpetuate alcohol use

Drinking escalated at 21 years old; going to bars nightly took mind off other problems and provided stress relief; Daily drinking became the norm; abstinence became unthinkable.

FIGURE 9.4.   Development of Jim's alcohol-related problems.

heavier drinking. At some point you went from drinking recreationally to self-medicating with alcohol. The more you drank, the more you
came to believe that drinking was the best, or perhaps the only, way to
reduce your stress, until eventually you couldn't imagine life without
alcohol.

JIM: I agree with what you're saying. It all makes sense.

This conversation, facilitated by the concept map in Figure 9.4, helped Jim
understand (perhaps for the first time) that multiple factors likely contributed to
his alcohol problem, beginning early in his life and developing over decades. This
exchange between Jim and his therapist provides an excellent example of psychoeducation. In this case the therapist linked Jim's past with his present behavior. For
many patients, this is a true "Aha!" moment.

Assisting Patients in Identifying Thoughts, Beliefs, and Feelings

Many patients initially find it difficult to identify their thoughts, beliefs, and feelings. They might say things like, "I don't have any thoughts," or "I wasn't thinking
anything." To address this problem, therapists might wait for patients to experience
emotional shifts in sessions and then ask, "What's going through your mind right
now?" When timed effectively, patients are likely to have access to their thoughts.
Patients might also be asked, "If you can't identify any thoughts, can you describe
what you are feeling?" In response they may actually report their thoughts; for
example, "I feel like I don't want to be here today." Therapists might choose to
accept these responses as feelings, but at a later point educate patients to make a
distinction between thoughts (e.g., "I don't feel like being here today"), and feelings
(e.g., anxiety, anger, sadness, shame, guilt, frustration, and so forth).

Some patients are inexperienced and therefore unskilled at labeling specific
emotions. They say such things as, "I feel like crap," or, "I feel awful." One method
to help patients label feelings is to encourage them to use the simplest terms possible to describe their feelings, for example, mad, sad, irritated, angry, frustrated,
hurt, ashamed, disappointed, or worried. Also, when patients say, "I'm upset,"
therapists can ask, "*Where in your body* do you experience this feeling of being
upset?" Patients may then report some physiological indicator such as tightness in
the stomach, tightness in the chest, stiff neck, and so on. Patients can be taught to
use these bodily sensation cues to ask themselves the important question: "What's
going through my mind right now?" With repetition, patients eventually come to
understand how to notice and modify their thoughts and beliefs, which will provide them with better control over their emotions and behaviors.

The CBT Process

As described throughout this text, cognitive-behavioral therapy is an active, structured, collaborative, goal-oriented approach to helping people solve problems and develop self-regulation skills. Patients appreciate when therapists effectively explain *how CBT is done*. Hence, we strongly believe in the value of orienting patients to the CBT process. We begin by asking questions of patients to determine how much patients already know about CBT, especially from past experiences, friends, family members, the Internet, and even social media. We have often been surprised by both *how much* some patients know and *how little* other patients know about CBT. For example, some have attended numerous CBT sessions while in prior treatment and found it to be helpful. Others have never heard of CBT or received any type of therapy. The following is a list of potential questions to determine how much patients already know about the CBT process:

> "What help or therapy have you received for your addiction in the past?"
> "What help or therapy have you received for any other past mental health problem?"
> "What did you find helpful or unhelpful about any past therapy you've received?"
> "How familiar are you with cognitive-behavioral therapy (sometimes called CBT)?"
> "What do you know about CBT?"
> "What questions or concerns do you have about CBT?"
> "How do you feel about practicing skills between sessions, especially if I refer to this practice as *homework?*"
> "Based on what we've discussed regarding CBT so far, what are your goals for therapy?"
> "Based on what we've discussed so far, what are your reservations, if any, regarding CBT?"
> "Before we start, do you have any general questions about our work together?"

Depending on the answers to these questions, cognitive-behavioral therapists orient patients by explaining the CBT process. For the most part, patients who have learned about CBT from past experiences might require little psychoeducation regarding the CBT process, while those who know little about CBT might benefit from more information about the CBT process. We have also encountered patients who were told in the past that they were receiving CBT, but whose descriptions of the interventions were not consistent with the process or content of CBT. For example, we have had patients say such things as, "I've been in CBT before, and all we ever did was fill out thought records," or

"I've been in CBT before and it felt like I was back in school listening to boring lectures."

It should be apparent by now that there are many possible topics and techniques available to therapists providing CBT. For example, therapists might focus on cognitive distortions, advantages and disadvantages of addictive behaviors, individual case conceptualizations, the craving scenario, emotion regulation, and so forth. But cognitive-behavioral therapists also differ in their personalities and therefore the manner in which they provide CBT. Hence, it is important to determine when patients have an accurate understanding of CBT and when they do not. We have generated a sample of possible statements that may be provided to patients, regarding the CBT process. Some of these statements might be relevant or helpful to some patients, while other statements might be relevant or helpful to other patients:

> "Cognitive-behavioral therapy, or CBT, is a structured, focused approach to therapy."
>
> "In every session we focus on your concerns, so I will ask you to be responsible for bringing these concerns, in the form of agenda items, to each session."
>
> "I ask the same questions at the beginning of every session: *What do you want to work on?* or *What do you want to put on the agenda?*"
>
> "Our meetings are collaborative and goal-oriented. We work as a team in every session to address problems you want to solve."
>
> "To the extent that you find it helpful, we will focus specifically on your addictive behaviors."
>
> "At times we may also talk about problems that impact or result from your addictive behaviors."
>
> "In order to stay focused, I may need to redirect our conversations. I hope you don't take this as disrespectful."
>
> "I will often focus on skills and techniques that have helped other people with similar problems, but sometimes I will simply be interested in learning about your thoughts, feelings, and behaviors."
>
> "I will often ask you for feedback during sessions, to make sure we're on the right track and accomplishing your goals."
>
> "My goal is to help you gain useful knowledge and skills in each session, so you leave each session thinking we spent the time well."

Thus far we have presented four categories of potential psychoeducation topics: (1) the science of addiction, (2) the science of recovery, (3) the CBT model of addiction, and (4) the CBT process. Again, these topics reflect *what* may be taught in CBT. In the section that follows, we discuss the psychoeducation *process,* and place emphasis on *how* psychoeducation is conducted.

THE PROCESS OF PSYCHOEDUCATION

Therapists generally focus on *what* patients need to know and do in order to live healthy, effective, fulfilling lives. Unfortunately, many therapists do not attend to the *processes* underlying the delivery of CBT—and especially the delivery of psychoeducation. In this final section we focus on the processes that underlie effective psychoeducation. Specifically, we discuss the importance of therapist style, listening skills, and timing. We also focus on patient readiness to change, cognitive flexibility, and psychological mindedness, as these relate to the psychoeducation process.

Therapist Factors Impacting the Process of Psychoeducation

Some therapists are mostly direct or authoritative when sharing their thoughts with patients; others are mostly indirect or tentative when sharing their thoughts. Some therapists regularly engage humor during therapy; others are more serious. Some therapists are more didactic; others are more conversational in therapy. No single therapist style is better than others, and no single style works best for all patients. Hence, therapists are strongly advised to recognize their own styles, especially as they relate to the process of psychoeducation. Direct or authoritative therapists appear bossy or overbearing to some patients, while the same therapists appear knowledgeable or insightful to other patients. Tentative therapists appear detached or disengaged to some patients, while the same therapists appear thoughtful or reflective to other patients.

The key to delivering effective psychoeducation (and CBT generally) is therapist awareness of their patients' and their own styles—and the ability to adapt to the needs of diverse groups and styles of patients. When Jim entered therapy, it was apparent that he wanted to learn as much as possible about himself and his addiction. When his therapist would offer to introduce or explain a concept Jim always appeared eager to learn as much as possible. Hence, Jim's therapist felt comfortable providing information and direction to Jim on a regular basis. In contrast, Jim's therapist also had patients who appeared uninterested in new information or advice, but instead preferred to draw their own conclusions about problems and solutions.

In sum, each cognitive-behavioral therapist has a unique personal style, and patients seeking help for addictions vary greatly in their personal styles and preferences for therapist styles. Hence, a vital therapist skill is the ability to vary style according to the needs of individual patients, understanding that some will respond best to some styles and not so much to others.

Therapist Listening Skills

The importance of listening skills cannot be overstated. As we reflect on the process of psychoeducation it is especially important to emphasize the importance of listening. Simply stated, psychoeducation is only effective when therapists listen well to their patients and know what, when, and how to deliver therapeutic information. When therapists listen well to patients, they are likely to know what their patients want, need, or are ready to learn. Listening well enables therapists to anticipate the optimal method and timing of psychoeducation. Additionally, people have an innate capacity to determine when others are (or are not) listening to them. When patients observe that therapists have not heard their concerns, therapist efforts to educate patients are likely to fall on deaf ears.

Effective listening requires therapist attention to patient verbal and nonverbal cues. When a patient is disinterested in what a therapist is trying to teach, the early warning signs are likely to be subtle. They may involve changes in eye contact, fidgeting, sighing, or any number of patient cues. The decision to provide psychoeducation on any topic should correspond with attention to these cues. For example, when the therapist asks, "Would you like to learn about the ABC model?" a lukewarm response (e.g., "I guess so") should indicate less-than-optimal patient enthusiasm. A therapist would be wise under such circumstances to ask whether an alternative course might be preferable.

There are times when patients are likely to benefit from information or psychoeducation about particular topics, but only after they resolve (or at least discuss) other concerns. As an example, Jim talked about strong feelings toward his father in a session. His therapist was about to introduce a concept map to diagram Jim's thoughts and feelings, but Jim seemed uninterested. Noticing Jim's lack of interest, his therapist stopped and said, "Jim, you feel strongly about your father." Jim became teary-eyed as he exclaimed, "My father just never did seem to care about me." Jim's therapist encouraged him to continue talking and eventually Jim said, "I've never said those words out loud. I appreciate your listening to me." And shortly thereafter, Jim was receptive to the drawing of a concept map.

It is important for therapists to elicit *feedback* following efforts at psychoeducation, especially since psychoeducation often involves the delivery of new information. Therapists who listen well know how and when to ask patients for feedback. Put simply, after explaining new concepts or skills to patients, therapists should follow with simple questions like:

"What are your thoughts about the ideas/skills we've been discussing?"
"How might these ideas/skills be helpful to you?"
"Under what circumstances will you use these ideas/skills?"
"How will you practice these ideas/skills?"

Answers to these questions provide therapists with valuable guidance moving forward. In other words, they enable therapists to determine whether their efforts at psychoeducation have been helpful and therefore how they might proceed.

Therapist Timing

In order for psychoeducation to be effective, it needs to be well-timed. Patients struggling with poor health, physical pain, unstable relationships, financial problems, difficult living situations, and so forth are less likely to be interested in discussing addictive behaviors than those who have more stable circumstances. It is important to remember that addictive behaviors are often used to reduce emotional distress. Patients often need to solve basic life problems before they are ready to abandon addictive behaviors that reduce or distract from the emotional distress associated with these problems.

We recently witnessed a timing problem during a therapy supervision session. In a video segment chosen by the therapist, he was helping a patient complete an advantages–disadvantages analysis. The therapist's supervisor stopped the video and asked the therapist about an earlier comment made by the patient, who had stated that his wife recently left him for another man. The therapist responded, "Yeah, he was really upset about that." The supervisor pointed out that the patient did not seem terribly engaged in the advantages–disadvantages analysis, and the therapist agreed. This gave his supervisor an opportunity to remind the therapist that CBT techniques work best when they are delivered in a timely manner. The therapist immediately understood that his efforts at psychoeducation would have been more successful if he had first helped his patient address his struggle with the relationship problem.

Patient Factors Impacting the Process of Psychoeducation

As discussed in several earlier chapters, it is important to pay attention to patient motivation, or readiness to change, throughout the therapy process (Norcross et al., 2011; Prochaska et al., 1992; Prochaska & Norcross, 2001). Therapists should ask themselves whether patients are considering change, preparing to change, just beginning to make changes, or well into a change. A patient who is not even contemplating change has little use for psychoeducation regarding relapse prevention, which is more appropriate for those who have already made changes. Furthermore, a patient who has maintained abstinence for years is unlikely to benefit from completing an advantages–disadvantages analysis.

It is well known that therapists, enthusiastic about helping their patients, are at risk for providing psychoeducation to patients who are not ready to receive information about making substantive changes. While techniques related to urge surfing and stimulus control make good sense to those who are actively making changes, these techniques are unlikely to hold the attention of patients in the pre-contemplation stage of change.

Patient Cognitive Flexibility

Some patients have more flexible cognitive and behavioral patterns, while others have more rigid patterns. According to Diamond (2014), *cognitive flexibility* involves "being able to adjust to changed demands or priorities; take advantage of sudden, unexpected opportunities; overcome sudden, unexpected problems; or even admit you were wrong when you get new information" (p. 8). Conversely, *cognitive and behavioral rigidity* involves "the tendency of an individual *not* to change" (Schultz & Searleman, 2002, p. 166). *Psychoeducation is most likely to succeed when patients are cognitively and behaviorally flexible.* Hence, it is important to attend to this dynamic when introducing patients to new ways of thinking and behaving.

A process related to cognitive and behavioral inflexibility is *overlearning*. Overlearning occurs when individuals repeat thoughts and behaviors beyond the point of maximization, until they are fully retained and automatic (Driskill, Willis, & Copper, 1992). It has been said that overlearning "hyperstabilizes" a behavior (Shibata et al., 2017). Overlearned thoughts or behaviors are difficult to change (see Chapter 10, regarding System 1 thinking). It is important to distinguish between inflexibility and overlearning, and to be able to explain these processes to patients. We have observed that most mental health problems are associated with overlearned cognitive and behavioral patterns, or habits. For example, people with depression tend to have overlearned beliefs about their inadequacy and unlovability, while people with anxiety tend to have overlearned beliefs about their vulnerability (to harm, failure, illness, suffering, etc.). Both depressed and anxious people tend to automatically avoid situations and circumstances they fear will validate these overlearned beliefs, until avoidance itself becomes overlearned. Along the same lines, people with addictions tend to have overlearned beliefs about their addictive behaviors, and especially beliefs about these behaviors decreasing negative states and increasing positive states.

A major aim of CBT psychoeducation is to facilitate the acquisition of new beliefs and behaviors that eventually become more salient than the original overlearned addictive beliefs and behaviors. For example, Jim had overlearned beliefs and behaviors associated with consuming alcohol to manage his stress. He had engaged in alcohol consumption so often that he did not even consciously think about going to a bar after a stressful day at work; he just got in his car in the parking lot and the next thing he noticed was that it was time to leave the bar and go home for dinner. In therapy Jim was able to learn and practice alternative beliefs and behaviors in response to stress that eventually became overlearned. Jim was able to change his overlearned habits because he was cognitively and behaviorally flexible. Unfortunately, many people are less flexible than Jim. These individuals might have argued that, "Drinking is my only way to reduce stress. I've tried everything else and it doesn't work."

When working with patients who have overlearned thoughts and beliefs, it is important to understand that some of these are relatively rigid, or inflexible. When psychoeducation reliably fails to benefit a patient, it may be helpful to determine whether the lack of benefit might be due to a larger pattern of cognitive and behavioral inflexibility. When this is the case, it is important to address the inflexibility prior to focusing on changing overlearned thoughts and behaviors themselves. For example, a therapist might say to a patient, "I notice that you struggle to find my explanations and recommendations helpful. Perhaps we should discuss whether it is generally difficult for you to adopt new ideas or behaviors."

Patient Psychological Mindedness

Most psychological constructs are abstract. For example, relationships among thoughts, feelings, and behaviors are abstract constructs. Patients vary widely in their levels of abstract thinking versus concrete thinking, and especially in their levels of psychological mindedness. *Psychological mindedness* is the "interest and ability to be in touch with and reflect on one's psychological states and processes" (Nyklicek & Denollet, 2009, p. 32). An ability to grasp concepts that are psychological in nature is quite helpful in CBT. However, when working with patients who are not psychologically minded, it is sometimes wise to pursue more behavioral interventions. Jim, the patient discussed throughout this chapter, has the benefit of being both psychologically minded and cognitively flexible. As a result, he is able to grasp concepts and consider behaviors that are different from his addictive behaviors. In contrast, we have worked with patients who are neither psychologically minded nor cognitively flexible. In fact, many patients have developed these deficits as a result of their addictive behaviors. When working with these patients, we find it beneficial to initially focus on stimulus control and behavioral activation. Specifically, we recommend that they avoid triggers and engage in rewarding substance-free behaviors (see Chapter 7 for details).

Patients who are not psychologically minded might appear disinterested in all or most therapist efforts at psychoeducation. When this is the case, therapists are encouraged to "meet patients where they are," and explore topics that are relevant and interesting to patients. In doing so, the therapist is likely to discover unexpected opportunities to relate patients' interests to CBT principles and practices.

SUMMARY

An important component of CBT is psychoeducation, defined as the facilitation of learning facts, principles, behaviors, and skills for improving psychological and behavioral functioning. It is important for therapists to ask themselves at least two questions as they practice CBT and provide psychoeducation: *What* can I teach my patient to facilitate recovery? and *How* can I teach so my patient hears what I have to say and learns from my efforts? Therapists may educate patients regarding the science of addiction and recovery, the cognitive model of addiction, and the process of CBT. But perhaps most fundamental to psychoeducation are the connections among life experiences, triggers, thoughts, beliefs, emotions, and addictive behaviors—all conveyed in a timely and collaborative manner.

CHAPTER 10

THOUGHTS AND BELIEFS

Kristen is a 31-year-old single mom who initially sought therapy for depression. After 8 weeks of CBT, feeling less depressed, she now wants to quit smoking cigarettes. Over the last 2 weeks Kristen has been trying to quit on her own but finds it exceedingly difficult to do so. In a recent session she told her therapist that she has five reasons for quitting. She wants to save money, be healthier, protect her 2-year-old daughter from second-hand smoke, be a good role model for her daughter, and stop feeling "a deep sense of self-loathing" every time she lights a cigarette. In this session she feels particularly exasperated:

THERAPIST: Kristen, what would you like to work on today?

KRISTEN: I want to figure out why it's so damn hard for me to quit smoking.

THERAPIST: Good agenda item. You want to better understand why you can't just quit.

KRISTEN: Yes.

THERAPIST: Anything else you want to put on the agenda?

KRISTEN: Yeah, I'd like to know the secret to quitting. Millions of people have quit smoking, but I just can't seem to do it. There's got to be some *secret.*

THERAPIST: Another good agenda item: You want to learn how to quit. I'd like to help you with both of these agenda items.

KRISTEN: Great, because I'm not doing well on my own.

During this exchange Kristen asked two fundamental questions related to addictive behaviors: *Why* can't I stop? and *How* can I stop? When patients ask these questions therapists have an excellent opportunity to offer support, psycho-education, and self-management skills. We recommend responding to questions like these by first focusing on the essential role of thoughts and beliefs in addictive behaviors. As noted in Chapter 2, thoughts are brief, spontaneous ideas and images that grow out of more enduring beliefs developed over time. In the section that follows we explain how certain specific thoughts and beliefs are associated with addictive behaviors, and in a later section we discuss cognitive processes associated with addictive behaviors.

THOUGHTS AND BELIEFS ASSOCIATED WITH ADDICTIVE BEHAVIORS

We have learned over the years that certain thoughts and beliefs are common across chemical and behavioral addictions. For example, most people who struggle with addictions wish they were better able to control their addictive behaviors. Most believe their addictive behaviors play an important role in regulating their emotions. Most have ambivalent thoughts about continuing their addictive behaviors. Many believe the suffering associated with reducing or stopping their addictive behaviors is virtually intolerable. Many believe their addictive behaviors are stigmatized by others. Hence, many believe it is best to keep their addictions a secret.

Kristen's discussion with her therapist resumes here. In this exchange, some of Kristen's most salient addiction-related thoughts and beliefs become apparent:

THERAPIST: Kristen, you sound frustrated.

KRISTEN: I'm very frustrated. I thought it would be a lot easier to quit smoking now that I'm not depressed, but that's definitely not the case.

THERAPIST: You sound like you're angry at yourself.

KRISTEN: Maybe I am. You've taught me . . . [*Pauses and takes a deep breath.*] When I feel like this I'm supposed to stop and ask myself, "What am I thinking?"

THERAPIST: Yes, and then what?

KRISTEN: I'm supposed to stop judging myself . . .

THERAPIST: Right.

KRISTEN: . . . and get back to the problem at hand.

THERAPIST: Yes. And the problem is?

KRISTEN: Damn it, I want to quit smoking. [*She sits up straight and gets a determined look on her face.*]

THERAPIST: How interesting: I can see your mood change when you shift your thoughts from judging yourself to problem solving. I've been impressed with how quickly you've learned to regulate your thoughts and feelings since starting therapy.

KRISTEN: Yeah, so am I. It surprises me.

THERAPIST: So, looking back at your successes in therapy over the past eight weeks, is there any reason to think you can't beat the smoking habit?

KRISTEN: I don't know. I've actually tried on and off for years and I just can't seem to stop.

THERAPIST: Okay, let's discuss your thoughts and beliefs about smoking.

KRISTEN: Like I told you earlier, I think cigarettes are gross and disgusting. Smoking is expensive, bad for my health, and it's bad for Lilly's health to be around smoke. I don't want her to see me smoking. I'm supposed to be her role model. Every time I light a cigarette, I hate myself.

THERAPIST: I understand that those thoughts make you want to quit. But what about the thoughts that keep you smoking?

KRISTEN: I don't know. You mean like the thoughts I have right before I give in and smoke?

THERAPIST: Exactly.

KRISTEN: Well, I still think it's gross and disgusting, but sometimes I smoke to calm my nerves. Other times it helps me stay alert, like when I'm up late at night trying to get chores done. When I try to quit, I can't stand the craving. At those times I think, "Just this one cigarette. I'll just quit tomorrow." Also, Lilly is asleep, so she can't see me smoking. When I'm bored at work I suddenly think I need a cigarette. And because I'm trying to quit and don't have one, I think, "I'll just bum one off a friend."

THERAPIST: Obviously you have a lot of thoughts and beliefs about smoking that make it hard to quit. Here, I've started a list of your thoughts and beliefs about smoking and quitting. [*Shows the list in Table 10.1 to Kristen* (see Form 2.1 in Chapter 2 for a blank version).]

KRISTEN: Wow, you got all that from what I just said?

THERAPIST: Yeah, these are your thoughts and beliefs. It's important to become familiar with them. They are vital to understanding why it's so hard for you to quit and what it will take for you to become a nonsmoker.

KRISTEN: What do you mean? How will this list help?

THERAPIST: It's only the beginning. By writing down your thoughts and beliefs they become more real and more tangible. I put them on paper so you could actually look at them. It's important to remember that certain thoughts and beliefs drive you *toward* smoking, while others drive you *away from* smoking.

TABLE 10.1. Kristen's Smoking-Related Thoughts and Beliefs versus Self-Control Thoughts and Beliefs

Addiction-Related Thoughts and Beliefs	Self-Control Thoughts and Beliefs
"Smoking calms my nerves."	"Smoking is gross and disgusting."
"Smoking helps me stay alert."	"It's expensive."
"I can't stand the craving."	"It's bad for my health."
"Just this one cigarette."	"Second-hand smoke is bad for Lilly."
"I'll just quit tomorrow."	"I don't want her to see me smoking."
"Lilly can't see me smoking."	"I'm supposed to be her role model."
"I'll bum a cigarette off a friend."	"I hate myself each time I light up."

KRISTEN: I see. [*Looking at the list.*] Thoughts in the left column drive me in the wrong direction—and thoughts in the right column drive me in the right direction.

THERAPIST: Yes.

KRISTEN: So why can't I just *replace* thoughts on the left side with thoughts on the right side?

THERAPIST: I promise I'll answer that question soon.

In this exchange, Kristen's therapist introduced the idea that there are thoughts and beliefs associated with both smoking and quitting. As noted earlier, some of these thoughts and beliefs are common across all addictions. In fact, therapists can practically replace the word *smoking* in Table 10.1 with any addictive behavior: "*Drinking* calms my nerves," "*Weed* calms my nerves," or "*Binge eating* calms my nerves."

Some patients find it helpful to organize their thoughts and beliefs into groups or categories, such as:

- *Anticipatory* thoughts and beliefs (e.g., "Engaging in my addictive behaviors will produce desired results.")
- *Relief-oriented* thoughts and beliefs (e.g., "Engaging in my addictive behaviors will make unpleasant feelings go away.")
- *Permissive* thoughts and beliefs (e.g., "I have *valid reasons* for continuing my addictive behaviors.")
- *Instrumental* thoughts and beliefs (e.g., "To engage in my addictive behaviors, I need to [call my dealer, drive to the liquor store, buy a pack of smokes, etc.]")

- *Change-related* thoughts and beliefs (e.g., "My addictive behaviors aren't working for me anymore. Maybe it's *time for something different.*")
- *Control-related* thoughts and beliefs (e.g., "I want to *modify* my addictive behaviors without necessarily stopping completely.")
- *Abstinence-related* thoughts and beliefs (e.g., "I plan to *completely stop* engaging in my addictive behaviors.")

These are just some of many possible categories for organizing thoughts and beliefs associated with addictive behaviors. Most of our patients find these categories helpful, but occasionally patients prefer their own categories. For example, many patients respond to the term *permissive beliefs* by saying, "Oh, you mean *excuses and rationalizations?*" Some prefer to use the term *stinkin-thinkin* for all thoughts and beliefs related to their addictive behaviors. As she reflects on her thoughts and beliefs, Kristen finds these categories to be helpful. In fact, she is able to easily place her thoughts into the categories described by her therapist:

THERAPIST: Kristen, what do you think of these categories?

KRISTEN: They make good sense. The left-hand column is full of anticipatory, relief, and instrumental thoughts and the right-hand column is full of change-related thoughts.

THERAPIST: So, which of these thoughts or beliefs are anticipatory?

KRISTEN: The first two: I anticipate that smoking calms my nerves and helps me stay alert.

THERAPIST: Excellent. How about the thoughts that are relief-oriented, permissive, and instrumental?

KRISTEN: "I can't stand the craving" is relief-oriented, since it will be a relief to smoke a cigarette. "Just one," "I'll quit tomorrow," and "Lilly can't see me" are all permissive, because they give me permission. And "I'll bum a cigarette" is instrumental because it's how I get the cigarettes I smoke.

THERAPIST: Excellent. And how about control-related thoughts?

KRISTEN: Everything on the right side of that list is about control, trying to change, and being abstinent.

THERAPIST: Again, excellent.

KRISTEN: It may be excellent, but I still don't know *how* to change.

At this moment in their conversation Kristen's therapist realizes it is time to shift from the *content* of her thoughts to the thought *processes* associated with her smoking. In the next section we explain how we focus on cognitive processes (i.e., *how* addicted patients think).

COGNITIVE PROCESSES
ASSOCIATED WITH ADDICTIVE BEHAVIORS

Our approach over the last couple of decades has been profoundly influenced by the work of Daniel Kahneman, recipient of the 2002 Nobel Prize in Economic Sciences. Kahneman and his colleagues (e.g., Kahneman, 2011; Kahneman, 1973; Kahneman & Frederick, 2002; Tversky & Kahneman, 1992) have studied complex cognitive processes, including attention, decision making, cognitive errors and bias, intuition, and (most relevant to our work) System 1 and System 2 thinking (see Table 10.2). System 1 thinking is automatic, spontaneous, effortless, intuitive, and impulsive. System 1 is what gets us through a typical day without having to calculate our every move and decision. System 1 enables us to brush our teeth and get dressed in the morning, go about our business during the day, and climb into bed at night without giving these activities much thought. System 1 enables us to make simple decisions like choosing to eat soup with a spoon rather than a fork and waiting to cross a street until traffic subsides.

Most System 1 thinking is possible because of overlearning. The more we engage in a behavior or set of behaviors the more automatic they become. For example, we learn to drive a car by repeating each necessary action over and over. When we first learn to drive, we need to focus on properly placing the key in the ignition, starting the car, engaging the transmission, checking for oncoming traffic, pulling away from the curb, using turn signals, clearing curbs on right turns, and so forth. But as time passes, all of these functions become automatic. In fact, after they become automatic we hardly notice the steps it takes to accomplish these functions. Again, most of our daily activities are governed by System 1 thinking.

In contrast, System 2 thinking is slow, intentional, deliberate, and conscious. System 2 thinking requires our full attention and substantial mental exertion. System 2 is activated much less often than System 1 in the course of a day. In fact, we

TABLE 10.2. Characteristics of System 1 and System 2 Thinking

System 1 thinking	System 2 thinking
Fast	Slow
Automatic	Methodical
Spontaneous	Intentional
Effortless	Effortful
Intuitive	Deliberate
Reflexive	Conscious
Impulsive	Mindful

do not typically activate System 2 unless System 1 runs into difficulties. System 2 is necessary when we rent a car that is different from the car we normally drive. System 2 is necessary when driving to a location that is completely unfamiliar. System 2 requires deliberate, careful attention. When studying a complex topic for the first time, learning a new skill, changing an old habit, or trying to modify an addictive behavior, we need System 2 thinking. Whereas System 1 is resilient and can withstand external clamor and activity (i.e., multitasking), System 2 is easily interrupted. This is why libraries are traditionally quiet and some people wear headphones or earplugs when they study. And this is why it is so difficult to change addictive behaviors; they become fully automatic and require deliberate, uninterrupted effort to change.

Kahneman (2003) additionally focused on *choice-making* and *decision errors,* which is another reason his model is applicable to addictive behaviors. By *choosing* addictive behaviors repeatedly, addiction-related thoughts become *intuitive* and *accessible,* rather than *rational* and the result of *careful consideration.* By default, *unhealthy choices* are erroneously assumed to be *best choices.* For example, people who smoke cigarettes or drink excessive amounts of alcohol to relieve stress *intuitively* reach for a cigarette or a drink, as if these choices are in their best interest. When this occurs *decision errors* have been made, since the long-term effects of addictive behaviors are life-threatening. Accordingly, patients will often describe their addictive behaviors as unconscious or involuntary. For example, they might say "I wasn't even thinking about smoking or drinking and suddenly I had a drink and cigarette in my hand." Kahneman (2003, 2011) also attributed decision errors to *familiarity* and *liking* (i.e., reward). The more rewarding a behavior, the more likely it will be chosen intentionally, until it becomes automatic and unintentional. When addictive behaviors first occur, they are unfamiliar, deliberate, and certainly not automatic. However, as they are increasingly liked, they are also increasingly familiar, until they have become fully automatic and are under the full command of System 1. Besides becoming automatic, effortless, and intuitive, System 1 thoughts become reflexively associated with certain events and activities, and these become their triggers.

The above descriptions of System 1 and 2 thinking clarify why it is so difficult to change addictive behaviors. It should not be surprising that so many individuals continuously make the error of engaging in addictive behaviors. Sometimes it takes years or even decades for System 2 to be called upon for help with change. And by that time, the amount of System 2 effort needed to make changes is considerable. These processes provide answers to the *why* and *how* questions asked by Kristen. So, let's return to Kristen. Her therapist is about to explain System 1 and System 2 thinking:

THERAPIST: Kristen, you asked two important questions: "*Why* can't I stop?" and "*How* can I stop?" Now that we've talked about *what* you think, let's talk about *how* you think.

KRISTEN: Okay. This is a lot to take in. Can we take some more notes?

THERAPIST: Sure. [*Picks up the same notepad where Kristen's thoughts are written.*] Have you ever noticed that most of what you do throughout the day is automatic and effortless?

KRISTEN: I hadn't really noticed, but now that you mention it . . .

THERAPIST: Exactly. You hadn't noticed *because* these behaviors have become automatic and effortless.

KRISTEN: When I was depressed everything felt like a huge burden. Now that I'm not depressed my daily activities are starting to feel normal again.

THERAPIST: For example?

KRISTEN: Like getting out of bed in the morning and getting dressed.

THERAPIST: Yes, these behaviors have become automatic because you've done them repeatedly, over the course of your entire life. When you were depressed, your helpless and hopeless negative thoughts and beliefs were automatic and predominant—so you didn't even think you could get out of bed.

KRISTEN: That's right. So, where do we go with all this?

THERAPIST: Now I can explain why it's so hard to change addictive behaviors and how you can make the change you want to make—quitting smoking, that is.

KRISTEN: Please do.

THERAPIST: Okay, I'm going to explain what is known as System 1 and System 2 thinking. [*While talking, Kristen's therapist makes a new list on her note pad* (this list closely resembles Table 10.2).] System 1 thinking is what enables you to get out of bed in the morning and get dressed—without really giving it much thought. System 1 thinking is fast, automatic, spontaneous, and effortless. It just seems to happen. Some people refer to System 1 thinking as intuitive thinking. It happens almost like a reflex. You might also think of System 1 as impulsive.

KRISTEN: I think I know where you're going with this.

THERAPIST: Good. Where?

KRISTEN: That's how smoking a cigarette is for me. I don't even think about it anymore. There have been times when I'll be smoking a cigarette and I don't even remember lighting it. Or I'll see a lit cigarette in an ashtray and ask myself, "When did I light that?"

THERAPIST: These are perfect examples of your System 1 thinking at work. Your anticipatory, relief-oriented, permissive, and instrumental thoughts about smoking are mostly running on System 1. These thoughts are like little voices in your head that you don't consciously hear.

Kristen: So that's what makes it so hard to quit smoking?

Therapist: Yes.

Kristen: So, what's the secret to quitting?

Therapist: Now we'll talk about System 2 thinking. System 2 thinking is much slower and is activated when you encounter something that System 1 can't handle, like when you want to solve a complex problem or are in an unfamiliar situation. Actually, you probably use System 2 when you want to smoke a cigarette but doing so is inconvenient or prohibited. For example, when you are at dinner with a group of nonsmokers and you crave a cigarette, you might plan a way to sneak out and smoke.

Kristen: That's happened to me often. How'd you know?

Therapist: I've seen enough smokers, shivering outside restaurants at night, in the cold, smoking cigarettes while their friends and family are inside enjoying each other's company. Now let's talk about what it will take to quit.

Kristen: Okay.

Therapist: You will need to energize System 2 and put it on high alert, instead of low energy mode, to change your overlearned System 1 thoughts about smoking. System 2 is slow, methodical, intentional, effortful, deliberate, conscious, and mindful.

Kristen: That's a long list.

Therapist: I've written these words down for you. [*He shows her the new list on the notepad.*] As we work on this together, your thoughts and beliefs about smoking and quitting are going to become more methodical, intentional, effortful, deliberate, conscious, and mindful.

Kristen: So that's the secret?

Therapist: I guess it's not a secret anymore.

Kristen: It sounds like what I did to overcome the thoughts and beliefs that made me depressed.

Therapist: Exactly.

In this segment, Kristen has been introduced to System 1 and System 2 thinking. Her therapist has described these systems and given Kristen a list of the characteristics of each system. But it will take more than one discussion for Kristen to fully understand and adopt a pattern of System 2 thinking to overcome her existing System 1 thinking processes. So, Kristen's therapist is patient. He fully recognizes that Kristen's change might be slow, especially given that System 2 thinking is so easily sidetracked.

HELPING PATIENTS
CHANGE THOUGHTS AND BELIEFS

In this chapter thus far, we have identified thoughts, beliefs, and cognitive processes that support addictive behaviors and behavior change. In this section we present a systematic strategy for applying this knowledge with patients who wish to change addictive behaviors. We find it convenient to organize this strategy into five steps: (1) eliciting thoughts and beliefs that underlie addictive behaviors; (2) facilitating patients' recognition and understanding of addiction-related thoughts and beliefs; (3) developing and maintaining thoughts and beliefs that support change; (4) anticipating roadblocks to changing thoughts and beliefs; and (5) practicing strategies that increase the salience and durability of new adaptive thoughts and beliefs. These steps are not actually discrete or orderly in practice. Instead, each step ideally continues even after subsequent steps have begun.

Step 1: Eliciting Thoughts and Beliefs
That Underlie Addictive Behaviors

Everyone has thoughts and beliefs, but few people think carefully about what or how they think. The first step in helping people to change addictive behaviors involves learning about the thoughts and beliefs that underlie their addictive behaviors. This process of thinking about thinking, sometimes called *metacognition,* does not come naturally or automatically to most patients or therapists. As previously discussed, thoughts and beliefs (including thinking about thinking) must be repeated over and over to become automatic. Experienced therapists, who have been conducting CBT for a long time, (hopefully) find themselves asking questions like, "What were your thoughts right before you lit that cigarette?" or "What did you think as you entered the bar where you always used to drink?"

Knowledge of patients' thoughts and beliefs is vital to understanding the foundation on which their addictions are developed and maintained. By eliciting patients' thoughts and beliefs, therapists are able to understand essential themes and patterns underlying patients' addictive behaviors. For example, some heavy drinkers believe they cannot possibly socialize or function in their careers without drinking (e.g., "I'll have no friends," or "Everyone in my industry drinks"). Many cigarette smokers believe they will feel prolonged tension and irritability if they quit smoking (e.g., "I'm a miserable person without my cigarettes," or "My family can't stand me when I quit smoking"). Some daily marijuana smokers believe they cannot relax without smoking every day (e.g., "It's how I chill out," or "Weed is the only thing that keeps my anxiety at bay"). During Step 1, therapists have an opportunity to develop a deeper understanding of their patients by learning all they can about patients' private thoughts and beliefs.

Unfortunately, many clinicians who identify as cognitive-behavioral therapists minimize this vital first step in the therapy process. Rather than focusing
on thoughts and beliefs, they focus exclusively on behaviors. To some extent this
occurs because patients themselves tend to focus on behaviors instead of thoughts.
For example, patients may reflect exclusively on actions that lead to relapse, as follows: "I was at work and it was time to take our lunch break. We all went outside.
Mary lit a cigarette and so did Amy and Chelsea. When Mary offered me one, I
said yes, and she fired up her lighter. I ended up smoking the whole thing. It all
happened so fast."

When patients share narratives in this fashion, therapists have opportunities
to refocus on patients' thoughts and beliefs. Such questions like "Right before you
took your work break, what did you think about being around smokers?" or "As
you watched everyone light their cigarettes, what went through your mind?" By
repeatedly asking such questions, eliciting patients' thoughts and beliefs, therapists
teach patients to pay attention to their own thoughts and beliefs. The following
is a list of some additional open-ended questions for eliciting thoughts and beliefs
about addictive behaviors:

"What were your thoughts immediately before you chose to [smoke, drink,
    gamble, binge eat, etc.]?"
"What did you hope to accomplish by [smoking, drinking, gambling, binge
    eating, etc.]?"
"After you finished [smoking, drinking, gambling, binge eating, etc.], what
    thoughts went through your head?"
"What did you imagine it would be like to experience a lapse and return to
    [smoking, drinking, gambling, binge eating, etc.]?"
"Now that some time has passed since you [smoked, drank, gambled, binge
    ate, etc.], what do you believe about your ability to change?"

As patients respond to these questions, therapists pay close attention to
thoughts and beliefs that appear most pertinent to patients' addictive behaviors.
To further illustrate this process, we return to Kristen's session with her therapist:

THERAPIST: I'm interested in hearing more of your thoughts and beliefs
    about smoking.

KRISTEN: What do you want to know?

THERAPIST: I'd like you to choose a particular day this past week, perhaps
    when you were most concerned about your smoking, and I'll ask you
    some questions about that day.

KRISTEN: Oh, that's easy. Yesterday sucked. I blew through a full pack of cigarettes. Today I woke up feeling like crap. It was like a cigarette hang-over.

THERAPIST: Let's review your thoughts and beliefs from yesterday. When did you smoke your first cigarette and what were you thinking right before you smoked?

KRISTEN: It wasn't until around 10:00 A.M., which is later than usual. I actually woke up thinking "This is the day I quit smoking."

THERAPIST: Okay, you had the thought, "I'll quit today." But then you smoked a cigarette at 10:00 A.M. You must have had some motivating thoughts that led to smoking. Do you remember what they were?

KRISTEN: I was on the phone, talking to my ex-husband about his late child support check, and he hung up on me. He's such a jerk!

THERAPIST: So that was obviously a very stressful situation. What were you thinking, besides that he's a jerk?

KRISTEN: I was thinking I was really pissed off at him. And I didn't want Lilly to see me so angry at her father.

THERAPIST: So, your thoughts were . . .

KRISTEN: "I need to calm down." "I need a cigarette."

THERAPIST: And then what were your next thoughts?

KRISTEN: "I need a cigarette *now*."

THERAPIST: And then?

KRISTEN: I remember thinking, "I just can't handle this without a cigarette."

THERAPIST: That thought, "I just can't handle this," reminds me of thoughts that contributed to your depression.

KRISTEN: Oh yeah. You told me that my thoughts were all about helplessness. You said it was a pattern or a theme that I'd need to change.

In this exchange Kristen and her therapist began to determine that her helpless thoughts about smoking are similar to helpless thoughts that led to her depression. Her therapist was encouraged, given that Kristen was effective at addressing many of the helpless thoughts that led to her depression.

The process of eliciting thoughts and beliefs should continue until therapy is terminated. Patients gain substantial benefits from identifying their thoughts and beliefs throughout the course of therapy. However, the process of eliciting thoughts and beliefs is particularly vital during the earliest stages of CBT, when therapists first begin to conceptualize their patients and help their patients conceptualize themselves in new, adaptive ways.

Step 2: Facilitating Patients' Recognition and Understanding of Addiction-Related Thoughts and Beliefs

In Step 1 thoughts and beliefs are elicited, while in Step 2 thoughts and beliefs are mirrored back to patients with emphasis on their impact on emotions and behaviors. In Step 2, therapists provide considerable psychoeducation by teaching patients to recognize and understand their thoughts and beliefs. As mentioned earlier, entering into Step 2 does not mean that therapists stop eliciting thoughts and beliefs. Instead, it means that patients are repeatedly reminded that many of their thoughts play a role in the maintenance of their addictive behaviors. As he elicits Kristen's thoughts and beliefs, her therapist actually writes them on their notepad so Kristen can begin to recognize them and realize their significance.

> THERAPIST: Kristen, have you noticed that most of my recent questions are about your thoughts?
>
> KRISTEN: Yeah, that's how you helped me with my depression.
>
> THERAPIST: You learned to recognize and understand that your depression was largely due to your negative thinking. Now I'm asking about thoughts related to your cigarette smoking because I want to help you identify the thoughts that cause you to smoke. Without thoughts and beliefs about smoking, you wouldn't smoke. Smoking would never enter your mind. People who have never smoked cigarettes never think they need cigarettes to handle stress.
>
> KRISTEN: That makes sense.
>
> THERAPIST: All of your thoughts about smoking that involve hopelessness and helplessness put you at risk for smoking. For example, "I can't quit," "I'm not capable," "I'm not worth it," "I never do anything right," and so forth. These kinds of thoughts also put you at risk for depression.
>
> KRISTEN: Those *are* the same kinds of thoughts, aren't they?
>
> THERAPIST: Yes. You see the pattern.

This process of guided discovery (described in detail in Chapter 6) continues throughout the course of therapy. As long as Kristen puts smoking cessation on the agenda, her therapist asks detailed questions about her successful and unsuccessful efforts to quit. When she describes lapses, or times she has smoked, the therapist helps her identify triggers. But equally or more important, the focus turns to thoughts and beliefs activated by these triggers.

When Kristen describes *success* at resisting urges to smoke, her therapist highlights the specific thoughts and beliefs that enable her to resist smoking. At these times, Kristen's therapist emphasizes that Kristen must initially activate System 2 thinking to resist urges to smoke. She is reminded that deliberate, intentional thinking enables her to abstain from lighting up. Kristen is reassured that this effortful System 2 thinking will eventually become automatic through repetition, as it evolves into System 1 thinking. We elaborate on this process in the next section.

Step 3: Developing and Maintaining Thoughts and Beliefs That Support Change

As patients recognize and understand the role of thoughts and beliefs that underlie their addictive behaviors, they begin to associate these with opposing (i.e., change-related) thoughts and beliefs. For example, as they realize that thoughts like, "I can't possibly quit right now," perpetuate their smoking, they also realize that *this is just a thought,* and perhaps they *can* quit right now. A common error that occurs when helping patients with addictions is that they are prematurely urged to change their thoughts and beliefs, often by well-meaning clinicians, without regard for their readiness to make such changes. Perhaps a more common error is that changes are recommended without regard for the powerful influence of automatic System 1 thinking.

Working with and Explaining Ambivalence

Ambivalence occurs when individuals have contradictory thoughts and beliefs about matters of importance to them. Most people experience ambivalence while trying to change or abstain from addictive behaviors. For example, an individual might simultaneously think, "I love getting high," while also thinking, "This is killing me." Ambivalence is most common during the contemplation stage of change, but it also manifests during the action stage of change. In fact, many people in recovery move from contemplation, to preparation, to action, enthusiastic about change, only to become ambivalent as their old automatic addiction-related thoughts creep in. They may find themselves, for example, waking up in the morning thinking "Today's a great day to quit." But by noon they may think, "Today's not such a good day to quit." And by evening they may be using again.

We recommend that therapists think of ambivalence as *the inevitable cognitive bridge between addiction and change.* Therapists can validate and explain ambivalence (rather than fight it) by understanding and teaching patients that ambivalence is their *change-related thinking* (System 2) battling their automatic *addiction-related thinking* (System 1) for dominance.

Kristen has only recently become committed to becoming a nonsmoker, and her lapses reflect substantial ambivalence. Until recently, many of her thoughts and beliefs about smoking were consistent with the themes of helplessness, weakness, and inadequacy. These thoughts existed before she became clinically depressed, and they were magnified when she was fully depressed. It was only after she began to recover from depression that she became ready to develop more resilient thoughts and beliefs about her ability to make changes in her life. Kristen's therapist begins to focus on these thoughts and beliefs in the following exchange:

THERAPIST: Now that you recognize the thoughts and beliefs that lead to smoking, it's important to establish thoughts and beliefs that support the change you want to make.

KRISTEN: That's nice in theory, but how do I get these new thoughts to knock out the old ones?

THERAPIST: Like we've discussed in the past, the new thoughts need to be repeated over and over until they are under the control of System 1 thinking. Let's start by talking about this battle between your old thoughts and your new thoughts.

KRISTEN: What do you want to know?

THERAPIST: For example, you told me that you woke up one morning thinking, "Today's the day I quit." And then after talking to your ex-husband you started smoking again. You explained that your thoughts revolved around controlling your emotions, and not wanting to be angry in front of Lilly.

KRISTEN: That's right.

THERAPIST: When you first woke up, what led you to think "Today's the day I quit"? What prior thoughts caused you to draw that conclusion?

KRISTEN: I remember it was a beautiful day. I had fun plans to take Lilly to the park. I couldn't imagine how smoking a cigarette would make the day any better. I even thought, "How could anyone want to smoke a filthy, dirty cigarette on such a pretty day?" I thought, "I can do this!"

THERAPIST: You had lots of change-related thoughts that morning, before 10:00 A.M. Let's write them down [*He gives the writing pad to Kristen, who writes as he talks*]: "It's a beautiful day." "I'm going to the park with Lilly." "Smoking a cigarette couldn't possibly make this day any better." "I don't want to smoke a filthy, dirty cigarette." "I can do this!"

KRISTEN: [*Looking down at the words written on her pad.*] These are some empowering thoughts.

THERAPIST: Yes, but they still haven't won the battle over your old automatic thoughts about smoking. You are still ambivalent about quitting smoking.

KRISTEN: Ambivalent?

THERAPIST: That's when you have thoughts about cigarette smoking that are both pro and con, for and against.

KRISTEN: Yeah, I guess I still have both.

THERAPIST: You've gotten off to a good start by writing down thoughts that support the change you want to make. We want to fully establish these new thoughts in your mind, until you're no longer ambivalent.

KRISTEN: What if I write them on sticky notes and put them all over my apartment—and even in my car?

THERAPIST: That's a terrific idea. We want them to be so well established that they are primary—as in System 1—instead of secondary—as in System 2.

KRISTEN: So that's the secret. Move the new thoughts into System 1 so they are automatic . . . and louder than the old thoughts about smoking. This all makes good sense.

Guided Discovery and Psychoeducation in Action

As noted earlier, Kristen's therapist used guided discovery and psychoeducation to help Kristen make sense of her recent slip and her ambivalence about smoking and quitting. They worked together to establish thoughts and beliefs that support change, and her therapist reflected on cognitive processes (System 1 and System 2 thinking) that operate while she feels ambivalent.

Guided discovery should be continuously used to elicit patients' addiction-related thoughts and beliefs and replace them with more adaptive, change-related thoughts and beliefs. Regardless of the particular addiction, guided discovery stimulates patients to examine their addictive thoughts and beliefs and begin to replace them with change-related beliefs. Some specific questions that introduce new change-oriented beliefs are the following:

"What are the negative consequences of your [addictive behavior]?"
"How else can you think about your [addictive behavior]?"
"What would you do if your [addictive behavior] weren't available?"
"What else can you do to achieve the same results, instead of your [addictive behavior]?"

Earlier it was noted that addictive behaviors almost always involve thinking errors. Guided discovery can also be used to help patients examine evidence for and against their addictive behaviors. Examination of addiction-related beliefs involves asking patients probing questions that test the validity of these beliefs. The following are examples of questions appropriate for this process:

"How confident are you in that thought or belief about your [addictive behavior]?"
"Where did you learn that thought or belief?"

"How do you know that your thought or belief is true?"
"What is your evidence for that thought or belief?"
"What are some other ways to think about your situation?"

These questions are helpful in challenging addiction-related thoughts and beliefs, as well as supporting change-related thoughts and beliefs. They enable patients to realize that many of their addiction-related thoughts and beliefs are unfounded, while many of their change-related thoughts can come true.

Imaginal Exposure

Programmed practice in sessions, via imaginal exposure, is another tool for helping patients establish and maintain change-related beliefs. In this practice, patients are encouraged to imagine a situation associated with addictive behaviors. As this situation evokes craving in patients, they are helped to activate change-related beliefs to reduce urges and craving. The following dialogue between Kristen and her therapist illustrates this technique:

THERAPIST: Let's try a brief activity. I would like you to go back in your mind to the moment when your ex-husband hung up on you.

KRISTEN: Do I have to? Just kidding, I know that I need to get better at this.

THERAPIST: Alright, can you remember again what you thought and felt?

KRISTEN: [*Sits up straight in her chair.*] As if it just happened.

THERAPIST: What are you feeling and thinking right now, as you recall that scene?

KRISTEN: Like I said earlier, I feel angry and I'm thinking a cigarette will calm me down.

THERAPIST: And what are you thinking and feeling next?

KRISTEN: Like I want to smoke.

THERAPIST: What does that feel like?

KRISTEN: It's like a powerful urge. Like an intense craving.

THERAPIST: On a scale from one to ten, how strong is the feeling of craving?

KRISTEN: After I slam the phone down, it's a four or five. I'm just really pissed.

THERAPIST: And then?

KRISTEN: I can feel the urge grow. It gets bigger and bigger.

THERAPIST: And how big, from one to ten?

KRISTEN: When I finally decide to smoke, it's a full-blown ten.

THERAPIST: Can you feel that now?

KRISTEN: Yeah, I'm starting to crave a cigarette just sitting here thinking about it.

THERAPIST: Now let's try this. I want you to start talking to yourself, using the change-oriented language we discussed earlier.

KRISTEN: You mean the thoughts that are supposed to keep me from smoking?

THERAPIST: Yes.

KRISTEN: [*Thinks for a while.*] Okay, smoking is gross and disgusting. It's bad for me and Lilly. I don't want to model smoking for my daughter. I'm better than that. She deserves better. [*She starts to get teary-eyed.*]

THERAPIST: What are you thinking and feeling right now?

KRISTEN: You probably think I'm getting sad, but I'm actually picturing Lilly and thinking about how much I love her. In a way it feels really good. [*Points to her eyes.*] These are tears of joy.

THERAPIST: How strong is that craving you started to feel earlier?

KRISTEN: What craving? [*Laughs.*]

This process of imaginal exposure with change-oriented responses is repeated several times over the next few sessions with Kristen. And of course, she is encouraged to practice this exercise as homework, whether or not she is tempted to smoke. In each subsequent session, she reports that she has done her homework and it is quite helpful.

Automatic Thought Records and Advantages–Disadvantages Analyses

Another strategy for examining and testing addictive beliefs is the automatic thought record (ATR; Chapter 7). The ATR is a standardized form for listing and modifying addiction-related thoughts. Regardless of the addiction, it is useful for examining and modifying thoughts and beliefs that might lead to any step in the addiction process. For example, it can be used to realize the potential risk related to spending time with friends with addictions, or it can be used to realize thoughts that stop addictive behaviors just before they occur. Specifically, the ATR has five columns: situations; automatic thoughts or related beliefs; emotions; alternative thoughts, beliefs, or responses; and outcomes (see example of ATR in Figure 7.3). When patients experience an urge or craving, they list automatic thoughts and beliefs that precipitate them. Then, in the alternate beliefs column they list change-oriented beliefs. For example, if the addictive belief is, "I can't stand the stress without [drinking, smoking, gambling, etc.]," the change-oriented response might be, "Yes, I can. In fact, there are many days when I feel better because I don't [drink, smoke, gamble, etc.]."

Another strategy for developing control beliefs is the advantages–disadvantages analysis (ADA; Chapter 7). The purpose of the ADA is to redirect the patient's attention to the advantages and disadvantages of engaging in their addictive behaviors. Patients are helped to construct a four-cell matrix where the advantages and disadvantages of two alternative decisions are compared (see Form 7.1). In most cases, this exercise enables therapists and patients to highlight the advantages of change and the disadvantages of continuing addictive behaviors.

Step 4: Anticipating Roadblocks to Changing Thoughts and Beliefs

Changing thoughts, beliefs, and ultimately addictive behaviors, is difficult. In just moments, confidence can turn into ambivalence, ambivalence can turn into a lapse, and a lapse can turn into a relapse. In fact, patients will encounter numerous triggers that will activate old addiction-related thoughts and beliefs. Hence, roadblocks can certainly involve triggers. But we consider System 1 addiction-related thoughts and beliefs to be the primary roadblocks to changing thoughts and beliefs. In other words, we consider patients' automatic, spontaneous, reflexive, and impulsive addiction-related thoughts to be the most likely barriers to change.

Patients' understanding of System 1 and System 2 thinking helps them prepare for and respond to roadblocks to change. Faced with stressful, complex, difficult, or novel circumstances, patients learn that their System 2 battle against old addiction-related thoughts is necessary for maintaining abstinence from addictive behaviors. Hence, we continually discuss these thinking processes and help patients imagine how they will use System 2 thinking in their recovery. The following is an exchange between Kristen and her therapist, occurring several minutes into one of their sessions. This discussion begins with Kristen reporting that she has not smoked for an entire week, but abstinence has not been easy:

KRISTEN: It's been a roller-coaster of a week.

THERAPIST: Explain.

KRISTEN: I haven't smoked, but it hasn't been easy.

THERAPIST: What's made it difficult?

KRISTEN: At times, the craving has been excruciatingly painful.

THERAPIST: Congratulations on abstaining for an entire week. What made the craving so painful?

KRISTEN: I'm not sure. I got rid of all my cigarettes, lighters, and ashtrays, so it would be impossible to just start smoking, but I really wanted to.

THERAPIST: Can you recall a particularly difficult time?

KRISTEN: Yeah, of course. I sat down to pay my bills Wednesday night, and realized that I wouldn't have enough money to pay them this month. I could feel my heart starting to pound in my chest as I got more and more worried, trying to decide which I could pay and which would have to wait.

THERAPIST: And then?

KRISTEN: Of course I thought, "I need a cigarette."

THERAPIST: Keep going. Tell me more about your thoughts.

KRISTEN: I went back and forth. I thought I wanted one and then I told myself I didn't want one. I realized that I didn't have any cigarettes, so I started to think about how I'd get my hands on a pack of cigarettes. I told myself I would just take a few puffs and throw the rest of the pack away. Lilly was sleeping. I even thought about taking a quick trip to the convenience store to buy a pack.

THERAPIST: You had lots of thoughts about smoking: relief-oriented, instrumental, and even permissive thoughts. And all these thoughts were doing battle with your fresh, new thoughts about staying healthy and being a good role model for Lilly. But then, somehow, the fresh, new thoughts won out. How'd that happen?

KRISTEN: First, I walked around my apartment, reading my sticky notes and remembering why I'm not smoking anymore. Then I looked into Lilly's bedroom and saw her there, sleeping safely and peacefully, and that's when it really hit me. It suddenly felt like a matter of life and death. And I chose life.

THERAPIST: Wow! In response to intense anxiety about not being able to pay your bills, you were flooded with System 1 thoughts about smoking, and you used your best System 2 thinking to win the battle!

KRISTEN: I guess that's what happened.

THERAPIST: Kristen, you're living proof that some triggers, like your financial challenges, are inevitable and can't necessarily be avoided. You're learning that your efforts to be a nonsmoker will run into roadblocks when you encounter triggers. But the real roadblocks are not the triggers themselves; they are the old automatic thoughts and beliefs that still tell you to smoke. You exerted a lot of deliberate effort to get around these roadblocks and win that battle. Congratulations!

As noted in this exchange, the actual roadblock that Kristen overcame was her stubborn System 1 addiction-related thinking. The trigger, anxiety related to financial problems, was unavoidable in her case, so the solution had to be an effective coping response. In a recent therapy session, she anticipated that there would be System 1 roadblocks interfering with her new, healthy thinking, so she prepared for these by posting System 2 reminders around her home. She also activated her most powerful System 2 thought: "I love Lilly more than I love cigarettes."

Step 5: Practicing Strategies That Increase the Salience and Durability of New Adaptive Thoughts and Beliefs

Repetition is the key to moving new System 2 thinking (e.g., "I am no longer a smoker.") into the position of System 1 thinking. Hence, practice is necessary for increasing the salience and durability of these new adaptive thoughts and beliefs. As patients identify new thoughts and beliefs, they are encouraged to choose various methods for remembering these and committing them to System 1. In an earlier dialogue, Kristen suggested that sticky notes, posted in prominent places, might serve this purpose. Other patients might consider the creation of flashcards to activate and reinforce these newly developed beliefs. For example, patients might consider writing addiction-related beliefs on one side of a card, and change-related beliefs on the opposite side.

The most important consideration in choosing techniques is the degree to which the patient appears invested in the techniques that are eventually chosen. This can be determined in session as various techniques are discussed. Patients should be asked, "Can you think of any activities that might help you to remember these new thoughts and beliefs that support change?" Depending on the answer, therapists might either suggest techniques (when patients say they cannot think of any), or they may simply reinforce ideas offered by patients. Given that most people carry and use smart phones, many techniques for establishing and maintaining change-related thoughts are likely to involve electronic media.

Homework provides the best opportunity for rehearsing change-oriented thoughts and beliefs. Hence, patients are continually reminded to notice triggers in their lives and pay attention to their reasons for making changes. Homework may involve any activity that enables activating change-oriented beliefs in the face of tempting high-risk triggers. As mentioned earlier, people who have struggled with addictions cannot possibly avoid all triggers for the rest of their lives. Kristen, for example, is unlikely to improve her finances in the near future, so she is encouraged by her therapist to review her bills on a daily basis, observe her anxiety without panicking, and remind herself that smoking will not make the bills go away. In fact, she can remind herself that cigarettes cost money, and now more money is available for paying her bills. As explained in Chapter 5, homework is assigned at the end of each session and reviewed at the beginning of each session. Initially, homework is quite structured. For example, patients are instructed to complete ATRs on a daily basis. Later, however, homework can be less formal, as the patient develops new, more adaptive, patterns of thinking.

SUMMARY

In this chapter we have discussed the importance of focusing on specific thoughts and beliefs when working with people who struggle with addictions. We have explained that certain thought *processes* play a role in developing, maintaining, and changing addictive behaviors. But perhaps more importantly, we described two thinking patterns, or *systems,* that profoundly influence how people become addicted, stay addicted, and then struggle to end addictive behaviors. These two systems operate in all people to accomplish and regulate human functioning. System 1 is responsible for day-to-day activities. It allows us to develop habits, so it is not necessary to deliberate about every action we take. Life would be terribly difficult if System 1 thinking did not exist. System 2 thinking is available on standby to address the more complex problems that System 1 thinking is not equipped to solve. System 2 is ready and waiting to be activated when System 1 fails to meet our needs.

Walking, talking, sitting, standing, waving at a friend, hugging a loved one, and lending an immediate helping hand to someone in need are all examples of actions that are possible thanks to System 1 thinking. These behaviors, like countless others, require no conscious, deliberate processing. Unfortunately for people who struggle with addictions, the many behaviors associated with their addiction reside in System 1. At some point in their lives, most eventually conclude that it's time to make changes. However, upon doing so they quickly discover that their addictive behaviors have become so automatic that a strong, sustained, deliberate effort is needed to overcome their addictions.

Therapists who work with people with addictions need to understand this process in order to be helpful. They also need to explain this process to their patients, who want to know *why* it's so hard to change addictive behaviors and *how* they can make changes. Both therapists and patients need to understand System 1 and System 2 thinking in order to be patient as System 2 chips away at System 1 habits. There are techniques and exercises that facilitate System 2 thinking. With much repetition, System 2 thinking transitions into System 1 thinking. Instead of addiction-related thoughts being in charge, new thoughts are in charge that make life without addiction possible. When this occurs, therapists get to congratulate their patients for a job well done.

CHAPTER 11

MODES AND
ADDICTIVE BEHAVIORS

Phil is 46 years old. He lives with his wife, Laura, and two daughters, Molly and Cyndi. Many people in his community know Phil and admire him. He is a successful businessman, widely respected for his generous support of worthy local causes. He is on the boards of several nonprofit organizations, including the county homeless shelter and community food pantry. Besides being successful, Phil is known to be warm, friendly, and gregarious. His friends describe him as a *Renaissance Man*.

But Phil has a secret. He has been a heavy drinker for most of his adult life, desperately afraid of turning out like his father who died as a result of cirrhosis. Phil has often tried to stop, or at least cut down on his drinking, but he has been unsuccessful at doing so. He has tried reducing the number of days he drinks and the number of drinks he consumes daily but neither effort has been successful. Besides being concerned about *how much he drinks* Phil is worried about *how he behaves when he drinks*. He vividly recalls that his father was "an angry drunk" and Phil often feels angry when he drinks. Sometimes he jokingly admits, "The apple doesn't fall far from the tree." Phil is not the only one concerned about his drinking. Laura, Molly, and Cyndi have all become increasingly frustrated with Phil as he drinks every night, becomes irritable, and finds reasons to complain about a wide range of issues.

A THEORY OF MODES

It is common for individuals with addictions to think, feel, and behave differently when they are engaged in addictive behaviors versus when they are not. Recently, Dr. Beck has written about his theory of modes (Beck, Finkel, & Beck, 2021), a particularly useful approach to conceptualizing differences in people when they

206

are engaged in addictive behaviors versus when they are not. Dr. Beck began to formulate his theory of modes years ago as he observed the differences between patients when they were depressed or anxious versus when they were not depressed or anxious. He even noted that people with schizophrenia would shift from being socially withdrawn, psychotic, and aggressive to being "energetic, communicative, friendly, and totally in touch with reality" (p. 393). Dr. Beck identified the various patterns of functioning in the same individual as their different modes.

A *mode* is a pattern, or thread, of human functioning that involves cognition, affect, motivation, behavior, and corresponding physiologic responses. Phil, described above, clearly has two modes of functioning. When Phil is not drinking, his mode is highly *adaptive*. For example, when he is at work his thoughts are generally positive. As a result, his affect is cheerful, he is motivated to do good, his behaviors are engaging, and he feels physically at ease. In contrast, when he arrives home a variety of triggers (e.g., the time of day, bourbon in the liquor cabinet, the absence of social validation, and internal restlessness) activate his thoughts about drinking—and quite automatically he begins to drink. Upon doing so, he reverts into a *maladaptive* mode: one characterized by negative thoughts, irritable feelings, counterproductive motives, unpleasant behaviors, and physical tension.

Beck et al. (2021) have explained that modes are activated automatically, and when individuals risk entering into maladaptive modes it is a *superordinate cognitive process* that keeps these modes from being activated. For example, entry into an angry mode might be met with a higher order set of thoughts that sound something like, "Don't go there. Anger will only make things worse." Beck and his colleagues have further explained that these superordinate processes may be impaired by substance use. Beck has recently stated explicitly that people who are engaging in addictive behaviors "make maladaptive decisions that defy logic or reason. This may be due to the inability to access one's cognitive resources and take part in reflective, adaptive thought processes as well as a loosening of inhibition" (Beck et al., 2021, p. 395).

Origins and Manifestations of Phil's Two Modes

After a particularly difficult evening with his family, Phil finally decided to discuss his alcohol concerns with a health care professional. He visited his family physician, who recommended a cognitive-behavioral therapist specializing in addictions. In their initial visit the therapist inquires about Phil's family history. In doing so he uncovers Phil's concern about becoming like his father:

THERAPIST: You have mentioned your father several times. Tell me more about him. What was he like?

PHIL: He would come home from a long day at work, give us all a quick hello, and head for the kitchen. I would hear the clinking of ice in his glass, the opening of the liquor cabinet, liquid pouring from a whiskey bottle, and the splash of water from the faucet, and I knew he'd be heading for his favorite chair in the living room.

THERAPIST: And then?

PHIL: At first, he'd be fine. If any of us were around he would start out pleasant. And then, with each refill, he'd become increasingly surly.

THERAPIST: Surly?

PHIL: Yeah, he'd become grumpy. We'd all know when it was time to leave him alone and do our own thing.

THERAPIST: Tell me more about your father.

PHIL: Like what?

THERAPIST: Like what was he like when he wasn't drinking?

PHIL: He was different. On the surface he was a friendly, outgoing guy. He didn't know any strangers. Everyone was an instant friend.

THERAPIST: How do you understand your father's different personalities? His good and bad dispositions, besides the alcohol?

PHIL: He had a rough upbringing. His dad, my grandfather, was a nasty drunk most of the time. Dad once told me, after he'd had a few drinks, that my grandfather made it hard to be a kid . . . that there were even times when my dad got pretty depressed.

THERAPIST: So, your dad may have occasionally struggled with depression. And he had two modes: one when he was drinking and the other when he wasn't drinking.

PHIL: Yeah, I guess you could call them modes.

THERAPIST: I wonder if he drank to self-medicate. You know, as a way of warding off depression.

PHIL: That makes sense.

THERAPIST: But the drinking itself actually caused the opposite to happen. Instead of making him feel better, it allowed the other mode to set in: the one that was grumpy. Or even miserable.

PHIL: I get where you're going with this. You're describing me, aren't you?

THERAPIST: I'm asking you to describe your father so I can better understand what you might have witnessed and ultimately learned from him.

PHIL: [Looking down at the floor.] You're making me realize my worst fear.

Phil's therapist is beginning to understand that Phil and his father have had two predominant modes. One is friendly, outgoing, and sociable. The other is unhappy, sullen, and detached from others. In fact, Phil and his father developed both adaptive and maladaptive modes over time. Phil's adaptive mode is activated in validating social situations, particularly when he is not drinking. His maladaptive mode is activated in situations that are less validating, and especially when he has started to drink. Phil's wife and daughters love him, but they do not shower him with the recognition that he receives from the community. And in addition to the recognition, Phil experiences a great deal of intellectual stimulation through his community activities. He certainly does not experience a similar level of stimulation at home, especially after he begins to drink. In fact, the opposite occurs. Rather than feeling stimulated, Phil feels numb, and even bored, as he sits alone in front of the television with his bourbon and water. As he continues to drink, he is less able to deactivate thoughts about his own inadequacy, and he turns his self-loathing thoughts toward his family. This pattern continues until everyone in his home feels invalidated, including himself, his wife, and their two daughters.

As Phil's therapist identifies this pattern, he realizes that Phil needs to activate the same adaptive mode at home that he activates at work and in public. His therapist asks about his adaptive mode and then helps Phil realize that he needs to consistently activate it at home. He helps Phil understand that his gregarious mode contributes to the positive outcomes he so enjoys in public and at work, and Phil needs to activate the same active, energetic mode with Laura and his daughters. Beck et al. (2021) explained, "In therapy, we call the elements that activate this energy and passion in individuals the 'sweet spot'" (p. 397). The following exchange demonstrates how Phil's therapist guides him to an understanding of the *sweet spot:*

THERAPIST: Phil, you really like being at work and out in the community, don't you?

PHIL: Yeah, you could say that.

THERAPIST: What happens when you get home?

PHIL: What do you mean?

THERAPIST: How is being at work different from being at home?

PHIL: I don't know. I guess I find work and friends to be interesting and stimulating. I'm around people who have lots of energy. They are enthusiastic about their work and what we're achieving together.

THERAPIST: And what about being at home?

PHIL: Uhhh . . . [*Pauses for some time.*] I don't usually compare the two like this. I guess when I get home I walk through the front door, try to relax, have a few drinks, open my mouth, and get myself into big trouble.

THERAPIST: So, the stimulation and validation seem to come to a screeching halt when you arrive home and you start thinking, "Time for a bourbon."

PHIL: Pretty much.

THERAPIST: Phil, it seems to me that you become energetic and passionate when you're engaged in stimulating activities where people appreciate you.

PHIL: That's right. That's when time just seems to fly by.

THERAPIST: This might sound like a funny term, but that's your *sweet spot*. It's when all the elements that activate your *best self* are present and your mode is most adaptive: typically, when you're engaged in stimulating activities and people appreciate you.

PHIL: Maybe I should never come home . . . just kidding. [*Laughs nervously.*]

THERAPIST: I have another idea. What if you came home and acted as energetic and passionate with your family as you do at work and with other people?

PHIL: My family would probably think my body was inhabited by aliens! [*Laughs again, but then pauses to more seriously consider what the therapist has just suggested.*] There might be some merit to that idea. But how would I do it?

THERAPIST: That's what we need to figure out together.

In this exchange, Phil and his therapist have begun to imagine a more adaptive mode when Phil comes home. His therapist has introduced the idea that Phil might have some agency in making his home a more stimulating environment. He has begun to assist Phil in extending this more positive mode by engaging in the same adaptive thoughts and behaviors at home as he does elsewhere. As they continue, Phil's therapist avoids confronting Phil about his drinking. Instead he guides Phil to realize that it will be difficult for Phil to activate his more adaptive mode while under the influence of alcohol:

THERAPIST: Phil, you seem on board with the idea of changing how you relate to your family when you arrive home.

PHIL: It's becoming more obvious that I'm my best self when I'm fully engaged with people, doing things I like to do, and doing them well.

THERAPIST: How might that happen at home?

PHIL: You mean what am I going to change?

THERAPIST: Yes, when you get home.

PHIL: Well, my wife Laura always asks how my day went, and I guess I could talk to her about it, though I don't know that I'd do it with energy and passion.

THERAPIST: That sounds like a good step—talking to Laura about your work. When was the last time you did something fun with her? or Molly? or Cyndi?

PHIL: It's been a while. [*Stops and thinks.*] They love going out for ice cream.

THERAPIST: What about you?

PHIL: Who doesn't love ice cream?

THERAPIST: When was the last time you did that?

PHIL: I can't even remember. Maybe I should put it on the calendar.

THERAPIST: On the calendar?

PHIL: Okay, maybe this week.

THERAPIST: Have you enjoyed going for ice cream with them in the past? And being in their company?

PHIL: Yeah. [*Pauses and looks down at the floor.*] I really suck at being a husband and father.

THERAPIST: Sounds like you're just out of practice. I notice that you haven't said anything about drinking.

PHIL: What do you mean?

THERAPIST: I mean you're thinking about going out with your family for ice cream after work this week, right?

PHIL: Yeah.

THERAPIST: Will you be drinking before you go?

PHIL: [*Looks surprised at the question.*] Definitely not. I never drink and drive.

THERAPIST: Are there other reasons for avoiding alcohol before going out to get ice cream?

PHIL: I get where you're going with this. I've been in a vicious cycle, where I come home, start to feel miserable, drink to feel better, feel worse, treat my family terrible, cause them to hate me, and then drink when I get home to avoid how much they hate me.

THERAPIST: I've never gotten the feeling that your family hates you. In fact, I bet they miss you. Let's see how your ice cream adventure goes, without alcohol, and see if they act like they hate you. This might even lead to a different mode.

PHIL: You mean like a *new* mode?

THERAPIST: No, actually I mean the mode you so enjoy outside of your home, but with your family instead.

PHIL: That would be great.

Phil's therapist has only just begun to explain modes to him. He has not yet provided any details about the dynamics of modes: the fact that they are patterns of thoughts, feelings, behaviors, and physiological responses that can be controlled by controlling a variety of processes. In the section that follows, we provide more strategies for working with modes.

WORKING WITH MODES

The term *mode* is useful in therapy as shorthand for certain thought, feeling, and behavior threads and patterns. For example, rather than explaining to a patient, "When you encounter certain stimuli, they tend to activate various thoughts, beliefs, and schemas, which ultimately lead to various physiologic responses, emotions, and behaviors," therapists might delay such complex descriptions and simply say, "It sounds like you get into an angry mode," or "It sounds like you get into a helpless mode." A more detailed explanation of these modes can then follow as patients learn to identify and label their own specific thoughts, feelings, behaviors, and physiological responses.

Addictive behaviors are often initiated, or begun, by individuals attempting to achieve desired modes (e.g., friendly, playful, relaxed, or courageous modes). That is, people choose to start drinking, smoking, gambling, binge eating, and so forth when they think any of these behaviors will make them feel and act in patterned ways that are rewarding, or at least satisfying. For example, adolescents might start smoking or drinking to get into a *popular* mode. College students might start using amphetamines to get into a *studious* or *partying* mode. Some people might binge eat highly palatable foods to get into a *comfort* mode. Some might start gambling in order to get into a *winning* mode. Some people might use certain drugs (e.g., opioids, benzodiazepines) or even online gaming to get into an *escape* mode. Others might start using certain drugs (e.g., methamphetamine, cocaine) to enter into a *power* mode or *productive* mode.

Problems arise when people continue to engage in these behaviors despite negative consequences: for example, when heavy alcohol use no longer results in popularity, gambling no longer results in net winnings, and drugs no longer provide escape. Rather than engagement resulting in a desired mode, it results in a highly undesired mode (e.g., a depressed, anxious, angry, or other uncomfortable mode). Among the reasons why this occurs is that most people become *tolerant* to addictive behaviors, needing increasing amounts to get the same effect, until eventually their originally desired mode is no longer achievable. This is referred to by many as "chasing the high." In the exchange that follows, Phil and his therapist discuss how this process transpired as Phil developed his alcohol use disorder:

THERAPIST: Phil, how old were you when you started drinking?

PHIL: I was around 16 years old. It was during the summer between my freshman and sophomore year of high school. A few of us would go to the beach and we would take turns supplying the alcohol, like a couple of six packs or a bottle of something. And someone would always bring a pack of cigarettes. I can almost remember how the booze tasted back then. We would all get drunk and smoke cigarettes, right on the beach. The booze was always cheap and gross. And I remember the cigarettes being really disgusting. I'm glad I never developed that nasty habit.

THERAPIST: If the booze and cigarettes were gross and disgusting, why did you partake?

PHIL: Oh, come on, you know the answer to that question: It was the cool thing to do.

THERAPIST: How would you have felt if you didn't drink or smoke with your friends?

PHIL: I would have felt like a freak ... like an outsider.

THERAPIST: So back then you wanted to avoid the *outsider* mode and get into the *cool kid* mode.

PHIL: Yeah, exactly. Doesn't every kid want to be cool?

THERAPIST: How long did the *cool kid* mode last? And how did it turn into the *angry* mode?

PHIL: I can't put my finger on a particular date or time, but I remember when I was old enough to go into bars even the smallest act of disrespect by a stranger would get me pissed off. I don't like to admit this, but I've been in more than a few bar fights.

THERAPIST: How do you think alcohol got you into an angry mode?

PHIL: It might have had something to do with how much I was drinking. When I first started to drink, just a small amount would get me tipsy and I'd have a good time. As I got older, I would drink more and more. It was like I lost control.

THERAPIST: It sounds like you developed a tolerance to alcohol and eventually started drinking so much that you could no long inhibit or hide from your unhappiness.

PHIL: Why would I be unhappy back then?

THERAPIST: You've told me that your father was a nasty drunk who would take his anger out on the family, including you. You've mentioned that depression runs in your family. It's very possible that your early drinking inhibited your feelings of depression and anger. It contributed to a happy *cool kid* mode. Then later, increasing amounts of alcohol had the opposite effect; it put you in an *angry* and maybe even a *depressed* mode. You know, alcohol does act like a depressant in a lot of people.

PHIL: That makes sense. Now that you mention it, I think I successfully inhibit a lot of anger when I'm *not* drinking.

THERAPIST: What do you mean?

PHIL: Everyone in my community seems to think I'm the most happy-go-lucky guy on the planet. They don't know that lots of little things irritate me.

THERAPIST: Like what?

PHIL: Like when people are late. Or when they promise to do things, but don't deliver.

THERAPIST: That's when you inhibit your anger?

PHIL: Yeah. I tell myself that it's okay . . . that it's not a big deal . . . that the world won't come to an end.

THERAPIST: And that's how you stay in a good, adaptive mode. When you're not drinking, you're good at talking yourself down instead of getting angry. So getting back to how your *angry* mode began. When you drank, small things would trigger angry, aggressive thoughts. At the time you'd have had too much to drink, and the *good guy* mode would certainly not prevail.

PHIL: That's when I must have started to become my father. These days I'll be sitting at home and my wife or daughters will do something really small and insignificant. I find myself feeling irritated, thinking, "That was stupid," and I get into an angry *mood*. Or as you call it, an angry *mode*. And sometimes I might drink more at home, thinking it will make me feel better, like mellow, but it never does.

THERAPIST: So, you're unable to maintain the *good guy* mode when you start drinking. And you have a lot of negative thoughts around your family.

PHIL: My family and just about anything else: religion, politics, social injustice, climate change. You name it and I'll let it bug me.

During this exchange, emphasis was placed on Phil's original motivation to drink, in order to escape feelings of anxiety and depression. His therapist helped him understand that drinking accomplished this at an earlier time in his life, until eventually he needed to drink so much (i.e., he became so tolerant to alcohol) that it no longer worked for him.

There are multiple benefits to focusing on modes in CBT. For example, most patients readily understand the meaning of the term *mode*. The term provides a convenient way for patients to identify and label salient thought, feeling, and behavior patterns (or *threads*). They can be used to help patients understand that their early experiences with addictive behaviors were largely aimed at achieving modes that are no longer achievable in their current relationship with addictive behaviors. Furthermore, people with addictions can be taught that adaptive modes can be activated in ways that do not require engagement in addictive behaviors. Rather than seeking comfort, power, popularity, or escape modes through addictive behaviors, patients might actually achieve healthier, more adaptive modes by developing coping skills, healthy lifestyles, and positive relationships. In the following exchange, Phil's therapist inquires about Phil's homework from the previous session (activating his adaptive mode during a family outing for ice cream):

THERAPIST: Phil, do you recall any homework from our last visit?

PHIL: I was supposed to take my family out for ice cream, and I did. It went much better than I thought.

THERAPIST: Tell me more.

PHIL: I got home and everyone was there. I suggested that we go out for ice cream after dinner, and just like I predicted, they looked at me like I was an alien—but of course they said yes. It was at that moment that I realized I wouldn't be able to drink for a couple of hours, since we needed to eat dinner before going for ice cream, and they all agreed to go.

THERAPIST: I want to hear how it all went.

PHIL: I was surprised at how pleasant dinner was. I thought it would be pretty hard, without taking even one drink, but it wasn't that bad. Nobody acted like they noticed that I wasn't drinking, but I'm sure they did.

THERAPIST: No one ever brought up the topic of drinking?

PHIL: No, should I have?

THERAPIST: Not necessarily. So, what happened at dinner and afterward?

PHIL: We talked about a bunch of things at dinner, there was some laughter, and before you knew it we were headed for ice cream.

THERAPIST: Phil, you're getting teary-eyed.

PHIL: I'm starting to realize how much I've been missing.

THERAPIST: What have you been missing?

PHIL: I've almost forgotten how beautiful my girls are. And Laura, too. [*Starts to sob, reaches for a tissue, and blows his nose.*]

THERAPIST: [*Begins after Phil has stopped crying and is able to focus again.*] It sounds like you may have learned a valuable lesson.

PHIL: Yeah, I've been a really crappy dad.

THERAPIST: Let's try to look at it a little differently. How about viewing this experience as the start of bringing home a new mode?

PHIL: And what would that mode be?

THERAPIST: Let's call it the *Awesome Sober Dad* mode.

PHIL: That sounds really good to me.

SUMMARY

Modes are patterns of functioning (e.g., thoughts, feelings, behaviors, and physiology) that manifest in individuals at various points in time, usually in response to certain environmental contexts (i.e., a variety of similar stimuli). For example, individuals may enter into an *adaptive* mode when receiving social validation and enter into a *maladaptive* mode when they do not receive validation or are alone. People with addictions often initiate addictive behaviors to achieve certain modes (e.g., sociable, numb, productive), but eventually the problems associated with addictive behaviors make these modes unachievable. In fact, maladaptive modes become the norm for most people with addictions, particularly while they are engaged in addictive behaviors.

Therapists and patients are likely to benefit from identifying adaptive and maladaptive modes. Such pattern recognition helps both to see the big picture regarding addictive behaviors. And as therapists explain modes and how they operate, patients can begin to set goals to change thought, feeling, and behavior patterns, in order to achieve adaptive modes without relying on addictive behaviors.

CHAPTER 12

GROUP CBT FOR ADDICTIONS

Six patients file into a conference room and sit silently around a table, avoiding eye contact as they wait for the start of their first CBT addiction group session. Tom's third DUI has convinced him that he needs to finally quit drinking alcohol. Rick recently violated probation by testing positive for marijuana, so his lawyer advised him to "get into rehab." Mary's physician says she will no longer prescribe pain medication unless Mary sees a therapist. Sarah struggles with binge eating. Bill's wife is threatening divorce after discovering that his gambling has depleted their children's college fund. And Kristen wants to quit smoking for the sake of her 2-year-old daughter. All eyes turn to Lois, the therapist, as she enters the room, sits down, and welcomes everyone to their first session.

Group therapy is central to the treatment of addictions, and most addiction treatment programs consider therapy groups essential to their efforts. In fact, hundreds, if not thousands, of therapy groups and mutual-help groups (e.g., SMART Recovery, 12-step approaches, moderation management, Women for Sobriety) meet worldwide each day to help people who struggle with addictions.

Group therapy is effective for most psychiatric conditions, including substance use disorders (Burlingame, Strauss, & Joyce, 2013), and group CBT is considered as effective as individual CBT for the treatment of alcohol and substance use disorders (Magill & Ray, 2009; Weiss, Jaffee, de Menil, & Cogley, 2004). The Center for Substance Abuse Treatment (CSAT; 2005) describes potential benefits of group therapy as follows:

> Groups can support individual members in times of pain and trouble, and they can help people grow in ways that are healthy and creative. Formal therapy groups can be a compelling source of persuasion, stabilization, and support. In the hands of a skilled, well-trained group leader, the potential healing powers

inherent in a group can be harnessed and directed to foster healthy attachments, provide positive peer reinforcement, act as a forum for self-expression, and teach new social skills. In short, group therapy can provide a wide range of therapeutic services, comparable in efficacy to those delivered in individual therapy. (p. xv)

CSAT (2005) lists five effective group therapy models: (1) psychoeducational groups, (2) skill development groups, (3) cognitive-behavioral or problem-solving groups, (4) support groups, and (5) interpersonal groups. They acknowledge that actual real-world therapy groups draw upon each of these models. Throughout this text and elsewhere (e.g., Liese, 1994; Liese, 2014; Liese & Beck, 1998; Liese & Franz, 1996; Liese & Tripp, 2018) we emphasize the importance of five components of CBT: structure, case conceptualization, collaboration, psychoeducation, and standardized techniques. When effectively combined, these five CBT components produce CBT groups that offer knowledge, problem-solving skills, emotional support, and interpersonal processing—per CSAT recommendations. Ideally, group members who attend well-run CBT sessions come to realize the following beliefs:

"I am gaining an understanding of my thoughts, feelings, and behaviors."
"I am acquiring important skills."
"I am learning to solve problems instead of avoiding them."
"I feel valued and supported in the group."
"I am realizing that I can care for, get along with, and relate to people."

ORGANIZING CBT ADDICTION GROUPS AND ENROLLING NEW PATIENTS

We have been developing, reviewing, and revising our *cognitive-behavioral therapy addiction group* (CBTAG; Liese et al., 2002; Wenzel et al., 2012) for more than 20 years. CBTAGs ideally have between five and eight members and sessions generally run 90 minutes. Some groups have had as many as 12 members, and these groups obviously require more time per session. Group sessions typically occur weekly, though as demand grows some group facilitators offer sessions more frequently. Group members with chemical and behavioral addictions are referred by community agencies and clinicians familiar with the value and benefits of CBTAGs. And of course, many group members are self-referred or referred by group members who have benefited from CBTAGs. Therapists may also refer their own individual therapy patients to groups they facilitate. Many such therapists work with patients in *both* group and individual therapy, finding that individual and group sessions potentiate each other. Specifically, individual sessions provide an opportunity to process what has occurred in group sessions, and group sessions provide an opportunity to practice skills learned during individual CBT sessions.

We encourage facilitators to offer *open enrollment* groups, so members may come and go as they wish. We have found that people seeking help for addictions benefit most from services that are readily accessible, rather than those that impose a waiting period (Liese & Monley, 2021). We have also found that some group members exit the group when they need it most (e.g., during relapses and other crises). Open enrollment enables them to return when they are ready to get the help they need. When we began offering open enrollment, we were concerned that group sessions would lack continuity. Fortunately, we were wrong. We have since learned that current group members consistently welcome new and returning members and appreciate opportunities to review basic CBT principles and skills along with new members.

Inclusion Criteria, Exclusion Criteria, and Screening

We have carefully considered group inclusion and exclusion criteria for many years. As noted earlier, group members include individuals with substance use disorders and behavioral addictions, and it is common for people with other problematic habitual behaviors (e.g., binge eating and problematic sexual behaviors) to join CBTAGs. Group members also tend to have coexisting mental health problems (e.g., depression, anxiety, PTSD, personality disorders, bipolar illness). As a result, CBTAG members tend to be quite diverse.

As we will discuss in detail later, group members are likely to have an assortment of reasons for attending CBTAGs. Some sincerely wish to change their addictive behaviors. Some initially feel ambivalent about changing addictive behaviors and being in the group. And some state directly that they have no desire to change and are only in the group to meet some mandate. *The primary inclusion criterion for a CBTAG is a willingness to be an engaged participant.* By engaged, we mean at least *willing to share concerns and be supportive of other group members.* While many involuntary (i.e., mandated) participants initially resist being in group therapy, an effective facilitator and supportive group members can engage even the most recalcitrant group members.

It is rare for a patient to be excluded or dismissed from a CBTAG. *The only exclusion criterion is that a group member is, or has the potential to be, disruptive in the group.* Examples of potentially disruptive behaviors include intimidation or aggression toward other group members, repeatedly breaking group rules (e.g., by perpetually giving advice, being defensive, externalizing personal issues), and refusing to participate in group processes. We have been offering CBTAG for more than 20 years and few patients have ever become so disruptive that they were transferred out of the group.

All group members are screened by the facilitator prior to entering the group. Ideally this occurs in person, though sometimes new group members are screened by phone or video conferencing. Careful screening is vital to the well-being of the group. It offers an opportunity for potential group members to learn about group norms, processes, activities, expectations, and rules. A primary facilitator responsibility is to protect group members from potential psychological harm that might occur as a result of being in a therapy group that does not meet its members' needs. Screening is the first step toward offering that protection. Consider this exchange between Lois and Rick (from the group introduced at the beginning of this chapter), as she screens him for entry into the group:

LOIS: Rick, I understand you are interested in attending our addictions group. Tell me about yourself and particularly your interest in the addictions group, so we can be sure it's a good fit for you.

RICK: There's not much to tell. I got in trouble last year for cocaine possession, ended up on probation, and then had a dirty urine. My lawyer said I should get into rehab, even though it was only weed.

LOIS: Rick, we offer a cognitive-behavioral therapy addiction group here, rather than a rehab program. Is that what you're looking for?

RICK: It's all the same to me. I just need to start something.

LOIS: You don't sound very enthusiastic about getting help.

RICK: Should I be?

LOIS: I'll tell you about the group and you can decide for yourself. I have been offering group cognitive-behavioral therapy for years because I find it an extraordinary resource for patients. Group members come to learn about and change their addictive behaviors, but they also become sources of support and encouragement to each other. Each time we meet, group members share the current status of their addictions, their goals, and related concerns. As I listen, particularly to their goals, I decide which skills might be most relevant at each session. It's kind of like individual therapy, but I focus on skills that will benefit *all* group members, rather than just one individual. In your case, it might help to focus on skills to keep you from getting in the kinds of trouble you've been in.

RICK: Like what kinds of skills? I've never been in any kind of therapy.

LOIS: I don't know you well enough to say for sure, but it might help to focus on skills like decision making, impulse control, or problem solving.

RICK: That's fine. Just tell me how to get into your group.

LOIS: The first thing you need to do is decide whether you're willing to be *an engaged participant.*

RICK: What does that mean?

LOIS: It means you attend each week, or as often as you can, and be an active member of the group. Speak honestly about your difficulties and listen well to others, even if you think you can't relate to their problems.

RICK: I've come this far, so I might as well give it a try.

LOIS: Does that mean you are committed to being *an engaged participant?*

RICK: [*Sighs.*] I'll do my best to be an engaged participant.

Following this exchange, Lois asks more about Rick's history and determines that he would likely be appropriate for the group. She then explains the rules of the group (described in the next section) and tells Rick that all group members commit to these rules prior to attending meetings.

GUIDELINES AND STRUCTURE OF CBT ADDICTION GROUPS

Among the most important facilitator responsibilities are the safety, privacy, and productivity of the group. Groups are safe, private, and productive when members fully understand and follow group guidelines and rules. Over the years we have put considerable effort into deciding which rules are necessary and important and which are not. Prior to entering as group members, potential participants must agree that they will:

1. Protect each other's privacy and confidentiality by never discussing other group members outside of the group
2. Not give advice to other group members, though they may share what has worked for them in the past as long as they identify it as their own strategy
3. Be receptive to feedback, including other group members' perceptions of them (i.e., not be defensive)
4. Not be confrontational or aggressive toward other group members
5. Discuss only their own personal thoughts, feelings, circumstances, and behaviors, rather than philosophizing, politicizing, intellectualizing, and so forth
6. Not form subgroups or cliques outside of the group, since doing so is likely to make other group members feel alienated

Group facilitators vary in how they review and enforce these rules during actual sessions, though all facilitators should fully describe these rules as part of the consent process. Some facilitators choose to share these by providing printed copies of them at each group visit. Some write these rules on a whiteboard at the front of the room. Most gently remind group members about rules when they are violated.

The First Session

During the first CBTAG session it is especially important to spend time reiterating guidelines, goals, structure, and rules of the group. In the group introduced above, all members are new to the group and will benefit from such an introduction. Lois, the facilitator, begins by introducing herself:

> LOIS: Welcome everyone, my name is Lois, I'm a cognitive-behavioral therapy group facilitator, and I will be facilitating this group. I have spoken to each of you prior to enrolling in this group, so you understand how we function and the basic ground rules. But just to review, this group is for people with any addiction. Some of you struggle with drinking, some with smoking, some with prescribed medications or other drugs, some with food, and some with certain behavioral addictions, like gambling. We can all meet together in a single therapy group because the processes that drive addictions are common across addictions. Whether your problem is drinking, smoking, eating, gambling, or some other behavior, you have probably tried to make changes and found it very difficult to do so. You have probably felt remorse for things you've done, hidden certain behaviors from others, and wished you could be like other (nonaddicted) people when it comes to your addictive behavior.

> RICK: I have a question. How long are these groups? Like what time are these sessions over? Sorry to interrupt, but I promised my girlfriend I'd text her, to let her know what time I'd get to her place.

> LOIS: Our sessions are 90 minutes long, so we'll be working together until 6:30. Your question reminds me to talk about logistics. As I just mentioned, we meet every week for 90 minutes, from 5:00–6:30 P.M. You are all here voluntarily, so you can attend as many or as few sessions as you like, but I ask all of you to do your best to come as regularly as possible so you can get to know each other and others can get to know and help you. If at all possible, please arrive on time, just as you all did today. If you need to use your cell phone for calls or texting, please walk into the hallway to do so. And for those of you who are new to our facility, the restrooms are just down the hall. Any questions so far?

> RICK: Thanks. I'll text her later. Sorry for interrupting.

> LOIS: That's okay. I'll share some more things about the group, and then the remainder of our session will be based on your introductions. Each of you will introduce yourselves by first name and then tell us the addiction

you wish to change, the status of your addiction, your goals for addressing that addiction, and any other issues that play a role in your addiction, like personal, family, legal, housing, social, or financial problems. You can disclose as much or as little about these things as you like, but the more open and honest you are, the more likely it is that you will benefit from this group. Sometimes, after you introduce yourself, we'll immediately move to the next person. Other times, I'll stop and ask whether other group members have had similar thoughts, feelings, or experiences. I usually do that when I think it helpful to relate your experiences to those of everyone else in the group. You'll soon see that your thoughts and feelings are quite similar. Most importantly, I'll do my best to help you understand cognitive-behavioral principles and skills that should help you reach your goals. Any questions?

During this introductory session, Lois presents the most basic elements of the group. If she were to continue to describe all rules, principles of CBT, typical topics discussed, and other details, her introduction would probably take too much time, and group members would likely become distracted, bored, and restless. Hence, she stops here and asks for questions. As group members begin to participate, rules are explained as they become pertinent. For example, Rick might ask whether his participation in the group will be reported to his probation officer. In response, Lois might say, "This would be a good time to talk about group privacy and confidentiality. The most important rule of this group is that we don't share information about anyone else in the group. Rick, I am bound by the same rules as group members. I won't be revealing anything about you or anyone else without your consent. And while we're on the topic of rules, I'd like to review some other rules with all of you."

Structure of a CBTAG

Structure is vital for keeping the group on track and productive. Too much structure can cause the group to feel rigid and impersonal, while too little can result in virtual chaos. Group members are encouraged to interact with each other throughout each session by asking questions and sharing their own relevant experiences with each other. And of course, while the CBT model is reviewed, or skills are being taught, members are encouraged to ask questions and share personal thoughts and experiences. It is often during these exchanges that group members get to know and care about each other and the group becomes cohesive. However, the facilitator is continually responsible for redirecting conversations back to the concepts being discussed or the skills being taught.

Interactions between group members also provide opportunities to learn and practice interpersonal communication skills. Group members naturally wish to help each other, and most are tempted to give advice and recommend their own problem-solving strategies. When this occurs, facilitators intervene and guide group members to communicate effectively (e.g., by asking open-ended questions, reflectively listening, and expressing empathy). At the same time, the facilitator is charged with maintaining the basic structure of the group and remaining focused on the agenda.

In each meeting the facilitator follows the same basic structure. However, depending on the problems, questions, and concerns raised by group members, more or less time may be spent on any of these elements:

- Facilitator introductions
- Member introductions
- Introduction and review of the CBT model of addictive behaviors
- Presentation of relevant cognitive, behavioral, and interpersonal skills
- Feedback from group members
- Summary and review

Each of these elements is described in detail in the following sections.

Facilitator Introductions

The amount of time needed for an overview of group aims, guidelines, and rules is dependent on several variables, including the presence of any new members and the length of time the group has been meeting. In the example above, Lois provides an extended introduction because it is the first meeting of this cohort. As group members get to know each other and understand the group processes, facilitator introductions take less time.

Occasionally, an incident takes place that may need to be revisited in the following session. For example, after one of our winter meetings a group member slipped on the ice while leaving the group and fell in front of our facility. Several members helped the member up and determined that he was not seriously hurt. The group member contacted the facilitator shortly afterward and recounted the event. During the facilitator's introduction at the following session, group members were thanked for helping the group member, the group member had an opportunity to thank those who helped him, and the group moved forward. On another occasion, a group member became extremely upset midsession and exclaimed (while crying), "Please excuse me, I just can't do this today." She then got up and left. Afterward, she informed the facilitator that her mother had recently become critically ill and she was terribly distraught about the situation. She said she would return to the group at some time in the future and asked the facilitator to explain her situation to the group. With the patient's formal consent to do so, the facilitator explained the situation to group members during her introduction at the following session.

Member Introductions

In every CBTAG session, group members introduce themselves by stating their names, addiction(s), status, goals, and any relevant or important issues in their lives. Most group facilitators find it useful to take notes on a group tracking sheet, such as the one in Figure 12.1.

The following excerpt from Lois's first group session provides a distinct example of member introductions:

LOIS: Who would like to introduce themselves first? Again, tell us: your name; your addiction or addictions; the current status of your addiction; your goals, especially regarding addictive behaviors; and any other issues pertinent to your addiction. And everyone, please feel free to ask questions or share thoughts related to anything other group members or I have said.

TOM: I'll go first and get it over with. My name is Tom. I'm 43 years old. My addiction is alcohol, I took my last drink 3 weeks ago, and my goal is to stay abstinent. [*Turns to Lois.*] What was that last thing on your list?

LOIS: Tell us about any other issues pertinent to your alcohol use.

TOM: I don't know if this is what you mean by other issues, but I got my third DUI recently and that's screwed up my life in a lot of ways. I don't need to go into detail about it today, but I'm determined to never drink again.

RICK: Three DUIs. Wow, that sucks. Why did you keep drinking after the first two?

TOM: When I was around your age, I quit for a year after my first DUI. I was on a diversion program and agreed to go to some classes and stop drinking. After diversion was over I started drinking again, and that's when I got the next one. You're right, it sucked. I lost my license, paid a big fine, spent some weekends in the county jail, got an interlock device on my car, and quit for years.

SARAH: What's an interlock device?

TOM: It's the thing you blow into that registers whether you've been drinking before you start your car. It doesn't let you start your car if there's any alcohol on your breath.

RICK: So how about the third DUI?

TOM: I own a small engine repair shop. At the end of the day I'd let my employees crack open beers and sure enough, I started drinking with them. Then just 3 weeks ago, I was driving home after work and got my third DUI. This time I'm done drinking for good. My lawyer says I'll probably spend some time in the slammer.

Name (age)	Addiction(s)	Status of addiction	Change goals	Other issues/context
Tom (43 y/o)	Alcohol	Quit drinking 3 weeks ago	Abstinence	Married; lives with wife; owns small engine repair shop; quit after arrest for third DUI
Rick (29 y/o)	Marijuana, cocaine	Marijuana—occasionally Cocaine—abstinent 6 mo.	Abstain while on probation; says "We'll see"	Single; lives with friends; legal problems (lawyer, probation) motivating abstinence and group
Mary (50 y/o)	Opioids (pain meds)	"Too much each day." Taking as much as physician will prescribe	Time to cut back—can't say how much right now	Married; chronic pain; lives with husband who smokes cigarettes and drinks heavily/daily
Sarah (34 y/o)	Binge eating	Last binge Friday night	Abstinence from binge eating	Single; obese; lives alone; lonely; depressed
Bill (59 y/o)	Gambling	Last time gambling lost $800 (1 month ago)	Abstinence from gambling; admits to ambivalence; says, "I think I can control"	Separated from wife; night manager at a fast-food restaurant; lives with elderly parents
Kristen (31 y/o)	Cigarette smoking	Currently smokes 1/2 pack daily; continually trying to quit	Abstinence from smoking	Single; lives with 2 y/o daughter (Lilly); has struggled with depression

FIGURE 12.1. Completed CBT addiction group tracking sheet.

SARAH: Wow, I'm sorry to hear about all that.

TOM: Yeah, me too.

RICK: [*After some silence.*] I'll go next. My name is Rick. I really don't think I need to be here. I only smoke weed and drink occasionally, and I've never gotten in trouble for doing either. My situation is complicated. I used to do a lot of cocaine but stopped when I got busted for possession. The problem is that I violated my probation by smoking weed the day before a random UDS. So, I got busted and now my lawyer says I have to come to these groups.

SARAH: I know I must sound stupid to all of you, but what's a random UDS?

MARY: Oh, I can tell you what UDS stands for. I get them all the time. It's a urine drug screen. It's how they know whether you've been taking drugs.

LOIS: Sarah, you don't sound stupid. I really appreciate when any of you jumps in with questions. I hope you will all ask questions and share your thoughts. That's a big part of how you get to know each other and realize how much you have in common.

SARAH: Okay, thanks.

LOIS: Rick, you were saying that you didn't think you belong here. I'm glad you're here. Group members often vary in how strongly they believe they have addictions. If it helps, when it's time for you to state your addiction, feel free to say you've used cocaine in the past and been a marijuana smoker and you're not sure if marijuana is causing you problems.

RICK: I can do that now. My name is Rick. I've used cocaine in the past and smoked a lot of marijuana, but am not sure it's a problem. My status is that I've stopped because I don't want to go to jail. And for now, I have no plans to start again. Like Tom, I have a few small legal problems to sort out. I live with some friends who smoke weed, but they know not to smoke around me, since I can't party with them right now.

MARY: [*After a pause.*] I'll go next, since I broke the ice with the UDS thing. My name is Mary, my addiction is oxys. [*Turns to Sarah and smiles.*] Oxys are oxycodone pills for my pain. They're considered narcotics and addictive. My doctor says I take too many each day. So that's my status: Apparently, I take too many each day. And I can't completely quit since I need them for chronic pain. I just need to keep them under better control and come to this group. At least that's what my doctor says. My other issues . . . [*Pauses.*] I live with my husband who smokes cigarettes all day and drinks too much. Sometimes I think I take pills to deal with him. A friend of mine has said that I probably take oxys for my mental pain as well as my physical pain and it's probably true. [*Pauses again.*] That's all I have for now.

SARAH: Okay, I'll go next. My name is Sarah. My addiction is binge eating. I heard about this group from a friend who quit drinking with the help of one of these groups. She told me that this group is for anyone with an addiction, and I binge eat like I'm some kind of a food addict. I've never actually done drugs, or even drank much, but I always recall this scene in a movie where this guy was doing cocaine. [*Looks at Rick.*] It was like watching one of my own feeding frenzies. I eat until I'm sick, and then I feel terrible for days. It's like a food hangover—made worse by how bloated, disgusted, and ashamed I feel for what I've done. My last binge was on Friday night. And my other issues? I'm single, live alone, feel lonely and depressed most of the time, and am sick of the way I'm living.

MARY: Sarah, I can relate to your feelings. I'm lonely even though I'm married. I often wish I was single, but I know it wouldn't make things better. If my husband was gone, I'd still be miserable. I always have been.

LOIS: [*After a silence.*] I hope it's becoming obvious that all of you have some important things in common. For example, you have all been suffering because of behaviors that initially brought you pleasure or relief.

MARY: That's for sure.

LOIS: There are still two people who haven't introduced themselves. Who wants to go next?

BILL: I'll go. My name is Bill. I don't drink, do drugs, or binge eat. My problem is gambling. My wife kicked me out of our house because of my gambling. My status is that I gambled a month ago and lost $800. My wife found out I was raiding the kids' college fund and said she was done with me. My goal is to get back on my feet, hopefully hang on to my marriage, and straighten my life out. When everything was crashing down around me I thought I'd quit gambling forever. But now some time has passed and I'm thinking I might be able to control it someday. I'm hoping I can go back to the casino with twenty or thirty bucks and leave when it's gone. But for the time being I'm not gambling. I don't have any money left, I live with my elderly parents, and I manage a fast-food restaurant.

TOM: You think you can eventually control your gambling?

BILL: Yeah. Now that I've stopped gambling, I realize I can quit any time I want. You know, in the future, before things get out of hand again.

TOM: That's what I thought before getting my second and third DUI: "I can control this." Boy was I dreaming.

LOIS: Bill and Tom, I'm glad we're talking about your thoughts and beliefs. After Kristen introduces herself, we'll be talking about the role of thoughts and beliefs in addictive behaviors. [*She turns to Kristen.*]

KRISTEN: I guess it's my turn. My name is Kristen. My addiction is cigarette smoking. I have been smoking half a pack a day and want to quit completely. I am single and live with my 2-year-old daughter, Lilly. Like a couple of you, I've struggled with depression, but I'm doing better with that. My therapist told me about this group and said he thought I'd get a lot out of it. I can already tell I will.

By the end of member introductions, Lois had completed her group tracking sheet (see Figure 12.1; a blank version of this tracking sheet is available in Form 12.1, at the end of this chapter, for use with clients). This sheet helps her to continually attend to problems and needs of each group member.

As we noted earlier, member introductions provide a kind of roadmap for the rest of the session. Lois knows she needs to introduce basic CBT principles to the group, and she is aware that members are most likely to understand and make use of these principles if they can apply them to their own lives. As members have introduced themselves, Lois has paid particular attention to thoughts and beliefs common to all group members. For example, all have expressed thoughts about the negative consequences of their addictive behaviors and have mentioned thoughts about their motivation to change.

Introduction and Review of the CBT Model of Addictive Behaviors

The CBT model is presented and discussed in each group session, with emphasis on thoughts, beliefs, emotions, and behaviors associated with addiction and recovery. As explained in detail in Chapter 2, the CBT model suggests that emotions, behaviors, and physiological responses are largely influenced by thoughts and beliefs (see Figure 12.2, repeated from Figure 2.2 in Chapter 2). Review and application of the CBT model occurs in some form during every group session, and sometimes multiple times during a single session. While the CBT model is often introduced or reviewed at the end of member introductions, it may also be reviewed any time it is relevant to a group discussion.

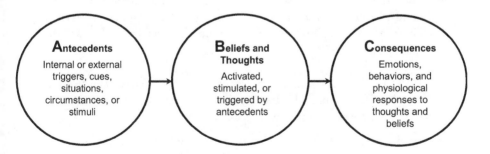

FIGURE 12.2. The ABC model.

Following member introductions above, Lois introduces the CBT model, as follows:

LOIS: I would like to explain the approach, or model, we use in this group to understand some dynamics, or processes, that underly your addictive behaviors. Let's start with the name of this group. We call it a cognitive-behavioral therapy group, or CBT group for short, because we focus on cognitive and behavioral processes to understand addictions. *Cognitive* is just a fancy word for thoughts, beliefs, and other similar mental processes. We emphasize that an understanding of your thoughts and beliefs is essential to understanding and changing your addictive behaviors. We place emphasis on thoughts and beliefs because it's possible to change these, but often impossible to change many things in the world around us. As you change your thoughts and beliefs, your emotions and behaviors will change. And as your emotions and behaviors change, so will your thoughts and beliefs.

Lois begins with this very basic explanation of CBT because this is the first time this group is meeting. She will likely repeat this explanation again when new members enter the group.

Next, Lois stands up and walks to a whiteboard in front of the room. She draws the circles containing letters *A, B,* and *C,* and arrows connecting them, as in Figure 12.2. She then asks group members to define the word *trigger* as it relates to addictive behaviors and relapse. As members offer definitions, she writes them on the board in the "A" circle. She then moves over to the "C" circle and explains that *C* stands for *consequences,* and she writes the words *emotions, behaviors,* and *physiological responses* in this circle. She explains that most people attribute their feelings, behaviors, and physiological responses (e.g., urges and craving) to triggers, events, situations, or circumstances outside of their control. She makes this discussion more relevant by using Tom's example of drinking again after a period of abstinence, as a result of his employees' drinking at the end of a workday. She then introduces the middle, "B" circle, by explaining that Tom's thoughts about drinking played a role in his drinking, as well as the trigger (seeing his employees drink). The following exchange between Lois and group members is provided to illustrate how she explains the ABC model:

LOIS: You can see that I've drawn three circles with letters, and two arrows between them. I'll be drawing these over and over in this group to help you understand the ABC process.

KRISTEN: I know this ABC stuff, because this is what my individual therapist has been teaching me. It's helped with my depression and he says it will help me quit smoking.

Lois: Thanks for sharing that, Kristen. I bet you'll have a lot more to share as we discuss the ABC model. So, I want to ask you all a question. What are some circumstances that trigger your addictive behaviors? What happens internally—inside of you—or externally—around you—that leads to drinking, smoking, eating, or using drugs? I'll write your triggers up here on the whiteboard.

Tom: Like I said earlier, I let my employees drink at my shop after work, and that led me to drink.

Lois: [*Writes on the board: "Other people drinking."*] Thanks, Tom. Anyone else?

Kristen: I want to smoke a cigarette whenever I feel uptight or when I'm tired and need to get chores done—mostly at night. The worst is when I get that physical craving.

Lois: [*Writes on the board: "Feeling uptight, tired, physical craving, mostly at night."*] Thanks for sharing, Kristen.

Rick: Most of my partying is social. All of my friends get high. When they're partying, I'm partying with them. I think that's normal for people my age.

Lois: [*Writes on the board: "Social, friends getting high."*] Thanks, Rick. Anyone else want to tell us about their triggers?

Sarah: For me it's my depression, which is most of the time.

Lois: [*Writes on the board: "Depression, most of the time."*] Thanks, Sarah. Now let's move to the "B" circle. Again, *B* stands for beliefs, thoughts, ideas, values, rules, standards, or any other mental processes. Most people find it difficult to identify their thoughts and beliefs, compared to identifying external triggers.

Kristen: I can tell you what I'm thinking because I've gone over this with my individual therapist a million times: "I want a cigarette," "I need a cigarette," "I'll feel better if I smoke," and lots more thoughts like that.

Lois: Excellent, Kristen, thanks for sharing these thoughts. [*She writes these on the board but leaves a blank where Kristen used the word cigarette.*] You'll notice I left a blank where Kristen said the word *cigarette*. Does anyone know why I did that?

Sarah: I can guess. Is that where we each need to fill in the blank with our own addiction? Like for me it would be food?

Lois: Exactly! How about the rest of you?

Rick: Well that's obvious. This is where I'm supposed to say weed. But I never feel like I *needed* to smoke weed, or that I'd *feel better* if I smoke weed. I guess I think, "I *want* to smoke weed."

Lois: Thanks, Rick. That sounds right: *Your* thought would be, "I *want* to smoke weed."

Lois continues this group discussion, and she helps all group members identify the triggers, thoughts, beliefs, emotions, behaviors, and physiologic responses associated with their addictive behaviors. She asks them to generate as many triggers and thoughts as they can think of. She next leads them into a discussion about strategies for gaining more control in their lives, by examining the extent to which they have successfully avoided or modified triggers and the thoughts that led to addictive behaviors in the past.

Discussions about the ABC model enable group members to see how similar they are to each other. They begin to understand that triggers and thoughts are comparable across addictions. For example, by listening to each other they learn that similar situations and emotions (e.g., boredom, restlessness, urges, craving, social events, excitement) trigger similar thoughts about addictive behaviors ("I want to . . ." or "I need to . . ."). Eventually they learn that the strategies, or skills, for addressing addictive behaviors are also similar.

Presentation of Relevant Cognitive, Behavioral, and Interpersonal Skills

The *presentation of CBT skills* has already begun with the introduction of the ABC model (described above). Applying the CBT model to addictive behaviors is a cognitive skill that requires substantial repetition to develop. The choice of other skills to be learned is based on member concerns shared during introductions and subsequent discussions during the session. For example, if it becomes apparent that several group members are struggling in relationships, the facilitator might focus on interpersonal skills (e.g., communication, empathy, conflict resolution). If group members are struggling with urges and craving, the facilitator might focus on the advantages and disadvantages of using, or delay and distraction skills.

As Lois listens to group members' concerns, she considers skills most relevant to their problems. While introducing the CBT model she emphasizes that all skills involve a shift in thinking from "I want to engage in [addictive behavior]" to "I want to use new skills to solve my problems." There are numerous skills that have the potential for helping people with addictions. Some of these include:

- *Refusal skills* that enable group members to say "no" to opportunities to use, typically in the midst of urges and craving
- *Emotion regulation skills* that enable group members to transform undesired emotional states (e.g., anxiety, depression, anger) into neutral or positive states (e.g., calm, relaxed, satisfied) without the use of familiar addictive behaviors
- *Impulse control skills* that enable group members to stop themselves when their old automatic responses to triggers are not in their best interest
- *Interpersonal skills* that enable group members to interact with others in ways that are effective and achieve their desired outcomes

- *Problem-solving skills* that enable group members to generate multiple options for solving problems, choose the best option, and then carry it out
- *Mindfulness skills* that enable group members to decenter their thoughts and deliberately attend to issues that truly matter to them, with fewer distractions
- *Acceptance and commitment skills* that enable group members to accept the things they cannot change, commit to changing what they can, and intentionally differentiate between the two
- *Behavioral activation skills* that enable group members to identify and organize their values, and turn them into daily action plans that correspond with these values

Given these multiple options, an important question becomes, "How does a CBTAG therapist choose the most appropriate skill to teach?" The answer is that *the chosen skill should be most relevant to the greatest number of group members at the time.* In reality, an effective group facilitator manages to make each of these skills relevant to a majority of group members.

After teaching group members about the ABC model, and hearing their concerns, Lois chooses to discuss emotion regulation as the first skill to focus on. She helps members understand that they all feel some tension prior to engaging in their addictive behaviors. This comes easy for Mary, Sarah, and Kristen, who all directly identify negative emotional states (e.g., depression, anxiety, anger) as triggers. Lois helps Tom, Rick, and Bill to notice that they feel a certain urgency to engage in drinking, smoking weed, and gambling, just prior to engaging in these behaviors. Lois then points out that they all have some degree of ambivalence prior to engaging in their addictive behaviors, and she explains that ambivalence is, by nature, a form of tension.

In later group sessions, Lois teaches the group about behavioral activation. She does so by helping group members recognize that they all lack certain pleasurable activities in their lives that align with their values. She again uses the whiteboard and has group members list values of greatest importance to them. The resulting list includes family, friendships, career, integrity, physical health, helping others, and other common ideals. Finally, she helps them commit to scheduling and engaging in activities over the next week that correspond with their values.

Feedback from Group Members

The facilitator invites feedback from group members at various times during each session, and some group members may even offer feedback spontaneously. For example, group members might state, "This [new skill or group discussion] is helpful to me because . . ." However, more often than not, the facilitator asks, "What are you all learning right now?" There are several benefits to asking this question.

The most obvious is that it helps the facilitator determine the extent to which the session is helping group members. A less obvious reason for asking this question is that it helps some members articulate what they are learning for the first time. It is assumed that they are more likely to commit to new ideas that they are able to articulate.

There are times when the question, "What are you learning?" becomes particularly salient. For example, it is always appropriate to ask this question at the end of a group session, as it comes to a close. In fact, most group facilitators leave at least 5 minutes at the end of sessions to ask this question. The most common response to this question is reiteration of a skill that has been discussed during the session. For example, at the end of a session where acceptance and commitment has been discussed a member might answer, "I've learned that I either need to accept that my mother is controlling, or I need to commit to learning and practicing communication skills in order to be more direct with my mother."

Another common response to the question, "What are you learning?" is to mention something that another group member said. For example, a group member might answer, "From listening to Bill, I recognize that I am most likely to relapse when I give myself permission to do 'just a little bit' of my old addictive behavior." Another typical answer to the question, "What have you learned?" is, "I'm not sure" or "What [another group member] said." When the group is almost over, and time has run out, the facilitator notes any questions that might need to be addressed in future sessions.

Another time to ask, "What are you learning?" is during a transition from one topic or skill to another. For example, if a group member is having difficulties with urges and craving, the group might review strategies for controlling these. This discussion might occur during member introductions and not last more than 15 minutes. The facilitator might transition at that point to the next member or topic by summarizing what has been said and asking group members what they have learned from their brief discussion about urges and craving.

Summary and Review

A *summary and review* at the end of the session is most effective when it is combined with the question, "What have you learned?" As group members answer this question, the facilitator reiterates important common themes from the group, and relates these to as many members as possible. The following is an exchange between Lois and group members as she brings her first group session to a close:

LOIS: We are nearing the end of our session, so I'd like to hear what you've learned during our first meeting together. I appreciate your participation in our discussion about the ABC model. I especially appreciate how you all applied the ABC model to yourselves when we talked about managing urges and craving. I'd like to hear any feedback you're willing to share about these activities or about this entire group session.

TOM: To be honest, I'm surprised that we have so much in common—even with different addictions. I've always pictured recovery groups to consist of a bunch of old drunks. I liked hearing that my problems aren't that different from the problems of people who eat too much, or gamble . . . or smoke whacky weed. [*Group members all chuckle.*] It's like we're all different—but we're all the same in some ways.

RICK: I'm surprised about how mellow this group is. I thought we'd be getting lectured for an hour and a half on the evils of pot smoking and doing drugs.

LOIS: Thanks, Rick. I'm glad it wasn't as terrible as you expected. Can you think of anything that was particularly helpful to you?

RICK: Yeah, like Tom, I am surprised that we have so much in common. That ABC model spelled it all out.

KRISTEN: This was just like my therapist said it would be. He told me we would learn about the ABC model, but more focused on my smoking than my depression. He also said I'd like the way the group is run, and I really do.

SARAH: [*After a brief silence.*] I will try to recognize what I'm saying to myself before I buy junk food or eat things I shouldn't eat. While shopping, I need to start asking myself, "Do I really need to eat *this?*" Or even better, I might start asking myself, "How will I feel tomorrow if I eat all these tortilla chips and queso tonight?"

MARY: This has given me a lot to think about. My pain scares me, but I know I need to make some changes so I don't have to take so much pain medication. I've liked our discussion, but I need to give it a lot more thought. I'm one of those people who doesn't think as fast as other people.

LOIS: Thanks for being so honest, Mary. You are certainly on the right track. Keep thinking about these things and we'll talk much more about them next week and in all future meetings. Bill, how about you? What have you gotten out of our meeting today?

BILL: I don't know. . . . Nothing personal. . . . I like all of you, but I'm not sure this group will help me. I don't know that my gambling is like any of your problems. For me, it's just like any other form of entertainment, but it also gives me a chance to win back my losses. I'll keep coming because I have to, but I'm not *feeling it* like everyone else is. Like Mary just said, I'll have to give it some more thought.

LOIS: Bill, as I said to Mary, thanks for being so honest. I appreciate that you'll give it more thought, and I'm especially glad that you plan to come back next week. [*Turns to the group.*] It's 6:30 everyone, so we'll end here. Hope to see you all next week.

SETTING GOALS IN THE CBTAG

The primary aim of the CBTAG is to help people abstain from addictive behaviors and effectively manage their lives without them. Nevertheless, *each individual group member sets their own unique goals, and individual goals vary from complete abstinence to continued engagement in addictive behaviors.*

Many factors influence group members' addiction-related goals. For example, some choose abstinence, anticipating that continued use will lead to serious legal or family problems. Some choose abstinence after learning that their health is in serious jeopardy. Some choose abstinence because they no longer want to be chemically or behaviorally dependent. At the other end of the motivation continuum are those who insist that abstinence is not for them. Some are mandated to treatment against their will. Some believe they are trapped in an oppressive system or relationship, unfairly forcing them to stop. Most of these individuals do not wish to have the goal of abstinence forced upon them by family members, group members, the judicial system, group facilitators, or anyone else. Nonetheless, it has been our experience that many of these individuals benefit from group therapy as they discover that CBTAG facilitators and members aim to help and support them, rather than judge their particular choice of goals.

It is important to emphasize that CBTAG therapists are not expected to, nor should they, be in a position where *they* choose or enforce patients' goals. When patients attend groups and say they plan to continue their addictive behaviors, it is not the therapist's job to tell them to do otherwise. In fact, many individuals attending CBTAGs are inspired to modify their goals as a result of participating in, and learning from, the group. An interesting dynamic exists when group members say they have no plans to quit and the rest of the group is of the opinion that they should. Since an essential group rule is that *group members do not give advice,* group members learn to ask questions, express concern, and self-disclose their own struggles with quitting. In the following group discussion, group members share their thoughts about Rick's reluctance to quit marijuana:

RICK: I still don't see how marijuana causes me any problems.

KRISTEN: Didn't you say you might go to jail because of your continued marijuana use?

RICK: I almost went to jail because of cocaine. And even with cocaine I don't think I had a real problem. Marijuana is different. People don't get addicted to marijuana. And it's legal in most of the country.

SARAH: How would you know if you had a problem with marijuana?

RICK: I wouldn't be able to quit.

SARAH: But you haven't quit, and you said that's why you might go to jail.

LOIS: Rick, it's apparent that group members are trying to understand your belief that you don't have a problem with marijuana. I appreciate your answering their questions. How do you feel about these questions?

RICK: I feel like I'm getting busted.

LOIS: What do you mean by that?

RICK: It's uncomfortable. It feels like pressure.

LOIS: Is it okay that other group members are questioning your goals?

RICK: It has to be, right? Do I have a choice?

LOIS: Rick, you're the only one here who gets to set your goals. We're all here to gain knowledge and skills, set goals, and help each other to achieve their goals. But the group is also here to provide support, so I want you to feel supported as you hear these questions. I also want to remind everyone that you all get to set your own goals. None of us will judge or manipulate you to adopt others' goals.

RICK: I guess that's what I'm here for. I signed up for this.

As it turns out, this was a turning point in Rick's attitude toward the group. Moving forward, Rick appeared more receptive to questions asked by Lois and group members. He even began to ask others about their goals and motives regarding addictive behaviors and was supportive toward fellow group members. It has been our experience that such shifts are among the great rewards associated with facilitating CBTAGs.

It is common for group members' goals to *seem* unrelated to their addictive behaviors when in fact their goals might actually be directly related to addiction recovery. For example, many group members attend group therapy in part to feel less lonely. When these members succeed at making positive changes, they often attribute their success to *being cared about by other group members*. In addition to feeling cared about, group members' goals for starting and continuing group CBT might include:

- Wanting to be with others who have experienced similar problems
- Hearing how others solve their problems
- Finding meaning in their lives

- Increasing control over their thoughts and feelings
- Improving their social or interpersonal skills
- Improving their coping skills
- Helping others

It is important to emphasize here that group members' goals are likely to evolve as they witness others achieving goals like those listed above. For example, Tom's only goal when he entered the group was to quit drinking alcohol. After attending only three sessions he announced to the group: "I have a new goal. I've begun to realize that I was drinking with my employees after work because I'm bored at home. Besides quitting alcohol, my new goal is to figure out what I can do with my wife after work that would be more fun, or at least interesting."

CHOOSING GROUP TOPICS AND TECHNIQUES

Over the years, many people have asked, "How do you choose topics and techniques while a group therapy session is underway?" The answer is relatively simple: Doing so is not much different from choosing topics and techniques during an individual therapy session. *Topics and techniques chosen for each group session are dependent on group members' problems, needs, and goals.* For example, it might become apparent in an individual therapy session that a depressed patient needs to learn emotion regulation skills. In response, the therapist might decide to focus on modifying the individual's thoughts and beliefs, increasing pleasurable activities, accepting what cannot be changed, or committing to changes that will improve the individual's life. The difference in group CBT is that the choice of a focal point (e.g., dealing with urges to use, regulating emotions, improving relationships, controlling impulses) is dependent on the needs of most group members, rather than the needs of just one individual.

We have mentioned several potential content areas for group sessions. The mutual-help organization SMART Recovery (*www.smartrecovery.org*) has identified four potential focal points for their CBT-based mutual-help groups: (1) building and maintaining motivation; (2) coping with urges; (3) managing thoughts, feelings, and behaviors; and (4) living a balanced life. SMART (Self-Management and Recovery Training) is a science-based program, grounded in CBT, offered throughout the world. The SMART Recovery program provides numerous "tools" for achieving goals in these four areas.

Other factors influencing the choice of group topics include the interests, training, skills, and experiences of CBTAG facilitators. For example, some facilitators identify primarily as cognitive therapists, some identify as rational emotive behavioral therapists, some identify as acceptance and commitment therapists, others identify as dialectical behavioral therapists. These identities are most likely influenced by training, experience, and practice, but they are also likely influenced by personal interests and preferences. Stated differently, most cognitive-behavioral therapists feel more at home with certain approaches than others, and their "home theory" will certainly influence their choice of skills to be taught in any group session.

In Chapter 7 we presented standardized techniques for helping people in both individual and group CBT for addictions. We developed these techniques more than 30 years ago and continue to implement them, as our patients tell us that they are pertinent and helpful. Among the most versatile of these techniques are the advantages–disadvantages analysis (ADA), automatic thought record (ATR), and daily activity schedule (DAS). In the exchange that follows, Lois introduces the ADA and implements it with her group:

LOIS: Several of you have expressed ambivalence about changing your behaviors. Rick, you've said on several occasions that you don't think marijuana or cocaine cause you problems. Bill, you've said that you might eventually return to gambling because you'd like to recoup your losses and believe you can stop gambling at any time. And Mary, you've mentioned that your physician, more than you, wants you to reduce your oxycodone use.

MARY: I get why my doctor wants me to take less pain medication; she doesn't want me to overdose and die. I don't know if I'm ambivalent or just afraid of the pain I'll feel when I cut back on my meds.

RICK: I'm not against quitting cocaine. I just don't think weed is a problem.

LOIS: Thank you, Mary and Rick, for clarifying those things.

BILL: I'm not ambivalent. I know I want to go back to gambling.

LOIS: Thank you, Bill. Based on the things you've all said, I'd like to introduce an exercise known as the advantages–disadvantages analysis. Here's how it works . . . [*Draws figure, based on Form 7.1, on a whiteboard at the front of the room.*] I've drawn a square and divided it into four quadrants, or sections. You can see I've written the words *advantages* and *disadvantages* along the horizontal axis, with *using* and *not using* along the vertical axis. Let's fill in these four quadrants with the advantages and disadvantages of using and not using your chosen behaviors. And let's see if we notice patterns across the behaviors that you've each talked about in the group so far. Let's start with the advantages of using marijuana, pain medication, alcohol, gambling, or any other behavior that might be addictive for some.

TOM: Are you asking for the advantages of drinking for me, or what I liked about it?

LOIS: Exactly.

TOM: That's easy, I like the way it makes me feel.

LOIS: How did alcohol make you feel?

TOM: Relaxed, mellow, comfortable hanging out with my coworkers and employees. It's a social thing.

LOIS: [*Writes "I like the way it makes me feel" and "It's a social thing" in the appropriate quadrant.*] Who else wants to share advantages of continuing their behavior? [*As group members respond, she continues to write their responses; see Figure 12.3.*]

MARY: For me, it takes the pain away, like I'm taking care of myself.

BILL: It's my only form of entertainment. And it's my chance to get back at least some of the money I've lost. [*Lois continues to write.*]

LOIS: Since we've mostly filled that quadrant, let's move to another one. Who wants to pick the next quadrant?

KRISTEN: I want to talk about the disadvantages of continuing to smoke. Can I start?

LOIS: Of course.

KRISTEN: Smoking is definitely causing me health problems. I'm not sick yet,

	Advantages	Disadvantages
Using (continuing)	I like the way it makes me feel It's a social thing It takes the pain away It feels like taking care of myself It's my only entertainment It's a chance to get back what I've lost	Health problems Impact on daughter and other family members Guilt, shame, despair Relationship problems Legal problems Tired of being dependent
Not using (stopping)	Won't have more legal problems Save some money Get along better with certain people Feel more freedom Be healthier Better self-esteem	No chance of recovering losses Can't hang out with friends No way to mellow out Nothing like it Go through withdrawal Dealing with urges and craving Feel deprived

FIGURE 12.3. Completed advantages–disadvantages analysis.

but I can't walk as far or climb stairs without getting out of breath. And Lilly, my daughter, is almost old enough to understand how bad smoking is and she'll worry about me. Or even worse, she'll eventually become a smoker like me. [*Becomes teary-eyed.*] I'm ashamed to admit to these things.

BILL: Actually Kristen, what you said there hit a nerve in me. I may not believe gambling is a problem, but family means a lot to me. That's why I'm here. I don't want to lose my family. It's really nice that you're thinking about your daughter's feelings. I probably should have been thinking about my kids' feelings before I started spending their college funds. Maybe if I'd thought about these things when they were as young, like your daughter, I wouldn't have gambled as much.

LOIS: Wow, Kristen and Bill, what a meaningful exchange. Thank you both for being so open. Besides focusing on the advantages and disadvantages of your behaviors, discussions like these contribute to wonderful group cohesiveness, or a sense of bonding.

As Lois acknowledged, structured group techniques can facilitate insight, but they can also lead to increased group cohesiveness. As group members open up and express vulnerable feelings, other group members begin to care about them. And as group members share vulnerable feelings they also serve as role models for other group members who are more likely to reciprocate and be vulnerable.

Lois continues facilitating completion of the ADA and group members continue to share the advantages and disadvantages of using and not using behaviors. As they do so, they become increasingly surprised at the similarities between their addictive behaviors. By the end of this exercise, group members have learned a great deal about each other and themselves, and the group feels even more cohesive and supportive.

GROUP PROCESSES AND PROBLEMS

Effectively facilitated CBT groups are warm, supportive, and interpersonally safe—as well as educational, stimulating, and pragmatic. Perhaps the best way to describe the processes of CBT groups and other group approaches is by explaining how certain *therapeutic factors* contribute to positive group outcomes. The first scholars to study therapeutic factors were Corsini and Rosenberg (1955). They reviewed approximately 300 articles on group psychotherapy and extracted terms that ultimately reflected 10 categories. Yalom (1975) focused on the most salient of these factors, and expanded on them. According to Yalom and Leszcz (2005), the 11 therapeutic factors of group therapy include:

- *Instillation of hope*—when group members gain inspiration or become more optimistic by observing the successes of others
- *Universality*—when group members discover that are not alone in their thoughts, feelings, behavior patterns, and (perhaps most importantly) their problems
- *Imparting information*—when group members realize the benefits associated with learning in the group
- *Altruism*—when group members discover the positive experience of providing support, encouragement, knowledge, skills, and the like to others
- *Corrective recapitulation of primary family group*—when group members receive nurturing, caring, support, knowledge from the group that was not received in their own families
- *Development of socializing techniques*—when group members acquire valuable social and interpersonal skills
- *Imitative behavior*—when group members learn from others in the group who possess valued knowledge or skills
- *Interpersonal learning*—when group members learn how they are perceived through the eyes of other group members
- *Group cohesiveness*—when group members feel support, trust, and a sense of belonging in the group
- *Catharsis*—when group members express strong vulnerable emotions without feeling ashamed, judged, or criticized
- *Existential factors*—when group members focus on important matters outside of (and "bigger than") themselves

We consistently find that these therapeutic processes are essential to all CBTAGs. Skillful CBTAG facilitators fully understand the importance of these therapeutic factors and they deliberately underscore their importance. For example, they emphasize that group members: are not alone in their struggles (universality), benefit from helping each other (altruism), have the capacity to learn and grow (instillation of hope), learn from each other (imitative behavior), and grow closer as a collective (group cohesiveness).

While most group therapists agree that therapeutic factors are essential, these factors are not always operative. Instead, there are times when various problems impede these processes. In some cases, problems can be linked to members who do not wish to be in the group. In other cases, they can be linked to members who lack resources to function cooperatively in the group. We have compiled a list of common problems we have noted in CBTAGs. These problems are most often triggered by members who:

- Are silent or withdrawn from the group
- Perpetually come late to, or are absent from, group sessions

- Monopolize group conversations
- Give direct advice to other group members, despite being reminded that advice is not helpful or productive in the group setting
- Are perpetually defensive
- Become emotionally activated in ways that consistently distract or disturb other group members

Earlier in this chapter we described inclusion criteria, exclusion criteria, and group rules established over the years. Most of these were developed in response to problematic patterns we witnessed. For example, as we learned that group members were distracted by members who sat in silence, we decided to screen new group members for their willingness to participate in group sessions by sharing their personal concerns and being supportive of other group members. As we discovered that even severely impaired group members could be helped by the group, we decided to include group members with serious mental illnesses.

Over a period of almost 30 years, we have only asked a few group members to transfer from our CBT group to different therapeutic modalities. In one case, a group member perpetually blamed all of his problems on his wife, and continually became defensive when asked to consider changes he might make, so we advised him to complete a course of marital therapy before returning to the group. In another case a group member was floridly paranoid, accusing group members of conspiracies to harm him. And in a third case, a patient with borderline personality disorder became furious in response to all efforts to help her, ironically exclaiming, "None of you cares about me or understands what it's like to be me." When these group members were asked to consider alternative services, discussions occurred privately, following group sessions. In each case the group member was surprised and unhappy with the recommendation, so the therapist made sure to supply them with appropriate referrals, support, and guidance, until they understood that this process was in everyone's best interest, and they would ultimately benefit from shifting to another modality.

We have established rules like "No defensiveness," "Personalize everything," and "No advice giving," as we have learned that such rules decrease the likelihood that there will be interpersonal problems in the group. Furthermore, by explaining these rules prior to entry into the group, group members need only reminders when they are philosophizing, being defensive, or giving advice to others. As a brief example of such a reminder, consider the exchange that follows. Sarah has just listened to the successful efforts of two other group members:

SARAH: You all make your recovery sound so easy. I get so depressed that I don't even think about doing the positive things that make your recovery possible.

KRISTEN: Sarah, the ABC model is a great way to change your thoughts if you want to change your feelings. You should work on changing the thoughts that cause you to feel depressed.

SARAH: That's easier said than done.

LOIS: Kristen, I appreciate how much you value the ABC model. And I can see that you're sincerely trying to help Sarah.

KRISTEN: Oh no, have I done something wrong? I'm sorry!

LOIS: It's not that you've done something wrong. It's that certain rules exist to help group members be more effective at helping each other. For example, did you hear yourself say, "The ABC model is a great way to change your thoughts if you want to change your feelings"?

KRISTEN: Oh yeah, I should have personalized that. More like, "Sarah, it really helps *me* to use the ABC model when *I* start to feel depressed."

LOIS: Excellent, thank you! And did you hear yourself tell Sarah, "You should . . ."

KRISTEN: I already know what I did wrong there. I shouldn't be saying *should* to another group member. I mean I shouldn't give advice.

LOIS: What might you have said instead?

KRISTEN: I might have said that it helps me to change my thoughts. . . . Sarah, I'm so sorry!

LOIS: Kristen, I think by apologizing you're saying that you care about Sarah.

KRISTEN: [*To Sarah.*] Yes, that's exactly what I'm saying. I do care about you and want you to get the kind of help I got.

SARAH: [*Becoming tearful.*] Thank you, Kristen. That means a lot to me.

LOIS: [*To Sarah.*] How helpful was the advice Kristen was giving earlier?

SARAH: To be honest, I've always just shut down when people tell me what to do. I've been told what to do my whole life.

LOIS: How helpful was it when Kristen personalized her thoughts, by sharing what worked for her and especially that she cares about you?

SARAH: It was very helpful. Thank you again, Kristen.

This example, between Kristen, Sarah, and Lois, is actually quite common in a well-run CBT group. Over the course of their lives, many group members learn to distance themselves from their feelings, in order to avoid vulnerability. They have experienced hurt feelings when others have dismissed their sadness, disappointment, loneliness, anxiety, frustration, despair, or worry. They have also felt regret after trying to help others by sharing their own pain. In the group, members are encouraged to share private thoughts and feelings, and to support others who do the same. The rules described above serve to increase the likelihood that exchanges like the one between Kristen and Sarah are rewarding and fulfilling.

SUMMARY

Group therapy can be profoundly challenging and rewarding for both group members and facilitators. When group sessions are well-facilitated, both patients and therapists develop and practice vital skills. Patients are especially likely to benefit from group therapeutic factors described by Yalom and Leszcz (2005). For example, some group members learn for the first time that they are not alone in their suffering. Some have their first experience helping others who struggle. Some receive caring, constructive feedback, as they have never received before. And some experience what it's like to be part of a caring "family" for the first time in their lives.

Many clinicians believe group therapy is much more difficult to facilitate than individual therapy. This may or may not be true, but the rewards of running an effective CBT group are well worth the effort. Cognitive-behavioral therapists who effectively practice individual CBT are encouraged to extend their skills to the group setting, where they will learn directly the professional and personal benefits of the group CBT process.

FORM 12.1.   CBT Addiction Group Tracking Sheet

Instructions: This form is completed by group facilitators at each session. The primary aim in using this form is to track participant attendance and progress from session to session. At each session patients are asked to introduce themselves by stating their name, age (optional), addiction(s), status of their addiction(s), goals for change, and any other issues relating to their addiction (e.g., the context in which they live). A secondary aim is to help facilitators maintain focus in each session.

Name (age)	Addiction(s)	Status of addiction	Change goals	Other issues/context

CHAPTER 13

RELAPSE PREVENTION AND HARM REDUCTION

Barb, 65 years old, has worked as a cook in a nursing home for 20 years. For most of these years she has longed to retire, but she now concedes that this dream is not likely to come true. She has serious financial problems, all due to gambling losses. She has maxed out all of her credit cards and spent all of her retirement savings on gambling. After trying and failing to quit countless times she wearily admits, "I'll probably always go back to gambling."

Larry, 48 years old, has just been told by his family physician that he has lung cancer. As a cigarette smoker this is the news he has dreaded all his adult life. Larry and his wife have two daughters in high school. For as long as he can remember they have begged him to stop smoking so he has tried to quit over and over again. Now Larry feels tremendous guilt and shame. He's not sure which is more terrifying: facing his mortality or facing his daughters with this news. Recalling the many times he has tried to quit and failed, Larry despises himself for not quitting sooner.

Lynn, 39 years old, weighs just over 350 pounds. She needs an electric scooter to get around because she is unable to walk more than a few feet without stopping to rest. Lynn describes herself as a "yo-yo dieter" who has battled binge eating her entire life. There have been times when she has lost as much as 100 pounds but then gained it all back. She often thinks, "My eating habits have destroyed my life." But she can't imagine her life without comfort foods.

Jim, 46 years old, has just regained consciousness in the intensive care unit of his local hospital. He looks up, recognizes his wife's face, sees the tears in her eyes, and hears her pained voice say: "You almost died from that damn pain medicine. How could you do this?" As Jim's head starts to clear, he recalls the many times he's tried and failed to reduce the amount of medicine he takes. He's asked himself hundreds of times, "Why am I doing this to myself?"

Barb, Larry, Lynn, and Jim have several things in common: All have struggled with addictive behaviors; all have all tried unsuccessfully to change these behaviors; all have suffered numerous lapses and relapses; and all might benefit from therapeutic approaches that focus on relapse prevention and harm reduction.

What do the terms *lapse, relapse, relapse prevention,* and *harm reduction* mean? A *lapse,* or *slip,* is defined as initial engagement in a behavior (e.g., gambling, smoking, binge eating, opioid misuse) following a commitment to abstain from that behavior. A *relapse,* on the other hand, is a full return to an addictive behavior. *Relapse prevention* is generally considered any therapeutic intervention aimed at reducing the likelihood of relapse. And *harm reduction* involves efforts to decrease harm or damage associated with addictive behaviors.[1]

Nobody wants to be addicted. While many people with addictions wish to continue their behaviors without experiencing harm, most do not want to feel compelled to use or be dependent on their addictive behaviors. The four people described above all wish they could continue their behaviors without harm. Barb wishes she could "just enjoy gambling like other people enjoy their hobbies." Larry wishes he could "just enjoy a smoke once in a while," Lynn wishes she could "eat just like everyone else." And Jim wishes that he could "take just enough medication to ease the pain." Hence, many patients feel frustrated as they try unsuccessfully to reduce or stop addictive behaviors. Unfortunately, it's not just patients who feel frustrated with their relapses. Friends, family, colleagues, and even therapists may feel frustrated as they care for those who struggle with addictions.

This chapter focuses on relapse prevention and harm reduction. We are guided by five main principles:

1. Relapse is intrinsic to the process of recovery.
2. Relapse episodes provide opportunities for learning.
3. Relapse-prevention practices facilitate learning.
4. When relapse is persistent, harm-reduction strategies should be considered.
5. Both relapse-prevention and harm-reduction strategies *meet people where they're at* and therefore enhance therapeutic relationships and long-term success.

It is relatively easy for people to stop unwanted behaviors momentarily; sustaining behavior change is much more difficult. As stated earlier, most people with

---

[1] It should be noted that the seminal work in both relapse prevention and harm reduction was done by Alan Marlatt and colleagues (Hendershot, Witkiewitz, George, & Marlatt, 2011; Logan & Marlatt, 2010; Marlatt, 1996; Marlatt & Gordon, 1985; Marlatt & Tapert, 1993; Marlatt & Witkiewitz, 2005). Alan Marlatt has been described by colleagues as a visionary and luminary (White, Larimer, Sher, & Witkiewitz, 2011), and we agree. In fact, this chapter is dedicated to the memory of Alan Marlatt, who passed away in 2011.

addictions have setbacks (i.e., lapses and relapses). Hence, a major goal of CBT for *patients* is to learn from these *setbacks,* while a major goal for *therapists* is to be patient, collaborative, and strategic as patients experience *setbacks.* It is hoped that lessons learned from relapse-prevention and harm-reduction practices will ultimately increase both therapists' and patients' knowledge, skillfulness, and tenacity.

In this chapter we discuss CBT approaches to relapse prevention, but more importantly we emphasize that relapse is an inevitable aspect of the change process. Patients are encouraged to label a relapse as such (rather than self-stigmatizing), review skills for avoiding future relapses, and practice these skills in the future. Moreover, we urge patients and therapists to view relapse as a natural part of recovery and an opportunity for learning and personal growth. We emphasize to therapists that people with addictions make changes on their own schedule, rather than on the schedules of their wishful therapists. And we stress that patients who are not ready to abstain from addictive behaviors should be helped to reduce harm associated with these behaviors.

Most relapse-prevention strategies employ the basic components of CBT: structure, collaboration, case conceptualization, psychoeducation, and structured techniques. And many specific relapse-prevention techniques have already been described in previous chapters (for example, see Chapter 7).

RELAPSE PREVENTION AND HARM REDUCTION FROM A CBT PERSPECTIVE

As we have discussed, addictions involve overlearned, automatic cognitive, behavioral, physiologic, and affective processes that get activated when individuals encounter addiction-related triggers. These triggers may be internal (e.g., negative and positive emotions, urges, craving, hunger, exhaustion, physical pain) or external (e.g., people, places, things associated with addictive behaviors). Early consequences of addictive behaviors are predominantly positive or at least desired, but eventually they become associated with unwelcome outcomes. Indeed, Barbara, Larry, Lynn, and Jim all enjoyed their addictive behaviors—until they did not.

As the advantages of addictive behaviors shrink and the disadvantages grow, most addicted individuals attempt to exert control over their addictive behaviors. In doing so, they become intimately familiar with the dynamics of relapse. In fact, most individuals seeking treatment have tried to make changes on their own, but after failing to do so and growing tired of relapsing, they decide to seek professional help. By the time they arrive at the therapist's office, they feel ambivalent about their addictive behaviors. They might say something like, "I really don't want to quit my [addictive behavior], but I'm at a point where I have to."

Larry, Lynn, Barb, and Jim have all reached the point where the scales have tipped from "I *can* live with my addiction" to "I *can't* live with my addiction."

Barb is worried about finances, Larry is terrified by his cancer diagnosis and what it might mean to his family, Lynn wants to get around on her own and not be dependent on her scooter, and Jim wants to live more fully, as he did before getting hooked on narcotic pain medication.

Relapse Prevention from a CBT Perspective

Relapse prevention involves identification of the triggers, thoughts, feelings, behaviors, and consequences associated with relapse, and the development of skills that enable patients to resist relapse. Some patients are most at risk for relapse when they experience positive emotions, some when they experience negative emotions, some when they are exposed to external events associated with addictive behaviors, and of course many are at risk in all of these circumstances. Hence, some relapse-prevention strategies involve avoiding triggers, some involve learning cognitive and behavioral skills for coping with triggers, and some involve mastering meaningful activities that make the addictive behaviors themselves less seductive.

Harm Reduction from a CBT Perspective

Cognitive-behavioral therapists should always consider harm-reduction strategies when patients are not committed to abstinence. For example, people with alcohol use disorder might be helped by learning safe drinking limits and avoiding potentially hazardous activities (e.g., driving or operating potentially hazardous equipment) while under the influence of alcohol. People who smoke cigarettes might consider using nicotine replacement products, people with opioid use disorder might consider medications for treating opioid use disorder, and people who binge eat might agree to avoiding high-risk foods or eating small, healthy snacks between meals to feel less hungry at mealtime.

Focusing on harm reduction can feel like a slippery slope, particularly when patients are engaging in illegal or even life-threatening behaviors and talking to therapists about merely reducing these behaviors. Most therapists would prefer that patients never engage in such behaviors, and some wish their patients would not self-disclose these behaviors at all. The slope begins to feel slippery when patients say things like, "I'll try to use cocaine on weekends only," or "I'll drink less before driving my car." Upon hearing statements like these, therapists are advised to identify any positive steps that are being taken and discuss strategies for accomplishing these steps. Therapists who practice harm reduction realize that judgmental responses like the following may be ineffective or even counterproductive:

"You must stop your [addictive behavior] immediately."
"Don't you realize that your [addictive behavior] is unhealthy and/or illegal?"
"Your [addictive behavior] is likely to get you in a lot of trouble."

"There are better things to do with your time besides [addictive behavior]."
"It doesn't sound like you really want to change."

In contrast, effective therapist responses reinforce even small steps in the direction of harm reduction, for example:

"I understand that you want to make changes."
"That sounds like a good start."
"That would be a big change for you."
"Let's talk about how you'll make that happen."
"I'll be eager to hear how that turns out."

In addition to making reinforcing statements like these, therapists are encouraged to ask questions and initiate discussions about how such new behaviors might be accomplished. In order to succeed at harm-reduction strategies, therapists must shift their thinking from "Learn these skills and change now," to "Let's figure out a change plan that works best for you." Again, people with addictions change their behaviors on their own schedules (rather than on their therapists' schedules).

ORIENTING PATIENTS
TO HARM REDUCTION AND RELAPSE PREVENTION

We recommend that therapists consider introducing relapse prevention and harm reduction early in the CBT process (e.g., while orienting patients to CBT). The following exchange between Barb and her therapist, during their first meeting, provides an example of how this might occur:

THERAPIST: Welcome Barb. I'm glad to meet you.

BARB: Thanks, I'm glad to be here.

THERAPIST: What would you like to work on together?

BARB: My doctor told me to come talk to you. She thinks I'm depressed. I'm 65 years old and exhausted all the time. I work as a cook at an assisted living facility. I'm too old for this. Look at my hands. [*Holds out her hands for the therapist to see.*] I've cut and burned these hands more times than I can count. I thought I'd be winding down by now, but I'm really stressed about money.

THERAPIST: What do you mean when you say you thought you'd be "winding down by now"?

BARB: I'm 65 years old. I thought I'd retire right about now.

THERAPIST: You also said you're stressed about money . . .

BARB: [*Interrupts.*] Okay, before I chicken out, I need to just say it . . . [*Pauses and takes a deep breath.*] I'd have money for retirement if I hadn't spent it all on gambling.

THERAPIST: [*After another pause.*] Please explain.

BARB: It's not something I'm proud of. For starters, I live alone. Some years ago I had friends who would take me gambling. At first I didn't enjoy it, but then I started getting hooked. The actual gambling was only part of it. When I wasn't gambling, I found myself craving the sounds, the flashing lights, the people all around, the slot machines, and everything else you find in a casino. One day it suddenly hit me, and I thought, "I don't feel lonely when I'm here."

THERAPIST: So gambling, or at least being in a casino, met certain needs that weren't being met in your life.

BARB: Exactly. Until it started causing problems.

THERAPIST: What do you mean?

BARB: I didn't really admit it to myself right away. It was only when my credit card charges started getting denied that I realized I'd gone too far.

THERAPIST: Gone too far?

BARB: Yeah, it took a couple of years, but my gambling somehow ate through my savings and retirement account. And then I found myself at the end of my rope—financially that is.

THERAPIST: You must have been shocked by this realization.

BARB: Shocked? I was terrified.

THERAPIST: What efforts have you made to get your finances under control?

BARB: I knew I needed to stop gambling. I tried everything. I promised myself that I'd only spend so much money gambling. I'd only bring small amounts to the casino, like $20 or $30. I'd leave my credit cards at home. I'd promise to spend only so much time at the casino. It all failed. I broke all promises to myself.

THERAPIST: So, you've set all these goals and then relapsed over and over again. And now you find yourself here with me. Am I correct in assuming that you're looking for help for gambling addiction?

BARB: It feels like I don't have a choice.

THERAPIST: I'd like to help. Since you've struggled with multiple relapses, I'd like to discuss relapse prevention.

BARB: Relapse prevention. Is that a thing?

THERAPIST: Relapse prevention involves us working together to examine your relapses carefully, like under a microscope, to better understand all of the elements that lead you to relapse.

BARB: Elements?

THERAPIST: Yes. We'll spend time discussing what you've been thinking, feeling, and doing right before you go gambling. We'll look for patterns. For example, we'll try to figure out if you're typically at home or at work, feeling lonely or depressed, bored or anxious. We'll talk about how you plan your trips to the casino: whether they're impulsive or carefully planned . . . and much more. How does that sound?

BARB: It makes sense, but what do we do after we figure all that out?

THERAPIST: We figure out what you can change, to prevent or at least reduce the likelihood of relapse.

BARB: That sounds good, but what if I keep going back? What if this doesn't work? I'm really scared about being homeless.

THERAPIST: That's a good question. Another thing we'll focus on is harm reduction.

BARB: Harm reduction?

THERAPIST: Yes. That's where we talk about what you might consider doing to reduce the harm caused by your gambling.

BARB: You mean like bringing only small amounts of money to the casino and leaving my credit cards at home? I already know that doesn't work.

THERAPIST: That hasn't worked, so we'll try to figure out why. We'll also look for other possible harm-reduction strategies.

BARB: Hmmm. [*Pauses.*] I can already think of something I can change.

THERAPIST: What's that?

BARB: Because I've earned VIP status at the casino, I get a room in their luxury hotel at a really good price, so I often stay there overnight. Sometimes I'll even stay for a whole weekend. I get this beautiful room, perfectly decorated, with a hot tub, jacuzzi, and lots more. But I hardly spend any time in the room. When I try to climb into bed and get some sleep, I end up wide awake, craving more gambling. Eventually I get up, go back downstairs, and start again. It's rare that I get more than 2 or 3 hours of sleep when I'm there. And then I feel terrible for days afterward. It's like a hangover without drinking. When I'm honest with myself, I realize that I should never stay overnight at a casino hotel.

THERAPIST: Sounds like you might be willing to start a harm-reduction plan with no longer staying overnight at the casino. Is that right?

BARB: Yeah. I've been considering that for a long time anyway.

Barb and her new therapist have accomplished a lot in this brief exchange. Barb's therapist has introduced two important concepts, relapse prevention and harm reduction, and helped Barb reflect on these. Barb has openly shared her concerns about gambling (perhaps for the first time) and even expressed a willingness to consider changing one behavior pattern. Based on this interaction, it seems Barb and her therapist are off to a good start. In future sessions, Barb's therapist will go into much more depth, learning about the contextual, cognitive, behavioral, affective, and physiological processes involved in Barb's relapses. Barb and her therapist will also generate strategies for reducing the likelihood of relapse, or at least harm caused by relapses.

FUNCTIONAL ANALYSIS IN RELAPSE PREVENTION AND HARM REDUCTION

In Chapter 6 we described therapeutic processes for addressing addictive behaviors. Among the most important of these is functional analysis. In functional analysis, therapists and patients review and diagram the contextual, cognitive, behavioral, affective, and physiological processes associated with addictive behaviors. In doing so, both gain valuable knowledge about the factors influencing relapse, and they identify potential change targets. To illustrate, we share an exchange between Larry and his therapist during his first visit:

THERAPIST: Larry, I understand that you have been referred because you've been diagnosed with lung cancer and would like help with smoking cessation.

LARRY: Actually, I've quit smoking. It's been 10 days since I was diagnosed. As you might guess, I haven't smoked since that day.

THERAPIST: Congratulations on quitting. How are you coping with your diagnosis?

LARRY: I'm doing okay. I've taken leave from work to spend more time with my family, so it's been pretty easy to stay away from cigarettes. I worry more about my family than I do myself.

THERAPIST: I'm glad that you can take this time with them since they're so important to you. Given that you've quit already, what would you like to work on with me?

LARRY: I think I'll pull through the medical part okay. The doctors seem hopeful. They say we caught the cancer in its early stages. I want to make sure I never smoke again.

THERAPIST: Great. Tell me more about yourself, your family, your smoking, and whatever seems relevant today. We haven't met before so I'll be interested in just about anything you can tell me about yourself.

LARRY: Okay, I'm 48 years old, married, and I have two beautiful daughters in high school. I'm a senior partner at a law firm and until 10 days ago, my job kept me pretty busy. My wife, daughters, and I are very close and . . . [*He chokes back tears and trails off for almost a minute.*] I'm sorry . . . it's just that . . . that's what makes this so hard. . . . I never want to break their hearts like this again.

THERAPIST: Larry, there's no need to apologize. You obviously care deeply about your family. Would you like to talk more about these strong feelings toward them or continue talking about smoking? I'll let you decide.

LARRY: I'm really here to make sure I never smoke again. That's where I need your help.

THERAPIST: That's fine. Let's get back to your smoking. Tell me about your smoking and your efforts to quit.

LARRY: I'm sure you know the old adage: "Quitting smoking is easy. I've done it thousands of times." Well that's me. I've tried to quit thousands of times, but I only succeed for a few hours or days.

THERAPIST: So, you've repeatedly tried to quit and repeatedly relapsed.

LARRY: Yup, that's me.

THERAPIST: Let's look at your relapses more carefully. When you've tried to quit, what's happened? Try to recall the last time you tried.

LARRY: Oh, that's easy. I made the initial doctor's appointment, before I was diagnosed, because I had a cough that wouldn't go away. It was different from my daily smoker's cough, so I started to worry a little. After making that first appointment and being sent for all those tests and scans, I made a real effort to quit, but it was no use. I was so worried about the cough and getting the test results that I probably smoked twice as much as usual.

THERAPIST: So, your cough scared you and you decided to see your doctor about it. You tried to quit before the doctor's visit, but you found you weren't ready.

LARRY: That's exactly right.

THERAPIST: It sounds like your smoking gets triggered by stress, or tension.

LARRY: Yeah, that's right. My work is very stressful and demanding. If it's not one thing, it's something else. Every day there's a new challenge or problem. For some reason, I'm the guy everyone turns to when there's a big project or problem. Every time I've tried to quit smoking it seems that I get slammed with a big project. That's when I figure it's just not the right time to quit.

THERAPIST: I'm starting to understand. Do you mind if I draw your pattern out on paper?

LARRY: Of course not, go ahead.

THERAPIST: [*The therapist starts to draw the circles and arrows of a functional analysis.*] Your triggers for smoking are both internal, like feelings of stress or tension, and external, like extreme job pressure.

LARRY: That sounds about right.

THERAPIST: And these triggers activate certain thoughts, like "I need a cigarette."

LARRY: Yeah.

THERAPIST: That's when your urge to smoke begins and you crave a cigarette.

LARRY: Yes.

THERAPIST: And then you think, "I've quit. I can't smoke anymore."

LARRY: Yeah, and a lot of other thoughts that drive me nuts.

THERAPIST: Like what other thoughts?

LARRY: Like thinking, "I'll have just one more smoke."

THERAPIST: And then you smoke?

LARRY: That's when I light up and start smoking.

THERAPIST: Take a look at what I've drawn here. [*Shows the functional analysis in Figure 13.1 to Larry.*]

LARRY: Yeah, that's me. Seeing it on paper is helpful. [*Points at two of the circles.*] Those thoughts drive me nuts: "I've quit. I can't smoke." And then, "Just one more smoke."

THERAPIST: I can see how those thoughts would drive you nuts. There's a term for that, besides *nuts*.

LARRY: What's the term?

THERAPIST: *Ambivalence.* You feel extremely ambivalent about quitting smoking during those times.

After Larry's therapist draws the brief functional analysis in Figure 13.1, he explains that this the first of many functional analyses that they will construct together to reflect Larry's strings of thoughts, feelings, and behaviors. Larry's therapist explains that these functional analyses will help Larry be more aware and deliberate in his decision making, so he might make more conscious choices about whether or not to smoke, and how he might deal with his tension.

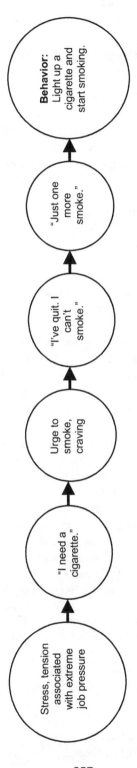

FIGURE 13.1. Brief functional analysis for Larry.

Identifying and Addressing Thoughts and Beliefs
That Lead to Addictive Behaviors

Larry's therapist will continue to help him identify thoughts that increase his risk of relapse, as well as thoughts that protect him from relapsing. For example, when Larry is craving a cigarette, he is most likely to relapse if he has *permissive thoughts*. Permissive thoughts (defined in Chapter 10) are a subset of addiction-related thoughts that involve patients' permission to use. Examples include the following:

"Just one more time."
"Today will be the last day."
"I'll start fresh tomorrow."
"I'll keep it limited."
"Nobody will find out."
"I'm not hurting anyone but myself."
"It's too late to erase the damage I've caused."
"Nothing else in my life makes me feel good."

Following a trigger, the onset of urges and craving, and the granting of permission, it is likely that an individual will *slip*. This slip, or *lapse,* then becomes a new trigger for the cycle to begin again. For example, after smoking that one cigarette, Larry might think, "I've totally blown it again." This belief might be followed by a cascade of additional automatic thoughts that lead to smoking another cigarette. When this occurs, it is likely that his craving for cigarettes will become stronger, and his smoking will increase again until he has had a full-blown *relapse* (i.e., a return to typical patterns of addictive behavior).

Ideally, therapists help patients view lapses and relapses as opportunities to practice adaptive ways of thinking and behaving. Larry's therapist might help him understand that there are more adaptive ways to deal with his tension at work. Rather than believing he is a slave to cigarettes and must smoke, he might focus on successful strategies for dealing with work pressure. Further, even if he does decide to smoke that single cigarette, he does not have to think he has failed and has no further control. Instead, he could practice reciting control thoughts that might help him to avoid a relapse. Such control thoughts might include:

"If I stop smoking right now, I show myself that I am stronger than cigarettes."
"Quitting smoking is the most loving thing I can do for my family."
"I'm a person who keeps his commitments."
"If I resist long enough, the craving will go away."
"I will endure this short-term pain for the long-term gain."

Many of these control thoughts are already familiar to those abstaining from addictive behavior. As noted above, the battle between addiction-related thoughts and control thoughts is best understood as *ambivalence*. Early in the process of recovery, patients are typically ambivalent about the changes they are making. Many find it helpful to learn that this ambivalence is caused by conflicting thoughts that are ultimately under their control. As they review their relapses, they learn to mistrust their addiction-related beliefs and further develop and trust their control-related beliefs.

PREDICTING, MANAGING, AND UNDERSTANDING RELAPSE

Entire books and hundreds of articles and chapters have been written on the topic of relapse prevention. Hence, we barely scratch the surface in this single chapter by making brief recommendations for predicting, understanding, managing and preventing relapse. In the following sections we discuss the identification and management of triggers, cognitive approaches to relapse prevention, behavioral approaches to relapse prevention, keeping a lapse from becoming a relapse, and social support approaches to relapse prevention.

Identifying and Managing Triggers

As described throughout this text, triggers include conditions that activate addiction-related thoughts, which in turn actuate addictive behaviors. Triggers may be internal or external. The following are common internal triggers:

- Negative emotional states (e.g., sadness, anger, worry, loneliness, frustration, disappointment, despair, boredom, restlessness)
- Positive emotional states (e.g., happiness, excitement, joy, pride, elation)
- Physical or physiologic states (e.g., hunger, pain, craving, tiredness, exhaustion, tension)

The following are common external triggers:

- Actual loss of some*thing* loved or valued (e.g., a pet, material possession, job)
- Actual loss of some*one* loved or valued (e.g., a friend, colleague, mentor, family member)
- Interpersonal conflict (e.g., a recent argument or a longstanding disagreement)
- Others who are using or encouraging use (e.g., friends, family, associates)
- Significant success or achievement (e.g., a major educational or career accomplishment, task completion, graduation, promotion, competitive win)
- Significant lack of success or failure to achieve something viewed as important

People who suffer from addictions inevitably encounter triggers. This is especially apparent when one considers the fact that all human beings experience some sadness, anger, worry, loneliness, or frustration (all internal triggers) at some time. The identification of internal and external triggers is an extremely important component of the relapse-prevention process, as it is not uncommon for people with addictions to lack an awareness of such triggers.

By increasing awareness of triggers, a person with an addiction may reduce the likelihood of exposure and reflexive reaction to them. In sessions, patients are encouraged to carefully review recent and remote memories of relapses in order to discover the full range of triggers that might lead to future relapse. The following is an exchange between Lynn and her therapist, who is helping her identify binge-eating triggers:

THERAPIST: Lynn, what circumstances are most likely to trigger your binge-eating or overeating episodes?

LYNN: I don't know. It's not like I need special circumstances. I just eat when I eat.

THERAPIST: Am I correct in assuming that you don't ever want to binge eat?

LYNN: Of course I don't *want* to binge eat! There have been so many times when I've looked at an empty potato chip bag or ice cream carton on my kitchen table and wondered how I could have eaten the entire contents. It makes me sick just thinking about it.

THERAPIST: I understand how that image bothers you. Let's work together to understand how that happens. My goal is to help you prepare and cope effectively at these times by determining what triggers these lapses.

LYNN: Yeah, I guess that makes sense: looking for triggers.

THERAPIST: Can we review your last binge? How did it begin?

LYNN: What exactly do you mean by a binge? How is a binge any different from overeating?

THERAPIST: Eating more than you had planned, feeling way too full when it's over, maybe feeling guilty afterward or disgusted with yourself. These are all symptoms of a binge.

LYNN: Oh, like last night.

THERAPIST: Tell me about last night.

LYNN: I'd eaten a perfectly healthy dinner around six-thirty. I made myself a salad with low-calorie dressing and a grilled chicken breast on top. It was really good, but then around nine o'clock I started feeling hungry again. I went into the kitchen and couldn't find anything healthy that would hit the spot. I looked through the cabinets and refrigerator: nothing. And then I looked in the freezer and saw the frozen pizza I'd bought in case I ever had guests over. You know, one of those big frozen pizzas from the grocery store with the crust that rises and all the meat and everything on it. I think they call it a Deluxe or Supreme. I thought, "That looks good."

THERAPIST: What happened next?

LYNN: What happened next? I took it out of the freezer, pulled it out of the box, threw it in the oven, and around forty-five minutes later, all that was left was a pizza box.

THERAPIST: And then?

LYNN: Like you said: I ate more than I'd planned, felt full and disgusted with myself, and woke up this morning feeling guilty and miserable.

THERAPIST: You said you were hungry by nine o'clock. Let's try to figure out what triggers may have influenced you to eat an entire pizza.

LYNN: Well I can tell you this: When I bought that pizza I knew it might not last in the freezer until I had guests.

THERAPIST: You're saying that the very presence of the pizza in your freezer was a trigger to cook and eat it.

LYNN: Oh yeah. The longer it sat in the freezer, the more I could hear it calling out to me.

THERAPIST: Calling out to you?

LYNN: Yeah, when I have anything like that in my house it's almost like it calls out to me. I can be sitting on my couch, innocently watching my TV shows, and it's like I hear a voice in my head calling out: "I'm in the freezer, waiting for you. I'll taste so good. Come and get me!"

THERAPIST: Like a real voice?

LYNN: No, of course not! It's my imagination acting up.

THERAPIST: So, the very existence of a pizza in your freezer is an external trigger. How about internal triggers?

LYNN: What do you mean by internal triggers?

THERAPIST: Like what are you feeling *emotionally* when you feel hungry again after eating dinner?

LYNN: Oh, that's easy. I'm bored, lonely, restless, and a lot of other bad feelings I know all too well.

THERAPIST: What keeps you from stopping when you've eaten enough pizza to be full?

LYNN: That's a good question. I eat, like, half the pizza, and then I look at the rest of it just sitting there and think, "I've really screwed up. Might as well polish it all off."

THERAPIST: I think you're telling me that the remaining pizza is another trigger. You see it in front of you and, even though you might be full, it triggers thoughts about finishing it off.

LYNN: Exactly.

In this exchange, Lynn described a fairly common scenario. *People with addictions are likely to be triggered by a combination of internal and external triggers.* In Lynn's case, she was initially triggered by boredom, loneliness, and restlessness. These feelings likely triggered physiologic changes that she experienced as a mild craving for something. Knowing that there was a pizza in the freezer, Lynn's craving took on a specific focus—on the pizza. She began to visualize the process of cooking, eating, enjoying, and getting momentary relief from eating the pizza. And before she knew it, the pizza was gone.

The process of identifying triggers is a vital one for therapists. Patients often engage in their addictive behaviors in such an automatic manner that they do not even realize when they have been triggered. When therapists and their patients identify, label, list, and categorize their triggers, it enables patients to anticipate when they will be vulnerable to relapse. As mentioned earlier, therapists can only help patients avoid or cope with triggers after they have been identified.

Lynn's therapist continues talking to Lynn about her triggers. They generate a list of internal and external triggers that Lynn can anticipate. In doing so, Lynn realizes her world has gotten "terribly small," with few rewards, which puts her at great risk for relapse. She also realizes she needs to avoid exposure to highly palatable (or "taboo") foods whenever possible. For example, if she decides to serve such foods to guests, she doesn't purchase them until the day of their visit. She might even consider purchasing only healthy foods for guests. She also agrees to bring only healthy snacks into her home (e.g., fruits, vegetables, and so forth), and leave less healthy foods at the grocery store for someone else to purchase.

Triggers vary greatly from person to person. Therapists need to evaluate triggers for each individual patient carefully. A useful method for doing so is self-monitoring homework. Specifically, the patient keeps a journal of craving in relation to internal and external events. This journal is then reviewed with the patient whenever it is relevant to do so. It is also prudent, prior to the end of each session, to anticipate specific triggers that might occur before the next session, and then ask patients to plan strategies for coping with such triggers.

Cognitive Approaches to Relapse Prevention

The significance of triggers is that they activate thoughts and beliefs that increase vulnerability to lapses and relapses. Thus, a fundamental cognitive strategy for relapse prevention is the development of *control* beliefs that reduce vulnerability to lapses and relapses. The following are examples of control beliefs that reduce vulnerability to lapses and relapses:

"I don't need [addictive behaviors] to feel good."
"My life will improve without [addictive behaviors]."
"I can cope with unpleasant emotions without using [addictive behaviors]."
"I have control over my own behaviors, including my [addictive behaviors]."
"Even if I slip, I don't have to continue using [addictive behaviors]."
"A lapse does not have to become a relapse."

Guided discovery, the most foundational of CBT strategies, is used to help patients identify addiction-related thoughts and beliefs and replace these with self-control thoughts and beliefs. The following exchange between Jim and his therapist demonstrates how this might occur:

THERAPIST: Jim, you said you woke up in the hospital and asked yourself, "Why am I doing this to myself?"

JIM: Yeah, I just don't get why I can't cut down on the pain medicine.

THERAPIST: One of the reasons it's hard to cut down is because you have so many thoughts and beliefs that support taking your medication.

JIM: I'm not sure I understand.

THERAPIST: There are two kinds of thoughts and beliefs I'd like to discuss with you: those that are addiction-related and those that help with self-control. The addiction-related thoughts lead to your excessive medicine use and the self-control thoughts—

JIM: [*Interrupts.*] Let me guess: help me get better self-control.

THERAPIST: Exactly. Do you mind if I write down your addiction-related and self-control thoughts on a piece of paper?

JIM: Not at all.

THERAPIST: Okay. [*Takes out a piece of paper.*] Tell me what goes through you mind right before you take your medicine.

JIM: You mean thoughts like, "I need my pain medicine"?

THERAPIST: Exactly. [*Writes "I need my pain medicine" under the heading "Jim's Addiction-Related Thoughts and Beliefs."*]

JIM: Oh, I have lots of thoughts. The pain is unbearable without my pain medicine. I can't function without it. I've tried everything else and it's the only thing that relieves my pain. [*Pauses.*]

THERAPIST: Other thoughts?

JIM: Yeah. Even the smallest amount of pain breaking through scares me into taking more medicine. Otherwise, the pain will knock me on my ass. Before I landed myself in the hospital, I thought I was being careful not to be one of those people who overdoses.

THERAPIST: Okay, I've written all those thoughts down. [*Shows Jim a list of his addictive thoughts.*]

JIM: Wow, you're a fast writer.

THERAPIST: Thanks. Now let's list some thoughts that will help you get better control over the amount of medicine you take.

JIM: Okay. This should be interesting. [*Pauses to think.*] I know it's not good for me to take as much as I do. I know it can kill me. And it terrifies my wife to know that I take so much pain medicine. I know there are people all over, dying from the same drug I take. I know I can do better.

THERAPIST: Keep going.

JIM: [*Pausing to think between each statement.*] I can take my medicine like my doctor tells me to. . . . My fear of pain, instead of the pain itself, is a powerful force that drives my medicine choices. . . . I'm afraid to feel the intense pain I felt before. . . . The doctors know what they're doing. . . . I can trust that they will help me control my pain. . . . I don't have to keep adjusting the dose myself.

THERAPIST: Well done. Now take another look at these two groups of thoughts. [*Shows Jim Table 13.1, a side-by-side list of his addictive and self-control-related thoughts;* a blank version of this table is available in Form 2.1 at the end of Chapter 2 for your convenience.] The first group contains thoughts that drive your current medicine-taking behaviors, while the second group might help to improve your control over your drug-taking behaviors.

JIM: It's really interesting seeing my thoughts written out like that. I think I get it.

THERAPIST: I'd like to keep working on identifying both sets of thoughts and beliefs: those that make it more likely that you'll take more medicine than prescribed and those that make it more likely that you'll take your medicine just as your doctors have prescribed.

JIM: I can agree to that, for sure.

In this example Jim was helped to recognize and list addiction-related and self-control thoughts and beliefs. In doing so, Jim can become more deliberate and intentional in his choices regarding thoughts and beliefs. Most people are not skillful at the processes of identifying and labeling thoughts. Upon learning this skill,

TABLE 13.1. Jim's Addiction-Related and Self-Control Thoughts and Beliefs

Addiction-Related Thoughts and Beliefs	Self-Control Thoughts and Beliefs
"I need my pain medicine." *"The pain is unbearable without my pain medicine."* *"I can't function without my pain medicine."* *"I've tried everything else and pain medicine is the only thing that relieves my pain."* *"Even the smallest amount of pain breaking through requires more medicine."* *"I need to take pain medicine as soon as I feel pain, or it will knock me on my ass."*	*"I am careful not to be one of those people who overdoses."* *"It's not good for me to take as much pain medicine as I do."* *"Too much pain medicine can kill me."* *"It terrifies my wife to know that I take so much pain medicine."* *"There are people all over, dying from the same drug I take."* *"I know I can do better."* *"I can take my medicine as prescribed."* *"My fear of pain, not the pain itself, drives my medicine choices."* *"I'm afraid to feel the intense pain I felt before."* *"The doctors know what they're doing."* *"I can trust that they will help me control my pain."* *"I don't have to keep adjusting the dose myself."*

patients are equipped to gain better control over their behaviors and abilities, in order to prevent lapses and relapses. Other cognitive approaches to relapse prevention include advantages–disadvantages analyses, daily thought records, and more. For details regarding these techniques, see Chapter 7.

Behavioral Approaches to Relapse Prevention

As patients learn to identify triggers, recognize addiction-related thoughts, and generate self-control thoughts, they are simultaneously encouraged to practice behavioral strategies for coping with triggers. The choice of one particular behavioral strategy over another depends largely on the trigger itself. Internal triggers involving emotional distress might call for behavioral strategies that reduce emotional distress. For example, behavioral activation strategies might be offered to patients who initiate addictive behaviors when they experience depression. Patients who initiate addictive behaviors when they feel anxious might be taught deep breathing and relaxation techniques. Internal triggers involving chronic physical pain might lead to relapse-prevention strategies involving physical exercise or yoga.

Internal triggers involving urges or craving might result in activities involving behavioral distraction techniques.

Perhaps the simplest of all approaches to relapse prevention is distraction. Specifically, patients are encouraged to compile lists of distracting activities that may be used when triggers are encountered. Distracting activities may include any non-addiction-related activity (e.g., exercise, talking to a friend, reading, writing, walking, gardening). Although distraction techniques are only a short-term coping device, they serve the all-important function of providing a delay between the onset of cravings and the act of seeking and engaging in addictive behaviors. Such delays may provide patients with time to think of the full negative ramifications of their addictive behaviors, as well as an opportunity to witness the diminishing of cravings if no addictive behaviors are actuated.

As Jim's therapist spends more time with him, he learns that Jim and his wife have a difficult marriage. Their children have grown up and left home, and they find themselves bickering almost every day. Jim eventually admits that he sometimes takes pain medicine to escape his marital problems. Upon learning this, Jim's therapist focuses on behavioral skills for improving Jim's marriage and reducing the likelihood of relapse. For example, Jim is assisted in developing and practicing methods for resolving conflicts with his wife. He is encouraged to think about ways to provide and ask for more emotional support. By communicating effectively with his wife, Jim is practicing problem-focused coping (i.e., effective communication) instead of avoidant coping (i.e., using pain medication). By doing so he reduces the likelihood that he will use pain medication inappropriately in the future. As Jim's case illustrates, relapse prevention necessitates that patients learn to cope with both general life stressors (e.g., marital discord) and discomfort that specifically is related to temptation to engage in addictive behaviors.

Keeping a Lapse from Becoming a Relapse

As mentioned earlier, lapses provide opportunities to apply cognitive and behavioral skills and promote further understanding of the mechanisms involved in relapse. Thus, a lapse is not necessarily perceived as bad; instead it is an opportunity to learn. An important theme of relapse prevention is helping patients keep lapses from becoming relapses.

There are many reasons why lapses occur. For example, people with addictions may choose to "slip" in order to test their ability to control their addictive behavior. They might think, "I'll try it just this once. It will prove that I am in control of my addiction." As we've mentioned above, some people "accidentally" or intentionally expose themselves to triggers without being prepared to respond cognitively or behaviorally to these triggers. Another reason for lapses may be that individuals again believe that the advantages of their addictive behaviors outweigh the disadvantages. Given the many reasons for lapses, an important component of relapse prevention involves the identification of decision points along the cognitive model of relapse. For example, did the lapse occur because of a failure to avoid external triggers (e.g., drinking buddies)? Or, did the lapse occur due to a lack of control beliefs for resisting inevitable triggers (e.g., a deadline at work)?

A lapse usually becomes a relapse as a result of underlying all-or-none beliefs; for example, "A lapse means I have no control," "This slip proves that therapy isn't working," and "A lapse is a failure." Marlatt and Gordon (1985) famously called this thinking process and the resulting relapse the *abstinence violation effect,* or AVE. An important strategy for relapse prevention, then, is to challenge such dichotomous thoughts about lapses so that they do not become relapses. When a lapse occurs, imagery techniques are useful to reconstruct the sequence of triggers, beliefs, thoughts, feelings, and behaviors leading to the lapse. Additionally, it is important to use post-hoc rehearsal of techniques at each decision point to prepare the patient for similar future circumstances.

Social Support Approaches to Relapse Prevention

Social and interpersonal processes are known to be associated with relapse. For example, Cummings, Gordon, and Marlatt (1980) found that 44% of relapse experiences are linked to interpersonal conflict. Loneliness, often associated with an absence of positive social support, is also a high-risk trigger for at least two reasons. First, loneliness itself is an uncomfortable emotion (i.e., internal trigger). Second, addictive behaviors often occur in social situations chosen specifically to avoid loneliness (e.g., bars, casinos, homes of friends who are still addicted). Hence, relapse-prevention efforts are likely to be enhanced by the acquisition of an addiction-free social support network.

It is important to understand that some patients have basic beliefs and automatic thoughts about relationships that influence their behaviors in these relationships. For example, some may believe "Only other people with addictions can understand me," "I will never be understood or accepted by people who haven't been addicted," "People who don't drink or get high are boring," and so forth. Obviously, such beliefs may result in social discomfort, or anxiety, and a certain degree of social avoidance. Patients can be helped by the therapist's understanding of this process, as well as by modification of such beliefs. Friends and family who do not struggle with addictions may be important sources of support to people with addictions. However, many people with addictions have avoided family members and friends for fear of judgment and rejection.

For many in recovery, mutual-help groups provide an addiction-free social support network vital to relapse prevention. As we've discussed, a mutual-help group is "a group of people sharing a similar problem, who meet regularly to exchange information and to give and receive psychological support" (Pistrang, Barker, & Humphreys, 2008, p. 110). Examples of mutual-help groups include 12-step programs

(AA, NA, OA, GA, etc.), Women for Sobriety, LifeRing Secular Recovery, and SMART Recovery (*www.SMARTrecovery.org*). Research on mutual-help groups generally find them to be beneficial (Grant et al., 2018; Kelly, Humphreys, & Ferri, 2020; Pistrang et al., 2008; Zenmore, Kaskutas, Mericle, & Hemberg, 2017). In fact, Pistrang et al. (2008) described two randomized trials that found mutual-help groups to be equivalent in outcomes to costly professional interventions. Mutual-help groups provide participants with private settings and people who support each other in their recovery. They also provide participants with structure, abstinence-based norms, role models, and coping skills (Moos, 2008). These mechanisms may operate even when mutual help is offered online or by telephone (Liese & Monley, 2021).

We encourage therapists to introduce mutual-help groups as part of the relapse-prevention process. Such introductions are best initiated by asking patients what they already know about mutual-help groups. Most patients will have heard of AA or SMART Recovery, and some will have already attended these or other mutual-help groups. It is recommended that therapists learn as much as possible about their local network of mutual-help groups and encourage inexperienced patients to sample each of the different available groups. By attending various groups, patients can decide which best fits their needs and personal tastes. They may also discover that there are benefits to attending both SMART Recovery and 12-step groups. Consider the following exchange between Barb and her therapist:

THERAPIST: Barb, when did you last gamble?

BARB: I think it's been about two weeks.

THERAPIST: Congratulations. How's it going?

BARB: I don't know. Okay, I guess.

THERAPIST: You don't sound very satisfied with your success.

BARB: It doesn't feel like success to me. It feels like punishment.

THERAPIST: How so?

BARB: I sit at home, feeling all the same crappy feelings I've always felt, and there's nowhere to go that makes me feel better. I told you that I feel lonely most of the time.

THERAPIST: Barb, have you ever heard of GA?

BARB: GA?

THERAPIST: Gamblers Anonymous.

BARB: Is that like AA?

THERAPIST: Yes, it's one of the 12-step programs.

BARB: Now that you mention it, I guess I have.

THERAPIST: How about SMART Recovery?

BARB: I'm not sure about that one either.

THERAPIST: These are two of the mutual-help groups that you can join that might help in your recovery from gambling disorder.

BARB: Mutual-help groups?

THERAPIST: Yeah, groups that meet regularly, don't charge for attending, don't require an appointment, and aim to help people with addictions. They aren't professional services. They are called mutual-help groups because the people who attend them all struggle with similar problems and they share what they've learned about addiction and recovery in order to help each other.

BARB: Sounds scary.

THERAPIST: Scary?

BARB: I'm not sure that kind of thing is for me. I don't think I'm comfortable telling a bunch of strangers about my problems.

THERAPIST: When you put it that way I completely understand. It might help if I tell you more about these groups. They are available all over the world, in communities big and small. You can even attend them online. You only share what you want to share, and you can take a pass on sharing if you just want to listen and learn. They are usually very welcoming.

BARB: I need to think about it.

THERAPIST: One of the reasons I'm recommending these groups is because you've said several times that loneliness is a problem for you. These groups are generally warm and supportive. My guess is that lots of people just like you attend them because it helps them feel less alone in their recovery.

BARB: Like I said, I'll think about it.

THERAPIST: Would you be interested in doing some more research on these groups before our next visit?

BARB: You mean like attend them?

THERAPIST: Not necessarily. I think it would be helpful for you to research them online. I'm sure you can find hundreds, or even thousands of Web pages on GA and SMART Recovery. You might even find other similar options online by searching for "mutual-help groups."

BARB: I could probably handle that.

THERAPIST: And then eventually, if you feel comfortable with doing so, you might visit a couple of these groups and decide if they might be helpful to you. You might consider trying a couple of visits to different groups in order to decide which is best for you.

BARB: Let's take this one step at a time.

THERAPIST: That makes good sense. Again, I believe these groups might help with both relapse prevention and the loneliness you feel.

During this exchange it became obvious that Barb was reluctant to join a mutual-help group. Most people in recovery feel just as Barb does. Most do not imagine it easy to jump into a group of strangers and share such deeply personal information. Barb's therapist is sensitive to Barb's concerns and encouraged Barb to take this step at a pace that was comfortable for her. Her therapist also recommended that she first research these options and sample more than one type of group.

Prior to ending this section on social support, it is important to emphasize that effective therapists are likely to become an essential part of patients' support networks. By providing warmth, acceptance, consistency, empathy, and wisdom to patients with addictions, it is likely that therapists will play an important role in relapse prevention. It is through such supportive relationships that people with addictions can develop strategies and learn skills that help them transition into a satisfying life of abstinence from addictive behaviors. In other words, therapists are likely to become part of the bridge from patients' life of addictions and relapses to much healthier, addiction-free lives.

TERMINATING THERAPY AND BOOSTER SESSIONS

When abstinence has been maintained for an extended period of time, patients and their therapists can become confident in their ability to refrain from engaging in addictive behaviors and formal therapy may be terminated. However, booster sessions are encouraged for some patients. Such sessions may include telephone calls, written correspondence, or face-to-face contact. This contact serves several purposes. First, it focuses the patient's attention on the need for vigilance in combating the relapse process. Second, the therapist's continued interest in the patient provides social support that motivates further abstinence. Third, the therapist can continue to provide expert guidance to a patient who may be at renewed risk for relapse.

Substantial gains may result from extended contact with the patient. Each booster visit or telephone call might decrease the likelihood that the patient will relapse, or at least will remind the patient that the therapist is a potential resource for coping with triggers. If a patient does relapse after therapy has been terminated, it is recommended that they be invited to return to therapy as soon as possible to work on improving coping skills. Again, careful review of each lapse and relapse provides the patient with an increased understanding and ultimately greater control over the relapse process.

SUMMARY

In this chapter, we have discussed relapse prevention and harm reduction. The primary aim of CBT for addictions is relapse prevention, or a reduction in the likelihood that patients in recovery will slip into lapses or lapse into relapses. The primary aim of harm reduction is to minimize the harm that may occur from continued engagement in addictive behaviors.

Throughout this text, strategies and techniques have been presented for predicting and reducing the likelihood of relapse. We have tried to emphasize that relapse prevention and harm reduction are as much about therapists' attitudes as they are about techniques. Therapists who are supportive and resourceful with patients who continue to struggle with addictions are most likely to help patients. These therapists are also most likely to experience fulfilment from working with patients with addictions—even when their patients struggle with lapses and relapses.

REFERENCES

12step.org. (2018). Recovery slogans. Retrieved from *https://12step.org/references/commonly-used/recovery-slogans*.

American Psychiatric Association. (2013). *Diagnostic and statistical manual of mental disorders* (5th ed.). Arlington, VA: Author.

Beck, A. T. (1967). *Depression: Clinical, experimental, & theoretical aspects*. New York: Harper & Row.

Beck, A. T., Davis, D. D., & Freeman, A. (Eds.). (2015). *Cognitive therapy of personality disorders* (3rd ed.). New York: Guilford Press.

Beck, A. T., Emery, G., & Greenberg, R. L. (1985). *Anxiety disorders and phobias: A cognitive perspective*. New York: Basic Books

Beck, A. T., Finkel, M. R., & Beck, J. S. (2021). The theory of modes: Applications to schizophrenia and other psychological conditions. *Cognitive Therapy and Research, 45*, 391–400.

Beck, A. T., Rush, A. J., Shaw, B. F., & Emery, G. (1979). *Cognitive therapy of depression*. New York: Guilford Press.

Beck, A. T., & Steer, R. A. (1993). *Beck Anxiety Inventory manual*. San Antonio, TX: Psychological Corporation.

Beck, A. T., Steer, R. A., & Brown, G. K. (1996). *Manual for the Beck Depression Inventory—II*. San Antonio, TX: Psychological Corporation.

Beck, A. T., Steer, R. A., Kovacs, M., & Garrison, B. (1985). Hopelessness and eventual suicide: a 10-year prospective study of patients hospitalized with suicidal ideation. *American Journal of Psychiatry, 142*(5), 559–563.

Beck, A. T., Wright, F. D., Newman, C. F., & Liese, B. S. (1993). *Cognitive therapy of substance abuse*. New York: Guilford Press.

Beck, J. S. (2021). *Cognitive behavior therapy: Basics and beyond* (3rd ed.). New York: Guilford Press.

Bevilacqua, L., & Goldman, D. (2009). Genes and addictions. *Clinical Pharmacology and Therapeutics, 85*(4), 359–361.

Bickel, W. K., Johnson, M. W., Koffarnus, M. N., MacKillop, J., & Murphy, J. G. (2014). The behavioral economics of substance use disorders: reinforcement pathologies and their repair. *Annual Review of Clinical Psychology, 10,* 641–677.

Bolton, J. M., Robinson, J., & Sareen, J. (2009). Self-medication of mood disorders with alcohol and drugs in the National Epidemiologic Survey on Alcohol and Related Conditions. *Journal of Affective Disorders, 115,* 367–375.

Bowen, S., Chawla, N., Grow, J., & Marlatt, G. A. (2021). *Mindfulness-based relapse prevention for addictive behaviors: A clinician's guide* (2nd ed.). New York: Guilford Press.

Brand, M., Laier, C., & Young, K. S. (2014). Internet addiction: Coping styles, expectancies, and treatment implications. *Frontiers in Psychology, 5,* 1–14.

Bromwich, J. E. (2020). This election, a divided America stands united on one topic: All kinds of Americans have turned their back on the destructive war on drugs. Retrieved December 28, 2020, from *https://www.nytimes.com/2020/11/05/style/marijuana-legalization-usa.html.*

Brorson, H. H., Arnevik, E. A., Rand-Hendriksen, K., & Duckert, F. (2013). Drop-out from addiction treatment: A systematic review of risk factors. *Clinical Psychology Review, 33,* 1010–1024.

Buckner, J. D., Ecker, A. H., & Welch, K. D. (2013). Psychometric properties of a valuations scale for the Marijuana Effect Expectancies Questionnaire. *Addictive Behaviors, 38*(3), 1629–1634.

Budney, A. J., & Higgins, S. T. (1998). *Therapy manual for drug addiction: Manual 2: A community reinforcement plus vouchers approach: Treating cocaine addiction.* Rockville, MD: National Institute on Drug Abuse.

Burlingame, G., Strauss, B., & Joyce, A. (2013). Change mechanisms and effectiveness of small group treatments. In M. J. Lambert (Ed.), *Bergin and Garfield's handbook of psychotherapy and behavior change* (6th ed., pp. 640–689). New York: Wiley.

Burns, D., & Spangler, D. (2000). Does psychotherapy homework lead to improvements in depression in cognitive–behavioral therapy or does improvement lead to increased homework compliance? *Journal of Consulting and Clinical Psychology, 68,* 46–56.

Casteneda, R., Galanter, M., & Franco, H. (1989). Self-medication among addicts with primary psychiatric disorders. *Comprehensive Psychiatry, 30,* 80–83.

Center for Substance Abuse Treatment. (2005). *Substance abuse treatment: Group therapy* (DHHS Publication No. (SMA) 05–3991). Rockville, MD: Substance Abuse and Mental Health Services Administration.

Clark, D. A., & Beck, A. T. (2010). *Cognitive therapy of anxiety disorders: Science and practice.* New York: Guilford Press.

Connors, G., DiClemente, C., Velasquez, M., & Donovan, D. (2013). *Substance abuse treatment and the stages of change: Selecting and planning interventions.* New York: Guilford Press.

Corsini, R. J., & Rosenberg, B. (1955). Mechanisms of group psychotherapy: Processes and dynamics. *The Journal of Abnormal and Social Psychology, 51*(3), 406–411.

Cummings, C., Gordon, J., & Marlatt, G. A. (1980) Relapse: Prevention and prediction. In W. R. Miller (Ed.), *The addictive behaviors: Treatment of alcoholism, drug abuse, smoking and obesity* (pp. 291–321). Oxford, UK: Pergamon Press.

Curreri, A. J., Farchione, T. J., & Wang, M. (2019). Fostering engagement in early sessions of transdiagnostic cognitive-behavioral therapy. *Psychotherapy, 56*(1), 41–47.

Daughters, S. B., Magidson, J. F., Anand, D., Seitz-Brown, C. J., Chen, Y., & Baker, S. (2018). The effect of a behavioral activation treatment for substance use on post-treatment abstinence: A randomized controlled trial. *Addiction, 113,* 535–544.

Daughters, S. B., Magidson, J. F., Lejuez, C. W., & Chen, Y. (2016). LETS ACT: A behavioral activation treatment for substance use and depression. *Advances in Dual Diagnosis, 9*(2/3), 74–84.

Diamond, A. (2014). Understanding executive functions: What helps or hinders them and how executive functions and language development mutually support one another. *Perspectives on Language and Literacy, 40*, 7–11.

Dimidjian, S., Hollon, S. D., Dobson, K. S., Schmaling, K. B., Kohlenberg, R. J., Addis, M. E., . . . Jacobson, N. S. (2006). Randomized trial of behavioral activation, cognitive therapy, and antidepressant medication in the acute treatment of adults with major depression. *Journal of Consulting and Clinical Psychology, 74*(4), 658–670.

Driskell, J. E., Willis, R. P., & Copper, C. (1992). Effect of overlearning on retention. *Journal of Applied Psychology, 77*(5), 615–622.

Enoch, M. (2011). The role of early life stress as a predictor for alcohol and drug dependence. *Psychopharmacology, 214*(1), 17–31.

Eubanks, C. F., Burckell, L. A., & Goldfried, M. R. (2018). Clinical consensus strategies to repair ruptures in the therapeutic alliance. *Journal of Psychotherapy Integration, 28*(1), 60–76.

Eubanks, C. F., Muran, J. C., & Safran, J. D. (2018). Alliance rupture repair: A meta-analysis. *Psychotherapy, 55*(4), 508–519.

Evans, K., & Sullivan, J. M. (2001). *Dual diagnosis: Counseling the mentally ill substance abuser* (2nd ed.). New York: Guilford Press.

Fergusson, D. M., Horwood, L. J., & Woodward, L. J. (2000). The stability of child abuse reports: A longitudinal study of the reporting behaviour of young adults. *Psychological Medicine, 30*, 529–544.

Gluhoski, V. (1994). Misconceptions of cognitive therapy. *Psychotherapy, 31*(4), 594–600.

Goldman, D., Oroszi, G., & Ducci, F. (2005). The genetics of addictions: Uncovering the genes. *Nature: Genetics Reviews, 6*, 521–532.

Grant, K. M., Young, L. B., Tyler, K. A., Simpson, J. L., Pulido, R. D., & Timko, C. (2018). Intensive referral to mutual-help groups: A field trial of adaptations for rural veterans. *Patient Education and Counseling, 101*(1), 79–84.

Griffiths, M. E. (2005). A "components" model of addiction within a biopsychosocial framework. *Journal of Substance Use, 10*(4), 191–197.

Hayes, S. C., Strosahl, K. D., & Wilson, K. G. (2012). *Acceptance and commitment therapy: The process and practice of mindful change*. New York: Guilford Press.

Hendershot, C. S., Witkiewitz, K., George, W. H., & Marlatt, G. A. (2011). Relapse prevention for addictive behaviors. *Substance Abuse Treatment, Prevention, and Policy, 6*(1), 17.

Higgins, S. T., Silverman, K., & Heil, S. H. (Eds.). (2007). *Contingency management in substance abuse treatment*. New York: Guilford Press.

Ilgen, M. A., Roeder, K. M., Webster, L., Mowbray, O. P., Perron, B. E., Chermack, S. T., & Bohnert, A. S. (2011). Measuring pain medication expectancies in adults treated for substance use disorders. *Drug and Alcohol Dependence, 115*(1–2), 51–56.

Kahneman, D. (1973). *Attention and effort*. Englewood Cliffs, NJ: Prentice-Hall.

Kahneman, D. (2003). A perspective on judgment and choice: Mapping bounded rationality. *American Psychologist, 58*(9), 697–720.

Kahneman, D. (2011). *Thinking, fast and slow*. New York: Macmillan.

Kahneman, D., & Frederick, S. (2002). Representativeness revisited: Attribute substitution in intuitive judgment. In T. Gilovich, D. Griffin, & D. Kahneman (Eds.), *Heuristics and biases* (1st ed., pp. 49–81). New York: Cambridge University Press.

Kazantzis, N., Whittington, C., & Dattilio, F. (2010). Meta-analysis of homework effects in cognitive and behavioral therapy: A replication and extension: Homework assignments and therapy outcome. *Clinical Psychology: Science and Practice, 17*(2), 144–156.

Kelly, J. F., Humphreys, K., & Ferri, M. (2020). Alcoholics Anonymous and other 12-step programs for alcohol use disorder. *Cochrane Database of Systematic Reviews*, Issue 3, Art. No. CD012880.

Kelly, J. F., Wakeman, S. E., & Saitz, R. (2015). Stop talking "dirty": Clinicians, language, and quality of care for the leading cause of preventable death in the United States. *American Journal of Medicine, 128*(1), 8–9.

Keyes, K. M., Hatzenbuehler, M. L., Grant, B. F., & Hasin, D. S. (2012). Stress and alcohol: Epidiologic evidence. *Alcohol Research, 34*(4), 391–400.

King, B. R., & Boswell, J. F. (2019). Therapeutic strategies and techniques in early cognitive-behavioral therapy. *Psychotherapy, 56*(1), 35–40.

Kosten, T. R., Rounsaville, B. J., & Kleber, H. D. (1986). A 2.5 year follow-up of depression, life events, and treatment effects on abstinence among opioid addicts. *Archives of General Psychiatry, 43*, 733–738.

Kroenke, K., Spitzer, R. L., & Williams, J. B. W. (2001). The PHQ-9: Validity of a brief depression severity measure. *Journal of General Internal Medicine, 16*(9), 606–613.

Leahy, R. L. (2017). *Cognitive therapy techniques: A practitioner's guide* (2nd ed.). New York: Guilford Press.

Lejuez, C. W., Hopko, D. R., Acierno, R., Daughters, S. B., & Pagoto, S. L. (2011). Ten year revision of the brief behavioral activation treatment for depression: Revised treatment manual. *Behavior Modification, 35*(2), 111–161.

Lejuez, C. W., Hopko, D. R., & Hopko, S. D. (2001). A brief behavioral activation treatment for depression. *Behavior Modification, 25*(2), 255–286.

Li, H. K., & Dingle, G. A. (2012). Using the Drinking Expectancy Questionnaire (revised scoring method) in clinical practice. *Addictive Behaviors, 37*, 198–204.

Liese, B. S. (1994). Psychologic principles of substance abuse: A brief overview. *Comprehensive Therapy, 20*(2), 125–129.

Liese, B. S. (2014). Cognitive-behavioral therapy for people with addictions. In S. L. A. Straussner (Ed.), *Clinical work with substance abusing clients* (pp. 225–250). New York: Guilford Press.

Liese, B. S., & Beck, A. T. (1998). Back to basics: Fundamental cognitive therapy skills for keeping drug-dependent individuals in treatment. In L. S. Onken, J. D. Blain, & J. J. Boren (Eds.), *Beyond the therapeutic alliance: Keeping drug-dependent individuals in treatment* (pp. 210–235). Washington, DC: U.S. Government Printing Office.

Liese, B. S., Beck, A. T., & Seaton, K. (2002). The cognitive therapy addictions group. In D. W. Brook & H. I. Spitz (Eds.), *Group psychotherapy of substance abuse* (pp. 37–57). New York: Haworth Medical Press.

Liese, B. S., & Esterline, K. M. (2015). Concept mapping: A supervision strategy for introducing case conceptualization skills to novice therapists. *Psychotherapy, 52*(2), 190–194.

Liese, B. S., & Franz, R. A. (1996). Treating substance use disorders with cognitive therapy: Lessons learned and implications for the future. In P. M. Salkovskis (Ed.), *Frontiers of cognitive therapy* (pp. 470–508). New York: Guilford Press.

Liese, B. S., & Monley, C. M. (2021). Providing addiction services during a pandemic: Lessons learned from COVID-19. *Journal of Substance Abuse Treatment, 120*.

Liese, B. S., & Tripp, J. C. (2018). Advances in cognitive-behavioral therapy for substance use disorders and addictive behaviors. In R. L. Leahy (Ed.), *Science and practice in cognitive therapy: foundations, mechanisms, and applications* (pp. 298–316). New York: Guilford Press.

Linehan, M. M. (2015). *DBT skills training manual*. New York: Guilford Press.

Logan, D. E., & Marlatt, G. A. (2010). Harm reduction therapy: A practice-friendly review of research. *Journal of Clinical Psychology, 66*(2).

Magidson, J. F., Young, K. C., & Lejuez, C. W. (2014). A how-to guide for conducting a functional analysis: Behavioral principles and clinical application. *The Behavior Therapist, 37*(1).

Magill, M., & Ray, L. A. (2009). Cognitive-behavioral treatment with adult alcohol and illicit drug users: A meta-analysis of randomized controlled trials. *Journal of Studies on Alcohol and Drugs, 70*(4), 516–527.

Marlatt, G. A. (1996). Harm reduction: Come as you are. *Addictive Behaviors, 21*(6), 779–788.

Marlatt, G. A., & Gordon, J. R. (1985). *Relapse prevention: Maintenance strategies in addictive behavior change*. New York: Guilford Press.

Marlatt, G. A., & Kristeller, J. L. (1999). Mindfulness and meditation. In W. R. Miller (Ed.), *Integrating spirituality into treatment: Resources for practitioners* (pp. 67–84). Washington, DC: American Psychological Association.

Marlatt, G. A., Larimer, M. E., & Witkiewitz, K. (2012). *Harm reduction: Pragmatic strategies for managing high-risk behaviors* (2nd ed.). New York: Guilford Press.

Marlatt, G. A., & Tapert, S. F. (1993). Harm reduction: Reducing the risks of addictive behaviors. In J. S. Baer, G. A. Marlatt, & R. J. McMahon (Eds.), *Addictive behaviors across the life span: Prevention, treatment, and policy issues* (pp. 243–273). New York: Sage.

Marlatt, G. A., & Witkiewitz, K. (2005). Relapse prevention for alcohol and drug problems. In G. A. Marlatt & D. M. Donovan (Eds.) *Relapse prevention: Maintenance strategies in the treatment of addictive behaviors* (2nd ed., pp. 1–44). New York: Guilford Press.

McLellan, A. T. (2002). Have we evaluated addiction treatment correctly? Implications from a chronic care perspective. *Addiction, 97*(3), 249–252.

McLellan, A. T., Lewis, D. C., O'Brien, C. P., & Kleber, H. D. (2000). Drug dependence, a chronic mental illness: Implications for treatment, insurance, and outcomes evaluation. *Journal of the American Medical Association, 284*(13), 1689–1695.

Meyers, R. J., & Squires, D. D. (2001). *The community reinforcement approach: A guideline developed for the Behavioral Recovery Management project*. Albuquerque, NM: Univerisity of New Mexico Center on Alcoholism, Substance Abuse and Addictions.

Miller, W. R., & Rollnick, S. (2013). *Motivational interviewing: Helping people change* (3rd ed.). New York: Guilford Press.

Moos, R. H. (2008). Active ingredients of substance use-focused self-help groups. *Addiction, 103*(3), 387–396.

Moyers, T. B., Manuel, J. K., & Ernst, D. (2014). *Motivational interviewing treatment integrity coding manual 4.2.1*. Unpublished manual, Albuquerque, NM.

Moyers, T. B., & Rollnick, S. (2002), A motivational interviewing perspective on resistance in psychotherapy. *Journal of Clinical Psychology, 58*(2), 185–193.

Nace, E. P., Davis, C. W., & Gaspari, J. P. (1991). Axis-II comorbidity in substance abusers. *American Journal of Psychiatry, 148*(1), 118–120.

National Institute on Drug Abuse. (2010). *Comorbidity: Addiction and other mental illnesses*. Washington, DC: U.S. Department of Health and Human Services.

National Institute on Drug Abuse. (2018a). Comorbidity: Substance use disorders and other mental illnesses. NIDA Drug Facts. Retrieved from *https://www.drugabuse.gov/publications/drugfacts/comorbidity-substance-use-disorders-other-mental-illnesses.*

National Institute on Drug Abuse. (2018b). Marijuana: NIDA drug facts. Retrieved from *www.drugabuse.gov/publications/drugfacts/marijuana.*

Newman, C. F. (2008). Substance use disorders. In M. A. Whisman (Ed.), *Adapting cognitive therapy for depression: Managing complexity and comorbidity* (pp. 233–254). New York: Guilford Press.

Nezu, A. M., Nezu, C. M., & Perri, M. G. (1989). *Problem-solving therapy for depression: Theory, research, and clinical guidelines.* Hoboken, NJ: Wiley.

Niaura, R. (2000). Cognitive social learning and related perspectives on drug craving. *Addiction, 95*(8, Suppl. 2), 155–163.

Nicolai, J., Demmel, R., & Moshagen, M. (2010). The comprehensive alcohol expectancy questionnaire: confirmatory factor analysis, scale refinement, and further validation. *Journal of Personality Assessment, 92*(5), 400–409.

Norcross, J. C., Krebs, P. M., & Prochaska, J. O. (2011). Stages of change. *Journal of Clinical Psychology, 67*(2), 143–154.

Norcross, J. C., & Lambert, M. J. (2018). Psychotherapy relationships that work III. *Psychotherapy, 55*(4), 305–315.

Nyklícek, I., & Denollet, J. (2009). Development and evaluation of the Balanced Index of Psychological Mindedness (BIPM). *Psychological Assessment, 21*(1), 32–44.

Petry, N. M. (2012). *Contingency management for substance abuse treatment: A guide to implementing this evidence-based practice.* New York: Taylor & Francis.

Pistrang, N., Barker, C., & Humphreys, K. (2008). Mutual help groups for mental health problems: A review of effectiveness studies. *American Journal of Community Psychology, 42*(1–2), 110–121.

Posner, K., Brown, G. K., Stanley, B., Brent, D. A., Yershova, K. V., Oquendo, M. A., . . . Mann, J. J. (2011). The Columbia–Suicide Severity Rating Scale: Initial validity and internal consistency findings from three multisite studies with adolescents and adults. *American Journal of Psychiatry, 168*(12), 1266–1277.

Prendergast, M., Podus, D., Finney, J., Greenwell, L., & Roll, J. (2006). Contingency management for treatment of substance use disorders: A meta-analysis. *Addiction, 101*(11), 1546–1560.

Prochaska, J. O., DiClemente, C. C., & Norcross, J. C. (1992). In search of how people change: Applications to addictive behaviors. *American Psychologist, 47*(9), 1102–1114.

Prochaska, J. O., & Norcross, J. C. (2001). Stages of change. *Psychotherapy: Theory, Research, Practice, Training, 38*(4), 443–448.

Ramsay, J. R., & Newman, C. F. (2000). Substance abuse. In F. M. Dattilio & A. Freeman (Eds.), *Cognitive-behavioral approaches to crisis intervention* (2nd ed., pp. 126–149). New York: Guilford Press.

Rees, C. S., McEvoy, P., & Nathan, P. R. (2005). Relationship between homework completion and outcome in cognitive behaviour therapy. *Cognitive Behaviour Therapy, 34*(4), 242–247.

Reynolds, B. (2006). A review of delay-discounting research with humans: Relations to drug use and gambling. *Behavioural Pharmacology, 17*(18), 651–667.

Safran, J. D., Crocker, P., McMain, S., & Murray, P. (1990). Therapeutic alliance rupture as a therapy event for empirical investigation. *Psychotherapy, 27*(2), 154–165.

Scholl, L., Seth, P., Kariisa, M., Wilson, N., & Baldwin, G. (2018). Drug and opioid-involved overdose deaths—United States, 2013–2017. *Morbidity and Mortality Weekly Report, 67*(5152), 1419–1427.

Schomerus, G., Lucht, M., Holzinger, A., Matschinger, H., Carta, M. G., & Angermeyer, M. C. (2011). The stigma of alcohol dependence compared with other mental disorders: A review of population studies. *Alcohol and Alcoholism, 46*(2), 105–112.

Schultz, P. W., & Searleman, A. (2002). Rigidity of thought and behavior: 100 years of research. *Genetic, Social, and General Psychology Monographs, 128*(2), 165–207.

Segal, Z. V., Williams, J. M. G., & Teasdale, J. D. (2013). *Mindfulness-based cognitive therapy for depression* (2nd ed.). New York: Guilford Press.

Shaffer, H. J. (2012). Introduction. In H. J. Shaffer (Ed.), *APA addiction syndrome handbook: Vol. 1. Foundations, influences, and expressions of addiction.* (Vol. 1, pp. xxvii–lx). Washington, DC: American Psychological Association.

Shaffer, H. J., & Hall, M. N. (2002). The natural history of gambling and drinking problems among casino employees. *Journal of Social Psychology, 142*(4), 405–424.

Shaffer, H. J., LaPlante, D. A., LaBrie, R. A., Kidman, R. C., Donato, A. N., & Stanton, M. V. (2004). Toward a syndrome model of addiction: Multiple expressions, common etiology. *Harvard Review of Psychiatry, 12*(6), 367–374.

Shapiro, F. R. (2014). Who wrote the Serenity Prayer? *The Chronicle of Higher Education, 4.*

Shibata, K., Sasaki, Y., Bang, J. W., Walsh, E. G., Machizawa, M. G., Tamaki, M., . . . Watanabe, T. (2017). Overlearning hyperstabilizes a skill by rapidly making neurochemical processing inhibitory-dominant. *Nature Neuroscience, 20*(3), 470–475.

SMART Recovery (2021, September). *SMART Recovery Toolbox. https://www.smartrecovery. org/smart-recovery-toolbox/*

Sobell, L. C., Sobell, M. B., & Nirenberg, T. D. (1988). Behavioral assessment and treatment with alcohol and drug abusers: A review with emphasis on clinical application. *Clinical Psychology Review, 8*(1), 19–54.

Spencer, J., Goode, J., Penix, E. A., Trusty, W., & Swift, J. K. (2019). Developing a collaborative relationship with clients during the initial sessions of psychotherapy. *Psychotherapy, 56*(1), 7–10.

Spitzer, R. L., Kroenke, K., Williams, J. B. W., & Lowe, B. (2006). A brief measure for assessing generalized anxiety disorder: The GAD-7. *Archives of Internal Medicine, 166*, 1092–1097.

Substance Abuse and Mental Health Services Administration. (2009). *Integrated treatment for co-occurring disorders: The evidence* (DHHS Pub. No. SMA-08-4366). Rockville, MD: Center for Mental Health Services, Substance Abuse and Mental Health Services Administration, U.S. Department of Health and Human Services.

Substance Abuse and Mental Health Services Administration. (2017). *Behavioral health barometer: United States, Vol. 4: Indicators as measured through the 2015 National Survey on Drug Use and Health and National Survey of Substance Abuse Treatment Services.* Rockville, MD: Substance Abuse and Mental Health Services Administration, U.S. Department of Health and Human Services.

Substance Abuse and Mental Health Services Administration. (2020). *Key substance use and mental health indicators in the United States: Results from the 2019 National Survey on Drug Use and Health* (DHHS Publication No. PEP20-07-01-001, NSDUH Series H-55). Rockville, MD: Center for Behavioral Health Statistics and Quality, Substance Abuse and Mental Health Services Administration. Retrieved from *https://www.samhsa.gov/ data.*

Tversky, A., & Kahneman, D. (1992). Advances in prospect theory: Cumulative representation of uncertainty. *Journal of Risk and Uncertainty, 5*, 297–323.

van Boekel, L. C., Brouwers, E. P. M., van Weeghel, J., & Garretsen, H. F. L. (2013). Stigma among health professionals towards patients with substance use disorders and its consequences for healthcare delivery: Systematic review. *Drug and Alcohol Dependence, 131*(1–2), 23–35.

Volkow, N. D., Baler, R. D., Compton, W. M., & Weiss, S. R. (2014). Adverse health effects of marijuana use. *New England Journal of Medicine, 370*(23), 2219–2227.

Volkow, N. D., & Koob, G. (2015). Brain disease model of addiction: Why is it so controversial? *The Lancet Psychiatry, 2*(8), 677–679.

Wampold, B. E. (2015). How important are the common factors in psychotherapy? An update. *World Psychiatry, 14*(3), 270–277.

Wampold, B. E., Baldwin, S. A., Holtforth, M. G., & Imel, Z. E. (2017). What characterizes effective therapists? In L. G. Castonguay & C. E. Hill (Eds.), *How and why are some therapists better than others? Understanding therapist effects.* (pp. 37–53). Washington, DC: American Psychological Association.

Weiss, R. D., Jaffee, W. B., de Menil, V. P., & Cogley, C. B. (2004). Group therapy for substance use disorders: What do we know? *Harvard Review of Psychiatry, 12,* 339–350.

Wenzel, A., Liese, B. S., Beck, A. T., & Friedman-Wheeler, D. G. (2012). *Group cognitive therapy of addictions.* New York: Guilford Press.

White, H. R., Larimer, M. E., Sher, K. J., & Witkiewitz, K. (2011). In memoriam: G. Alan Marlatt, 1941–2011. *Journal of Studies on Alcohol and Drugs, 72*(3), 357–360.

Wickwire, E. M., Whelan, J. P., & Meyers, A. W. (2010). Outcome expectancies and gambling behavior among urban adolescents. *Psychology of Addictive Behaviors, 24*(1), 75–88.

Witkiewitz, K., Marlatt, G. A., & Walker, D. (2005). Mindfulness-based relapse prevention for alcohol and substance use disorders. *Journal of Cognitive Psychotherapy: An International Quarterly, 19*(3), 211–228.

Witkiewitz, K., Montes, K. S., Schwebel, F. J., & Tucker, J. A. (2020). What is recovery? *Alcohol Research: Current Reviews, 40*(3), 01.

Yalom, I. D. (1975). *The theory and practice of group psychotherapy* (2nd ed.). New York: Basic Books.

Yalom, I. D., & Leszcz, M. (2005). *The theory and practice of group psychotherapy* (5th ed.). New York: Basic Books.

Young, J. E., Klosko, J. S., & Weishaar, M. E. (2003). *Schema therapy: A practitioner's guide.* New York: Guilford Press.

Zemore, S. E., Kaskutas, L. A., Mericle, A., & Hemberg, J. (2017). Comparison of 12-step groups to mutual help alternatives for AUD in a large, national study: Differences in membership characteristics and group participation, cohesion, and satisfaction. *Journal of Substance Abuse Treatment, 73,* 16–26.

Author Index

SUBJECT INDEX